MAYO CLINIC
ON ALZHEIMER'S DISEASE

Ronald C. Petersen, Ph.D., M.D.

Medical Editor

Mayo Clinic
Rochester, Minnesota

Mayo Clinic on Alzheimer's Disease provides reliable information about the diagnosis and treatment of and caregiving for Alzheimer's disease and other causes of dementia. Much of the information comes directly from the experience of health care professionals at Mayo Clinic. This book supplements the advice of your personal physician, whom you should consult for individual medical problems.

For bulk sales to employers, member groups and health-related companies, contact Mayo Clinic Health Solutions, 200 First St. SW, Rochester, MN 55905, or send an email to SpecialSalesMayoBooks@Mayo.edu.

Published by Mayo Clinic

© 2013 Mayo Foundation for Medical Education and Research (MFMER)

Library of Congress Control Number: 2013942610

First Edition

4 5 6 7 8 9 10

About Alzheimer's disease

Alzheimer's disease is the most common cause of dementia, a set of symptoms that robs you of memory, reason, good judgment and decision-making, communication skills and personality. The disease is progressive and irreversible. Other causes of dementia include frontotemporal degeneration, dementia with Lewy bodies and vascular cognitive impairment. All of these conditions are described in this book.

Although there is currently no cure and no known strategies to prevent Alzheimer's, impressive advances in brain research allows doctors to detect the condition in its earliest stages. This offers real hope for unraveling some of the most intractable mysteries surrounding Alzheimer's and may prove to be a turning point in the ongoing fight to stop the disease.

Armed with this knowledge and the capability of intervening earlier in the disease process, it is hoped that an effective treatment of Alzheimer's disease will quickly follow.

About Mayo Clinic

Mayo Clinic is the first and largest integrated, not-for-profit group practice in the world, providing health and wellness services to consumers and businesses across the globe. Joined by a philosophy that "the needs of the patient come first," more that 3,700 doctors and scientists from every medical specialty, and over 50,000 allied health staff work together to care for patients, conduct medical research, and train tomorrow's health care providers.

Each year, Mayo Clinic treats more than half a million people from all walks of life at its campuses in Rochester, Minn.; Jacksonville, Fla.; and Scottsdale/Phoenix, Ariz.; and via community-based providers in more than 70 locations in the Upper Midwest.

With its depth of knowledge, experience and expertise, Mayo Clinic occupies an unparalleled position as an award-winning health information resource.

Editorial staff

Preface

Alzheimer's disease may be the defining disorder of our generation. It is estimated that more than 5 million people in the United States have Alzheimer's disease today, and this number is projected to triple by the middle of the century. The costs to individuals, families and the healthcare system are incalculable. Moreover, public perceptions come into play. Surveys frequently rank Alzheimer's among the greatest health fears. At the same time, it's a misperception of many that Alzheimer's is a normal part of aging.

With this as motivation, the National Alzheimer's Project Act was signed into law in 2011. This legislation requires the federal government to generate a blueprint for dealing with Alzheimer's disease in the United States. The National Plan to Address Alzheimer's Disease, released in May 2012, is the cornerstone of a concerted effort in research, clinical care and services for fighting the disease. The overall goals of the Plan are to prevent and effectively treat Alzheimer's disease by 2025. These are ambitious goals but necessary ones to deal with this devastating disorder.

Mayo Clinic on Alzheimer's Disease is intended to help patients, caregivers, families and anyone interested in the disorder understand the underlying nature of the brain, the normal changes that come with aging, and the development of cognitive disorders, including Alzheimer's disease. Normal features of brain function are discussed as well as risk factors and treatments for several types of cognitive impairment. The Action Guide is designed to help people deal with many practical issues surrounding the disease. I would like to thank my many colleagues who helped in compiling this information, and hope that this volume will be useful to those who use it. Speaking for my colleagues, we are confident that we can treat Alzheimer's disease and reduce its burden on individuals and society.

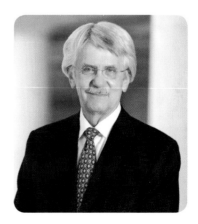

Ronald C. Petersen, Ph.D., M.D.
Medical Editor

Table of contents

Part 3: Causes of dementia other than Alzheimer's.................155

Part 1

Aging and dementia

Chapter 1

Typical aging

Mary feels great. The 67-year-old grandmother eats well, takes daily walks and tends a beautiful garden. She lives in her own home and prides herself on being independent.

Mary is noticing that her memory isn't what it used to be. She's been misplacing items, such as her purse and car keys. She forgot a doctor appointment last week, and when she came out of the grocery store today she couldn't remember where she'd parked the car. She worries that memory slips such as these may signal the end of her independent lifestyle.

John, 78, lives with his wife of 53 years in an apartment complex for seniors. He enjoys meeting with his morning coffee group and visiting family and friends across the country.

A former college professor, he's always considered his mind to be "sharp." But even though John continues to read extensively and listen to news, he's having a harder time recalling facts. Sometimes, in conversations, his thoughts hang in midsentence as he struggles to find the right word. For John, losing his ability to discuss current events threatens a part of his life that he takes great pride in.

Although Mary and John haven't mentioned their concerns to anyone yet, they both fear that these lapses may be indications of something more serious that's developing — something like Alzheimer's disease.

Alzheimer's disease (AD) is the most common cause of dementia and a fear of many adults, primarily those older than age 65. Dementia involves a sharp decline in memory and other cognitive skills that prevents people from being able to carry out the most basic tasks of daily living.

While some people worry obsessively about getting AD, others deny its existence. Yet, in almost every community, you can find someone who's providing care for a parent, sibling or friend who has dementia.

You regularly come across alarming news reports about Alzheimer's in print, radio, television and online. It's no wonder that you find yourself second-guessing minor memory lapses and wondering if these incidents aren't the first signs of the disease.

A common question

More Americans are reaching old age than ever before. In 2007, average life expectancy had increased to almost 78 years — which is 30 years more than Americans were expected to live 100 years ago. And this rising trend doesn't appear to be slowing down. While about 40 million Americans are older than age 65 today, the census data project that more than 88 million people will be in this age group by 2050.

This chapter addresses a common question that is asked by just about any individual reaching age 60 and older — years when the signs and symptoms of dementia typically occur: How does a person distinguish between the physical and emotional changes that are simply due to aging and those that could signal a potentially serious health condition or disease?

It's best to start by understanding the aging process. Certain changes are going to naturally occur as you age. Many physical and mental capabilities may gradually diminish or slow down — for example, your lung capacity, bone strength, reaction time or the rate at which you're able to process new pieces of information.

Some of the changes associated with aging are described in this chapter. Mention of them doesn't mean these changes are bound to happen to you, only that they're more likely to occur as you grow older. They're part of what may be described as typical aging.

Rest assured that many conditions associated with aging, such as AD, are still considered diseases and don't affect everyone. They're not "typical." Millions of people age with their physical and mental health intact.

What is 'typical?'

How do people age? When it comes to cognitive functions — thought, perception, memory, problem-solving, decision-making — what age-related changes are typical and what may be cause for concern? You may be surprised to learn that research into normal aging lags behind studies of abnormal aging. One reason is that, although most people assume they know what's typical, the answer isn't as straightforward as it seems.

For example, does "typical" apply to a woman in her early 90s whose mind is as sharp as a tack and who still lives at home, takes few medications, walks her dog every day and meets regularly with friends? People like this exist. But in terms of the actual number of people who age this way, it may not be typical. Experts refer to this as successful aging or optimal aging — the kind that most people would want to experience.

More often, aging is accompanied by illnesses and conditions such as heart disease, high blood pressure, bone fractures, and a reduction of hearing or vision. Many people consider slight forgetfulness, less energy and slower reaction times as common parts of aging, even though they may be caused by disease. The changes may be inconvenient and frustrating, but they aren't debilitating — for example, you can still live an active, independent life in spite of occasional memory lapses. The overall experience, with many variations, is known as typical aging.

The challenge lies in distinguishing characteristic elements of typical aging from abnormal changes that signal dementia and Alzheimer's disease. By being able to identify a disorder in its earliest stages, scientists hope to capture Alzheimer's when it may be most treatable. At the same time, researchers are exploring the concept of optimal aging and what can be done to promote lifelong health. Both tracks of research may provide valuable insight into the prevention of cognitive decline and the treatment of dementia in its different forms.

Physical changes with typical aging

Regardless of how healthy and injury-free you've kept yourself, wear and tear takes a toll on organs, muscles and other tissues in your body. You may notice this as early as your 30s and 40s, when it becomes just a little bit harder to bounce back from a cold or maintain a vigorous running pace.

Some of the physical changes of aging, such as graying or thinning hair, are visibly evident. With age, your skin may become thinner, drier and less elastic, causing it to wrinkle and sag. Your skin may bruise more easily, and age spots may appear.

Other physical changes may be less noticeable to other people (and even to yourself at first). As you age, your eyes and mouth may start to feel drier. Your lung capacity declines, which means you take in less air in a breath, making vigorous exercise more difficult. The walls of your bladder often become less elastic, so you have to go to the bathroom more often.

Some age-related changes are so subtle that you may not notice them until they're well established. Your digestive system naturally slows down, making bouts of constipation more frequent. Your immune system becomes less effective, making infections more likely. Kidney function declines, so it's easier to become dehydrated or retain fluid.

Many people learn to adapt to these changes as they affect physical appearance or function in everyday life.

Cardiovascular changes

Your cardiovascular system is key to the well-being of every cell in your body. This system comprises the heart and blood vessels, and it delivers oxygen and transports nutrients and waste products throughout the intricate vascular network.

With age, your heart muscle becomes less efficient, working harder to pump blood. In addition, your arteries thicken and stiffen, increasing your heart's workload. Over time, fatty deposits, or plaques, accumulate in the artery walls, obstructing blood flow.

Due to these changes, older adults are at higher risk of high blood pressure, coronary artery disease, congestive heart failure and stroke. The vascular disorders increase your risk of dementia.

Most older adults can still maintain an active life. Trouble develops when strenuous demands, such as heavy lifting or running, exceed capacity. That's when heart function can no longer meet the body's needs. After stressful events, it often takes longer for the system to return to normal levels.

Skeletal and muscular changes

As you get older, your bones shrink in size and become more porous and brittle. In addition, the gel-like disks that cushion your spinal vertebrae become thinner. Muscle mass decreases, and joints and tendons lose strength and flexibility. As a result, movement often becomes more limited with age. Your balance and coordination diminish. Most people adapt by performing everyday tasks just a little slower.

Sensory changes

Changes to vision and hearing are common as you age, which may make it more of a challenge to interact with other people within your surroundings. Sometimes these changes are subtle — often, other people are the ones who point them out to you.

Vision. Some of the first signs of aging are associated with poor eyesight. It's likely that by the time you're in your 50s, you'll need glasses, at least part of the time, for reading. That's because the lens of your eye loses elasticity over time. With age, you're at higher risk of cataracts, glaucoma and age-related macular degeneration.

Hearing. Hearing loss often results from damage to the delicate structures of the inner ear. Many things contribute to permanent hearing loss, including the wear and tear of aging, exposure to loud noises, certain medications, head injuries, and illnesses. Being male also works against you.

Metabolic changes

Metabolism involves thousands of chemical processes that help regulate your body systems, for example, food digestion and cell repair. Many changes associated with aging are the result of your metabolism slowing down. As you age, your levels of growth hormone and sex hormone decrease. You burn fewer calories than you once did, making it harder to lose weight. Not all hormone production decreases as you age — some levels remain unchanged, while other levels increase.

Your brain and typical aging

Not surprisingly, the process of aging brings changes to your brain. Weighing in at about 3 pounds, your brain is the most complex organ in your body — a master computer controlling actions you consciously think about, such as balancing a bank account or debating politics, along with actions you don't think about, such as swallowing food, experiencing pain or blinking dust from your eye.

In a healthy state, your brain monitors all vital functions and physical actions that your body undertakes. It's the repository for instincts, memories, intellectual analyses and creative thoughts. It organizes and shapes emotions. Most miraculously, perhaps, the brain enables you to do all of these things at the same time.

Consider something as simple as reading. In addition to absorbing the meaning of each word, you're likely holding a book or tablet upright, adjusting the distance from your eyes and turning pages when you need to. You're analyzing the information you read, recalling associated information you already know, and responding emotionally to the text. You're processing sounds and sensations from the environment around you, keeping an eye on the clock, and perhaps sipping from your coffee cup.

Your brain controls all of these actions. Simultaneously, your brain is managing vital functions unrelated to reading or other conscious activities — breathing air, maintaining body temperature and digesting food — that are necessary for life.

A tour of the brain

Your brain is composed of several distinct structures, and each structure performs a variety of tasks. These structures include:

Brainstem. Located at the base of your brain, the brainstem is responsible for some of your most basic survival functions, including breathing, digesting food and controlling the heart's pumping action. These actions are considered involuntary because they happen without you thinking about them or being aware of them. The brainstem connects to your spinal cord, which is the highway that carries messages back and forth between your brain and the rest of your body.

Internal structures of the brain

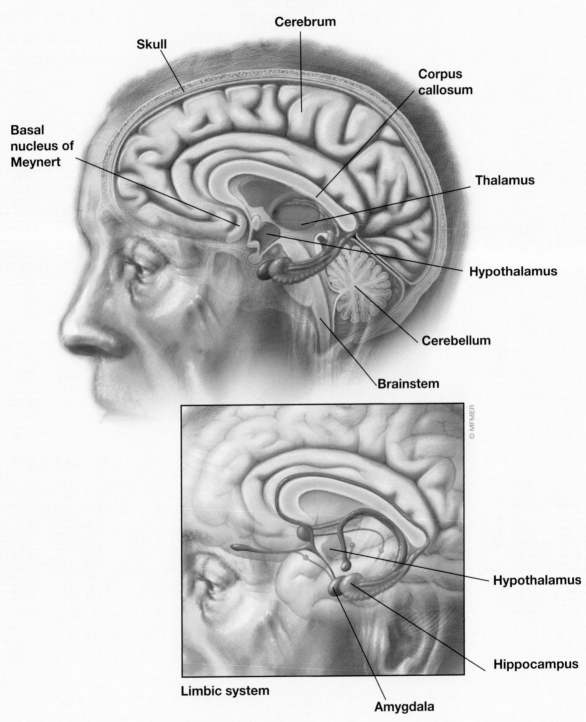

Skull

Cerebrum

Corpus callosum

Basal nucleus of Meynert

Thalamus

Hypothalamus

Cerebellum

Brainstem

© MFMER

Hypothalamus

Hippocampus

Limbic system

Amygdala

Cerebellum. The cerebellum, which sits at the back of the brainstem, is responsible for balance, movement and coordination. The cerebellum helps you do such things as stand upright, walk from one room to another and ride a bike.

Cerebrum. While the brainstem and cerebellum are busy handling involuntary actions in your body, your cerebrum performs the "thinking" functions. The cerebrum plays a central role in shaping who you are as an individual. Resting on top of the brainstem, it is the largest structure of the human brain and probably its most recognizable part.

A deep groove separates the cerebrum into left and right hemispheres. The hemispheres are connected by a thick band of nerve cell fibers called the corpus callosum.

Structures of the brain

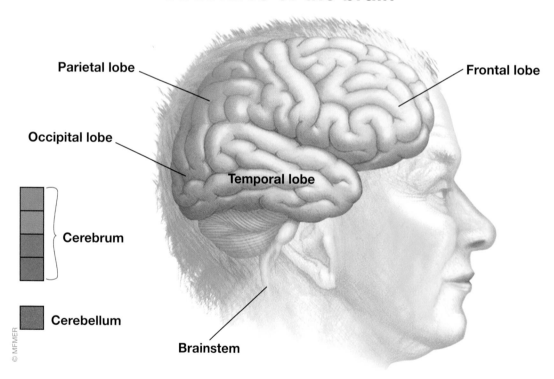

The cerebrum is divided into left and right hemispheres. Each hemisphere is divided into four sections, or lobes, separated from each other by surface grooves and connective tissue and by shape.

Each hemisphere of the cerebrum comprises four lobes (see page 20), and each lobe handles different functions (see page 22). For example, the frontal lobe is associated with planning, problem-solving, attention and behavior.

Behind the frontal lobe in each hemisphere is the parietal lobe, which handles sensory information such as pain, taste and touch. This lobe also supports visuospatial abilities — your readiness to move through your surroundings efficiently without bumping into objects or to assemble the interlocking pieces of a jigsaw puzzle.

The temporal lobe is situated at the side of your forehead, roughly at the location of your temple. It's vital for hearing and language comprehension and for perception and memory.

At the back of each cerebral hemisphere is the occipital lobe. You may know this lobe by another name, the visual cortex, because it's primarily responsible for your vision.

The outer surface of your cerebrum is a layer of tissue less than a quarter of an inch thick. Grayish brown and wrinkled in appearance, this layer is called the cerebral cortex, also known as gray matter. The cerebral cortex is where most of your intellectual operations take place — thinking, reasoning, analyzing, organizing, creating, decision-making and planning.

The grooves and folds of this layer allow for a greater surface area of the cortex to fit inside your skull, which increases the amount of information your brain can process. Underneath the cortex layer is a mass of white matter filled with nerve cells that control the communication that goes on among the various structures of your brain.

Limbic system. The limbic system comprises several small structures in the interior of your brain (see inset on page 19). It's associated with your emotional response to stimuli and your sense of motivation. Its job is to process the millions of messages bombarding your brain, both from within your body and from the outside environment. The limbic system includes the:

Hypothalamus. The hypothalamus (hi-po-THAL-uh-muhs) controls body functions such as eating, sleeping and sexual behavior. It regulates hormone levels and maintains a chemical balance in your body. It also controls body temperature — for example, telling you to sweat if you're too hot and shiver if you're too cold.

Functional areas of the brain

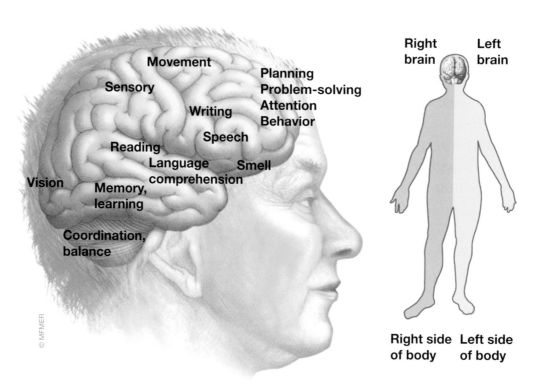

Higher cognitive functions, such as thinking, analyzing, memory and speech, as well as the processing of sensory information, are associated with specific lobes of the brain. Each side (hemisphere) of the cerebrum interacts with one half of the body, but the connections are crossed — the right hemisphere is connected to the left side of the body and the left hemisphere is connected to the right side.

Amygdala. The amygdala (uh-MIG-duh-luh) governs emotions such as anger and fear and triggers your response to danger, whether that response is confronting a situation or fleeing it (what is sometimes known as the fight-or-flight response). The amygdala assists you, for example, if you see a strange dog — you decide whether to run away, reach out to it or call for help.

Hippocampus. The hippocampus (hip-o-KAM-pus) is the central switchboard for your memory system. It's responsible for sorting pieces of information, storing them in different parts of your brain and recalling them when you need them. The hippocamous also transfers information between your recent and remote memory and helps you recall everything, from where you placed your car keys this morning to the resort town where you vacationed 20 summers ago.

Thalamus. Another structure in the brain's interior, located nearby but separate from the limbic system, is the thalamus. The job of the thalamus is to process information from your senses and relay this information to other parts of your brain.

In a healthy brain, all of these structures operate in a highly efficient, coordinated fashion. They're protected by the bony shell of your skull and cushioned by layers of membrane. An extensive network of blood vessels supplies the brain with food and oxygen in order for it to survive and function.

Brain-body communication

The brain and spinal cord make up your central nervous system — the primary channel through which all parts of your body communicate. Your spinal cord is a bundle of nerve fibers protected within a bony vertebral column.

Extending from your spinal cord is an intricate network of nerves branching out through your body tissues, all the way to the tips of your fingers and toes.

This network is called the peripheral nervous system. These nerves continually gather sensory information from inside and outside your body — such as pain, pressure, temperature change or muscle fatigue — and relay messages to your brain.

Your brain receives hundreds of messages from other parts of your body in

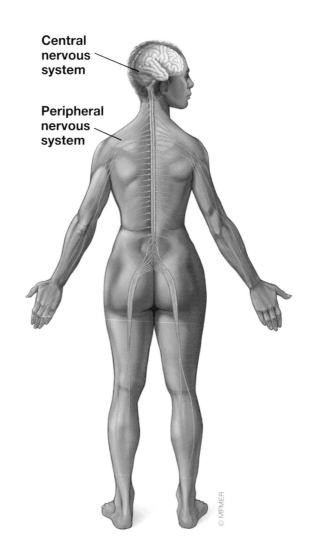

Central nervous system

Peripheral nervous system

an instant. As your brain interprets the messages, relevant bits of information may be kept for memory storage. When interpretation is complete, which can be a split-second process, the brain shoots back instructions to your fingers, legs, mouth, heart and other body organs on how to respond.

By rapidly interpreting, processing and responding to this barrage of incoming messages, your brain gives meaning to the world around you. The manner in which your brain performs these tasks — which may differ from the way any other person's brain responds — makes you the unique person you are.

Some of the changes associated with typical aging are a result of the brain's impaired ability to communicate. To understand this, it's necessary to focus on the nerve cell messengers that make the communication system work.

Neuron messengers

Nerve cells (neurons) are the basic units of your nervous system — you have about 100 billion neurons in your brain alone. The neurons generate messages (electric impulses), which allow your brain to communicate with other parts of your body.

Each neuron is designed to collect and process the messages, and then relay the information to other neurons. Branching out from the cell body (soma) are fibers called dendrites that receive incoming messages from the adjoining neurons.

The axon is a single branch extending out from a cell body that is larger than the dendrites. The axon has a different function from a dendrite — rather than relaying incoming messages, it relays outgoing messages. Wrapped around most axons is a fatty substance called myelin. Myelin helps insulate the axon and speeds up message transmission.

Linked by axon and dendrite connections, thousands of neurons form cellular pathways for messages to follow throughout the body. In order for one neuron to send a message, something must spur it to action. This may be an impulse relayed from another neuron, or it may be from external stimuli such as the pain of a pricked finger or the smell of morning coffee.

The electric impulse is picked up by a dendrite and travels like a wave through the neuron's cell body to the tip of the axon. Arrival of the impulse in the axon signals the release of certain chemicals (neurotransmitters) that are stored in the axon. The neurotransmitters enter a synapse, which is the narrow space separating the axon from an adjoining cell.

The released neurotransmitters cross the synapse to receptors on the receiving cell. This alters the membrane of the receiving cell in a way that recreates the impulse — and the process begins anew. In this way, impulses pass from neuron to neuron as messages travel to their intended destinations, which can be to your brain, heart or any other organ or muscle.

Think of this form of communication as a version of the telephone game that children play. A child whispers a message into the ear of the child sitting beside him or her, who turns to whisper the message into the next child's

Neuron structure

Billions of neurons, like the ones shown here, are the message carriers of your body. Neurons receive impulses from adjoining nerve cells through the dendrites and relay impulses via the axon.

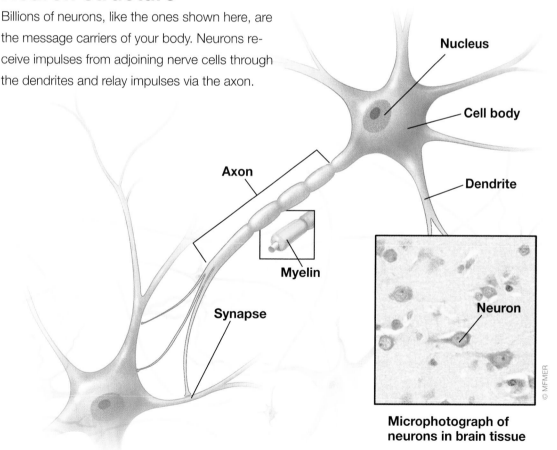

Microphotograph of neurons in brain tissue

ear, and so on, until an entire line of children has received the message — and can act on it together.

Only in your brain and nervous system, this communication process happens at lightning-fast speed and with far greater precision.

Making memories

Memory lapses are often a part of typical aging. They can trigger worry, anxiety and sometimes outright panic in older adults because memory loss is one of the earliest indications of dementia due to Alzheimer's disease.

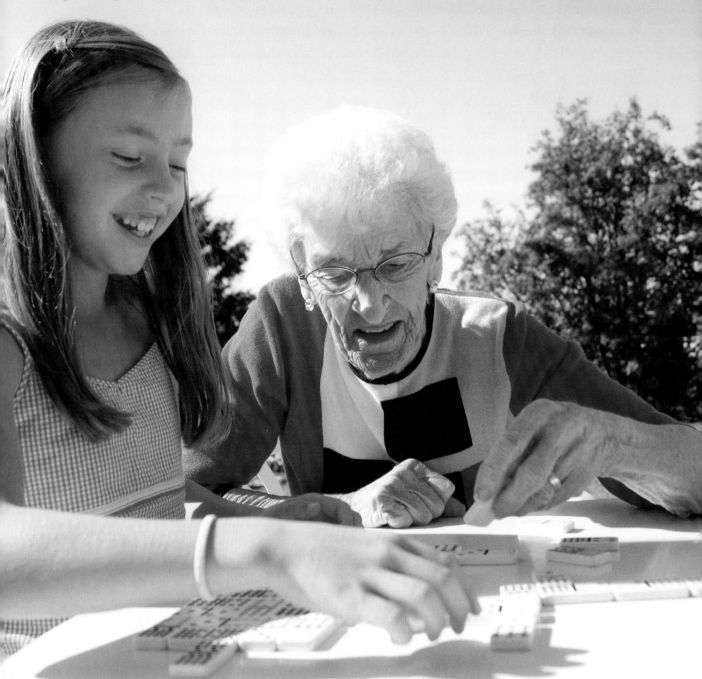

Memory is your ability to store, recall and reuse information. You might imagine that your brain is like a library filled with rooms of shelved books — or, in this case, memories — just waiting to be checked out and read.

But this analogy is only half true. Unlike a library's shelved books, your brain doesn't store an entire memory in a single place. Instead, the part of your brain called the hippocampus breaks memories down into pieces — such as how an object looks, smells, sounds and feels — then stores these pieces in different parts of your brain.

For example, the melody of one of your favorite songs may be stored in your temporal lobes, the areas of your brain that allow you to interpret sounds. What you know of the lyrics, on the other hand, may be stored in your frontal and parietal lobes. But there also may be, for example, certain emotions you associate with the song or information about the vocalist. This may be stored in other parts of your brain.

Whenever you hear the melody on the radio, your brain goes to work, reassembling a single memory from many different locations and — there you have it — you recognize the song and can sing along.

Your brain functions with two different kinds of memory: recent and remote. Your recent memory is for information that you need to remember for very short amounts of time. It's what you use for that interval between the time you look up a phone number and the time you dial the phone.

Recent memory has a high "turnover rate," meaning the bits of information are continually being replaced. Recent memory helps keep your brain clutter-free, allowing you to discard numbers and facts that you no longer need.

Remote memory, on the other hand, is stored in your brain for a longer time so that you can access this information when you need it — whether in 10 hours or 10 years. Your remote memory retains computer passwords, the directions to a friend's house and how you got a scar on your knee when you were 12 years old.

For a memory to become remote, it must go through a process called consolidation. When you learn someone's name, for example, that information forms a neural pathway in your brain. To become a long-term memory, the pathway must be strengthened. There are a variety of ways that this could happen: focusing your atten-

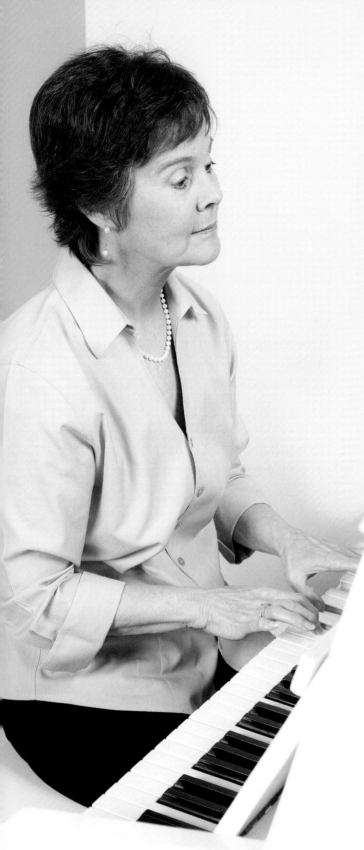

tion on the name when you first learn it, repeating or rehearsing the name afterward, or associating the name with more familiar knowledge. Any of these steps may help you remember.

Say you're learning to play the piano. You strike a skinny black key, and the sound of it vibrates briefly in your ears. That brief millisecond of recognition is your sensory register in action.

You note the location of that key among all the other black keys. Then your teacher points to a squiggle on the sheet music in front of you and says, "That's the note for an E flat." You hit the key again. The sound of the note and the information you've received are now registered in your recent memory.

If you go away and never play that note again, the information you learned will likely be forgotten. You will probably not remember which black key allows you to play an E flat note.

If, however, you practice regularly, associating the mark for E flat on the sheet music with the black key you're pressing, this information will pass into your remote memory.

Emotionally charged events often register in your remote memory without the need of consolidation. That includes first dates, marriages, vacations, job promotions, relationship breakups, accidents and even events, such as natural disasters, that you've had no part in. Many people vividly remember where they were and what they were doing at the instant of a faraway calamity.

Cognitive changes with typical aging

Starting around age 50, many people begin to notice subtle changes in their cognitive functions, such as memory, learning and decision-making skills. Their minds don't seem as nimble and sharp as they had once been. Although knowing these changes can happen may be unsettling, the reality is a little less forbidding than it seems.

It's true that as you age, the number of neurons in your brain decreases. This means there will be fewer neural connections and, potentially, less communication. Your brain actually shrinks (atrophies) as brain mass decreases.

But with billions of neurons and trillions of connections between them, your brain has a capacity that far exceeds what you'll probably ever require in your lifetime. Even better news is that living neurons continue to make new connections, replacing at least some of the ones that are lost.

Nevertheless, neuron loss from aging will affect your cognition to some extent.

What do these changes mean? For most people, it means becoming a little more forgetful — these are momentary lapses of memory often brought on by inattention or distraction. Forgetfulness is typical with aging. Aspects of forgetfulness include:

Difficulty with details. It may be harder to recall information that you feel you should know easily, such as the date of your best friend's birthday or the title of a book you finished reading recently. It's frustrating when you need to remember this information "on the spot."

Being absentminded. Being absentminded is often the culprit when you can't find your wallet or you overlook an appointment. It happens when you're too preoccupied with a single thought and overlook everything else. It also can result from doing too many things at once and not paying attention to any one thing.

What is cognition?

The term *cognition* comes from a Latin word that means "to know." It refers to all the processes of the brain that allow you to think and consciously act, to experience your surroundings, and to feel emotions. These mental processes involve awareness, perception, judgment, reason, learning and memory. Cognitive processes are in contrast to the many involuntary processes that your body undertakes, such as heartbeat and respiration — you don't have to think in order for those functions to take place.

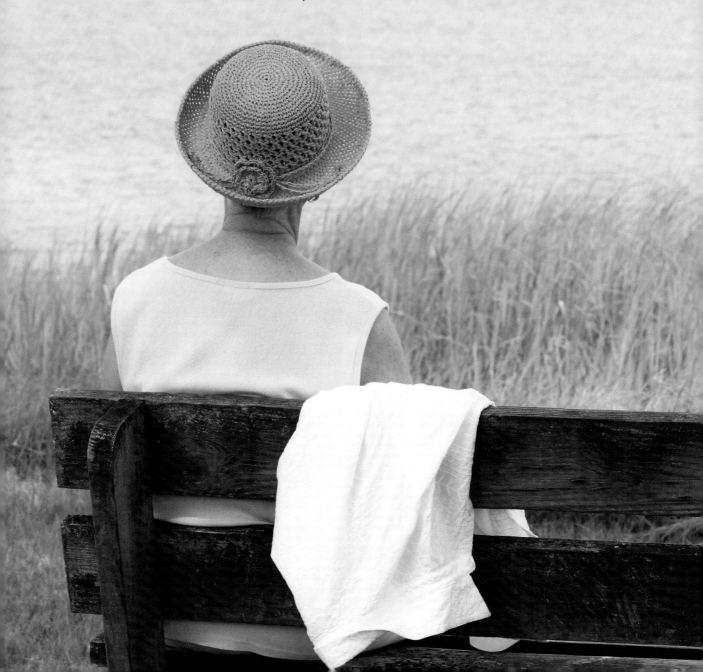

Weakened memories. Remote memories that you don't often call upon will fade with time. This is common sense: You remember the things you think about most often and lose track of the things you rarely need to recall.

Memory blocks. Do you ever have something to say but just can't think of the words to express it? Memory blocks may be the culprit if you find yourself saying, "The answer's right on the tip of my tongue!" This lapse can occur if you overconcentrate on what you want to say or if a persistent, deeply ingrained memory is blocking the concept you're after.

Besides memory (and forgetfulness), other cognitive functions are vulnerable to aging. Your brain may require more processing time for complex problems when compared with your 30- and 40-something counterparts. This may happen more frequently with input that's visually challenging and with complex construction tasks.

When given adequate time, older adults deliver accurate, effective solutions that are equal to those of younger adults. So if you're someone who enjoys solving complex puzzles, for example, you should be able to continue doing them well into old age — though you may find that the task takes a little longer to complete.

Making sense of new or unfamiliar information also may be more difficult as you age. Let's say you've waited to learn to drive a car until you were in your late 50s. While the instructions given in a driver's education class may "click" right away for teenagers, you may need a little more time — and maybe just a bit more instruction to master the skills.

This doesn't mean that you've lost intelligence or can no longer think for yourself. On the contrary, most people remain very capable as they age — it just may be a bit harder to make sense of new or unconventional information.

There are important cognitive functions that are hardly affected by the normal aging process. Your ability to focus, concentrate and create aren't diminished by age. Using a rich vocabulary and saying what you mean actually improve with each passing year.

Perhaps most importantly, age brings wisdom — the ability to enlighten others with the insight and knowledge that you've gained from a lifetime of experiences.

Some reassurance

Before reading further in this book, understand this: Minor memory lapses happen to almost everyone as they age. The lapses don't mean that dementia is just around the corner. While the possibility exists that any older adult can develop a form of dementia, such as the one due to Alzheimer's disease, having Alzheimer's should not be considered a typical part of aging.

The truth is that AD involves more than memory loss. Take the example of Mary at the beginning of this chapter. She's misplacing her purse and forgetting where she parked the car but, so far at least, she's not exhibiting other signs and symptoms of dementia, such as confusion, anxiety or inappropriate behavior. For John, the struggle to find words could mean the age-related slowing down of mental processing and not the onset of dementia.

The very fact that Mary and John are both aware of their forgetfulness suggests that they probably don't have Alzheimer's disease.

If a family member or friend is exhibiting memory loss, don't assume that he or she has dementia. Appearances can be deceiving — just because you think something looks like dementia, sounds like dementia and feels like dementia doesn't make it dementia. You need a specialist's careful interpretation of the signs and symptoms and study of the family history.

Sometimes, when older adults feel lonely, worried or bored, they exhibit signs and symptoms associated with dementia. For example, coping with emotional trauma or the death of a spouse can cause extreme changes in personality and behavior. Instead of jumping to conclusions, become more informed and talk with a doctor you trust about your concerns.

Chapter 2

Abnormal aging and dementia

Frank is 75 years old and proud to say that he's lived in a house for the past 40 years that he built with his own two hands. Though his wife died years ago, he feels like he's doing OK on his own and doesn't ask for a lot of help from family and friends.

For years, Frank liked to tinker in his workshop, fixing cars, lawn mowers, appliances — basically anything with a motor in need of repair. Almost every day, he dropped by a neighborhood diner to drink coffee and talk with other regulars. On weekends, he looked forward to visits from his grandchildren.

Months ago, people began noticing changes in Frank's behavior. Now, he's constantly misplacing keys, tools, glasses, food items and anything else he carries in his hands. Several times,

he's started out for the diner, only to become confused about where he was going and tried to turn back — unfortunately, remembering how to get back home also was a struggle for him.

Frank has become moodier. Sometimes, he'll ask the same question over and over again. He's having trouble counting out change. He just can't seem to finish workshop projects anymore. According to one grandchild, Frank insists that he's recently talked with his wife.

Family members are concerned about these changes, which appear to primarily affect Frank's cognition — his ability to reason, decide and remember. They're also disturbed by the changes to his personality. They worry that whatever is causing Frank's problems will only get worse.

Abnormal aging

How well people retain their cognitive skills as they get older varies widely. While some people begin to struggle with memory lapses in their 50s, other people retain good memory well into their 90s — and their reasoning and judgment stay sharp to boot. Regardless of degree, the changes that occur don't appear to disrupt everyday life, and cognition remains relatively intact. It's all part of typical aging.

But not all changes that occur later in life are typical. Some people, particularly after age 65, experience a sustained, severe decline in several aspects of cognition. They begin having trouble processing information, particularly new information. Memory problems and periods of confusion are

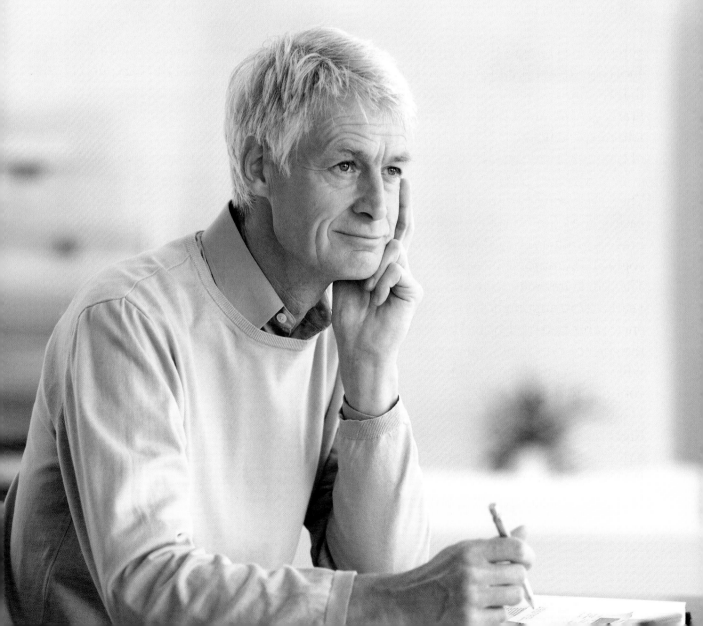

frequent. They struggle to keep their concentration, express ideas clearly, think abstractly and calculate numbers. They undergo personality changes, have trouble controlling emotions, and become paranoid or withdrawn.

Although these signs and symptoms are often associated with getting older, they should not be considered part of typical aging. Rather, these are signs and symptoms of abnormal aging.

Some of the changes that Frank is showing are abnormal, and it's unlikely that the problems are solely a result of Frank getting older. Not every older adult experiences cognitive impairment of this kind or to this degree.

There's a strong likelihood that disease-related (pathological) changes in Frank's brain are responsible for the cognitive symptoms he's experiencing. These changes may have started many years before anyone noticed a difference in his personality and behavior. As the disease progresses, the symptoms will worsen and Frank's cognition will continue to deteriorate.

Right now, Frank seems unaware that a problem exists because Frank lacks insight. He's unconcerned because he doesn't recognize his own failing memory and troubling behavior. Frank also doesn't appear to be depressed or withdrawn. But the symptoms are affecting his ability to carry out the tasks of daily living.

Family members are beginning to wonder whether a serious medical problem may be involved. And they're questioning whether it's still a good idea for Frank to be living alone. The best action that the family could take would be scheduling a visit for Frank with his personal physician or with a specialist in disorders of the nervous system (neurologist).

The cognitive spectrum

It wasn't that long ago specialists believed that clear boundaries existed between what would be considered normal cognition and impaired cognition. Either a person had no disease-related changes in the brain and was normal, or he or she had pathological changes in the brain, leading to severe cognitive impairment.

Using advanced imaging technology and other forms of testing, scientists have gained a better understanding of cognitive decline. They can identify minute changes in the physical struc-

Aging and cognitive change

This graph illustrates the different paths that cognition may take as people age. The vertical axis indicates the cognitive spectrum, with good cognition at the top of the axis and poor or impaired cognition at the bottom of the axis. The horizontal axis indicates years of age. Cognition levels range across the spectrum.

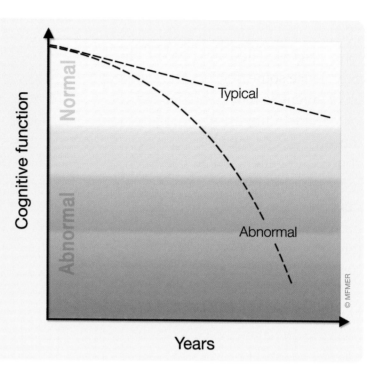

ture and chemical balance of the brain that may put you at increased risk of a neurodegenerative disorder such as Alzheimer's disease.

Just as important, scientists have learned that the physical and chemical changes in the brain can begin long before any signs and symptoms are evident — often, many years before. These findings have caused specialists to reconsider their approach. Cognition cannot be described strictly in terms of "either-or:" it's in either a normal state or an abnormal state.

It may be more accurate to describe a person's cognitive status in terms of a spectrum, or a wide, continuous range. On one end of the spectrum is normal function, a state in which cognitive skills are intact. At the other end of the spectrum is dementia, a state in which disease has severely disrupted cognitive skills. Between these extremes are many functional levels at which a person's cognition may shift back and forth between good function and poor function.

As the line graph on this page shows, age plays a major role in the cognitive spectrum. That's because people are at a higher risk of neurodegenerative disorders as they get older. The various disorders that can cause dementia are described later in this chapter.

The top line on the graph represents typical aging. These are people who experience some degree of cognitive impairment as they get older. Many factors, including disease, injury and trauma, genetic inheritance, substance abuse, and general wear and tear, may reduce or disrupt cognition. In a few cases, the cause of cognitive problems may be curable, for example, a serious infection such as meningitis that can be treated with antibiotics.

How much cognition is impaired varies. Some people may get a little more forgetful than they used to be but have no other symptoms. Other people may have trouble grasping new ideas or struggle to keep up with conversations, in addition to the memory issues. Regardless of a drop-off in cognitive function, people who "typically" age are still able to function well in everyday life.

A small pool of people, most of whom have been blessed with both good health and good genes, represent what may be optimal aging. They continue to enjoy good cognition as they grow old, including memory, reason, judgment, concentration, analytic skill, decision-making and language use.

The lower line on the graph represents abnormal aging, and with each passing year comes sharp cognitive decline. For example, the symptoms of Alzheimer's disease typically begin to appear in people in their mid-60s — causing cognitive function to drop deeper into abnormal levels. As the disease spreads in the brain, more cognitive skills become affected. The end of this degenerative process is marked by dementia, at which point people will have experienced severe impairment.

Dementia

If Frank's symptoms are caused by a neurodegenerative disorder, then the progressive changes in his brain will eventually impair his cognitive functions to an extreme degree. At this time, a neurologist or other specialist may diagnose Frank with dementia. If the physician believes that Alzheimer's disease is the condition responsible for this impairment, Frank's condition will be diagnosed as dementia due to Alzheimer's disease.

People with dementia may become dependent on others for personal care, such as eating, bathing, dressing and using the bathroom. They may lose their ability to use and understand language, either written or spoken. They

What's a syndrome?

A syndrome is a collection of signs and symptoms that occur in a consistent pattern — and the pattern often indicates a specific condition as a cause. For example, during a medical examination, if a doctor notes severe memory loss, confusion and personality changes, the doctor will likely suspect the condition is dementia due to Alzheimer's disease. With a different set of symptoms, the doctor may suspect a different condition as a cause, for example, dementia due to vascular cognitive impairment.

You may be aware of syndromes other than dementia. For example, many women regularly experience headache, fatigue, breast tenderness and irritability before their menstrual cycles in what is known as premenstrual syndrome (PMS). Other well-known syndromes include carpal tunnel syndrome and acquired immunodeficiency syndrome (AIDS).

may be unable to interact with other people or incapable of living independently. Some of these capacities may be retained longer than others.

Many people think of dementia as a disease. In fact, dementia is a syndrome, which means it's a collection of signs and symptoms caused by disease. The signs and symptoms vary according to what's causing the syndrome. A wide variety of diseases and conditions that can cause dementia are discussed in more detail later in this chapter. But regardless of its form, dementia means certain cognitive functions have become severely impaired.

Although a wide variety of signs and symptoms may be included in dementia, some of the most common are:

- Memory loss
- Difficulty communicating
- Inability to learn new information
- Inability to reason
- Difficulty with planning and organizing
- Difficulty with coordination and motor function
- Personality changes
- Inappropriate behavior
- Paranoia
- Agitation
- Hallucinations

Memory loss is a common symptom of dementia — in fact, it's a hallmark of dementia due to Alzheimer's disease — but memory loss by itself does not mean you have dementia.

Having dementia means you have significant problems with at least two different cognitive functions, one of which is memory. For example, dementia could be signaled by memory loss with impaired language use or with extreme personality changes (or with both). It's the combination of signs and symptoms that's critical for a diagnosis.

Scientists hope to detect different patterns of cognitive change — and therefore identify the cause of dementia — in the earliest stages. Many believe that the best time to treat dementia is when it is just beginning, before the condition is well established in the brain.

Scientists also hope to discover links between signs and symptoms and how fast or how far a person shifts through the cognitive spectrum from normal function to dementia. For example, why does memory stabilize for some people after mild to moderate loss while other people have severe decline? Due to the brain's complexity, questions such as these may be difficult to resolve with any certainty.

Common causes of dementia

Cognition refers to brain processes that allow you to think, reason and interact within your environment. If these processes become seriously impaired, the result is some form of dementia. Most cases of serious impairment are caused by neurodegenerative disorders (of the central nervous system) or vascular disorders (of the circulatory system) or a combination of both.

Current treatment options help ease the symptoms of dementia but cannot cure many of the causes. For a few exceptions, dementia may arise from conditions that can be treated, such as from medication side effects or infection.

Neurodegenerative disorders. Neurodegenerative disorders are those caused by the progressive loss of or damage to nerve cells (neurons) in the brain. There are four primary forms of neurodegenerative disorders that ultimately lead to dementia.

Alzheimer's disease. Alzheimer's disease (AD) is the most common cause of serious cognitive impairment and dementia. People with Alzheimer's begin losing functioning neurons in the interior part of the brain associated with memory and emotions. Those affected begin to experience memory loss and personality changes. As the disease progresses, the number of impaired cognitive skills increases and their severity worsens. Performing routine, everyday tasks becomes more difficult.

Over time, people with Alzheimer's can become disoriented, delusional, and possibly short-tempered or hostile. They may not recognize loved ones. Eventually, basic functions, such as speaking or chewing and swallowing food, may become seriously impaired or lost altogether.

Frontotemporal degeneration. Frontotemporal degeneration (FTD) actually refers to a group of brain disorders, and all are characterized by the extreme loss of neurons in the frontal and temporal lobes of the brain (see Chapter 10). Initially, people with FTD experience behavioral and personality disturbances. They may exhibit compulsive behavior, motor problems, and impaired speech and language. Memory loss typically occurs later in the disease.

Dementia with Lewy bodies. Dementia with Lewy bodies (DLB) gets its name from abnormal protein deposits, called Lewy bodies, that develop in the brain, primarily in the cortex (see Chapter 11). Similar to AD, signs and symp-

toms of cognitive impairment with Lewy bodies may include confusion, impaired memory, poor judgment and hallucinations. DLB may also mimic Parkinson's disease, with such signs and symptoms as a shuffling, unsteady walk and bent posture.

Parkinson's disease dementia. Parkinson's disease is a progressive neurodegenerative disorder that affects movement (see Chapter 13). It causes muscle tremors (shaking) and stiffness. People in the later stages of Parkinson's may develop dementia, but it may not always be the case with this condition.

Vascular disorders. Your vascular system involves the heart and a network of blood vessels that circulate blood throughout your body — from your head to your feet and everywhere in between.

Conditions such as high cholesterol, high blood pressure and atherosclerosis can put you at risk of cardiovascular disease, heart attack and stroke. Forms of dementia known as vascular cognitive impairment (VCI) occur when brain tissue is deprived of nourishing blood flow (see Chapter 12).

One of the most common forms of VCI results from a series of small strokes to the brain. These strokes damage brain tissue after the blood supply is blocked, creating areas of dead tissue called infarcts. The infarcts appear as lesions in the brain's white matter.

The onset of VCI may be sudden if the strokes are severe. And the condition may progress in a step-by-step fashion with each incident of an additional stroke. The symptoms may include cognitive impairment, loss of motor skills, and delusions or depression. Depending on where the infarcts are located in the brain, symptoms may be limited to just one side of the body or to a couple of cognitive functions.

Although damage to brain tissue from strokes cannot be reversed, factors that can increase the chance of future strokes, such as high blood pressure, can be treated, helping to prevent further damage.

Diagnosing a cause of dementia isn't as easy as checking off the entries on a symptoms list. The various neurodegenerative and vascular causes described here share many of the same signs and symptoms. Complicating the issue is the fact that, frequently, two conditions may develop in the same person at the same time, making it difficult to distinguish between them.

Other causes of dementia

Cognitive impairment may be a result of conditions that are not primarily neurodegenerative or vascular in nature. Some of these conditions you may have heard of, or even experienced, without being aware that dementia-like symptoms may result.

What distinguishes many of these conditions is that treatment can reverse the cognitive impairment or stop it from progressing. That's why it's important to contact your doctor if you're experiencing any significant problems with memory and concentration.

Other causes of cognitive impairment may include:

Infection. Inflammation of brain tissue from infections such as meningitis and encephalitis can damage brain cells and cause dementia-like symptoms as your body works to overcome the infection. Meningitis may cause confusion, impaired judgment and memory loss, but if caught early, both the infection and the resulting impairment can be cured.

Reaction to medication. The side effects from some drugs can cause temporary problems with memory and concentration.

Metabolic or endocrine imbalances. Diseases of the thyroid, kidney, pancreas and liver can upset the chemical balance of your blood, causing delirium or dementia.

Normal-pressure hydrocephalus. A buildup of cerebrospinal fluid can compress brain tissue even though the fluid pressure remains normal.

Brain tumors. Certain tumors may cause dementia symptoms, for example, if a tumor presses against brain structures that control hormone levels.

Subdural hematoma. The collection of blood between the brain's surface and its thin outer covering can cause dementia-like symptoms.

Heart and lung problems. Conditions such as heart disease, emphysema and pneumonia can deprive the blood stream of oxygen, causing cell death and possibly dementia.

Nutritional deficiencies. Deficiencies of nutrients, such as the B vitamins, may cause dementia-like symptoms.

Chronic alcoholism. The complications of chronic alcoholism, such as liver disease and nutritional deficiencies, can lead to dementia.

Substance abuse. Misuse of prescription drugs, such as sleeping pills and tranquilizers, may cause dementia symptoms. Street drugs, especially in high doses, can have a similar effect.

Poisoning. Exposure to toxic solvents or fumes without protective equipment can damage brain cells and ultimately lead to dementia.

Risk factors for dementia

What factors can put you at risk of dementia? Some, such as age and family history, are ones you can't avoid — they cannot be changed. Others, however, are lifestyle related, which means you may be able to minimize their impact or avoid them altogether.

As you review these factors, remember that if several apply to you, it's not a promise that dementia is in your future. Calculating risk is an inexact science — it estimates what your chances are of getting a disease over a certain period of time — and by no means is your risk result definitive.

Age. The risk of getting dementia approximately doubles every five years after you reach age 65. The risk is about 50 percent after age 85.

Family history. As a rule, people with a family history of Alzheimer's are considered at higher risk than are people without that family history.

Genes. Researchers have identified certain genes and gene mutations that increase your risk of dementia. Of course, rules are made to be broken — and some people with this particular genetic makeup never develop Alzheimer's. The bottom line: It's still not possible to predict the risk of dementia strictly based on genetic evidence.

Cardiovascular problems. There appears to be a connection between the health of your brain and of your heart. Risk of stroke and vascular cognitive impairment increases with the development of atherosclerosis and high levels of low-density lipoprotein cholesterol or high blood pressure.

Diabetes. Diabetes can damage blood vessels in the brain and increase the risk of vascular cognitive impairment. In addition, ongoing research is uncovering possible links between diabetes and Alzheimer's disease.

Smoking. Although somewhat controversial, some studies indicate that people who smoke have a higher risk of dementia. One reason for this may be that smokers have a higher risk of cardiovascular disease that, in turn, increases the risk of dementia.

Although there are still no definitive conclusions, accumulating evidence suggests that some lifestyle factors — such as physical activity, social engagement, and continuing to learn and challenge your mind — may actually have protective effects on the brain and help reduce the risk of dementia. You can learn more about these factors in chapters 14 and 15.

Causes of dementia-like symptoms

Sometimes you may worry that a loved one is showing signs and symptoms of dementia, when it's really nothing of the sort. For example, some people fear that mild memory loss is the first step to dementia, but it's likely to be a natural slowing down of mental processing. With some accommodation for forgetfulness, there's little cause for alarm.

More serious memory loss is associated with mild cognitive impairment (MCI).

This condition occurs when people experience cognitive problems beyond what's considered normal, age-related decline — but not so much that it interferes with their quality of life. Though MCI isn't dementia, people who experience it do have a significantly higher risk of developing dementia in the future. For more on MCI, see Chapter 6.

Two other conditions — depression and delirium — may mimic dementia, but both are treatable conditions.

Depression

People often use the term *depression* to describe a temporary low mood that comes from a bad day or bad feeling. But as a medical term, *depression* denotes a serious illness that affects your thoughts, emotions, feelings, behaviors and physical health.

People used to think depression was "all in your head" and that if you really tried, you could pull out of the mood. Doctors now know that depression is not a weakness and you can't treat it on your own. It's a medical disorder with a biological or chemical basis.

Sometimes, a stressful event, such as retirement or the death of a spouse,

triggers depression. Other times depression seems to occur spontaneously with no identifiable cause. Regardless, depression is much more than grieving or a bout of the blues.

Like those who experience dementia, people with depression may be confused, forgetful and slow to respond. The condition affects how they feel, think, eat, sleep and act.

Two hallmark symptoms of depression are an ongoing sense of sadness and despair and loss of interest in activities that once brought pleasure. Individuals often have difficulty concentrating, which may give them the appearance of having a dementing illness.

Other signs and symptoms of depression may include:

- Unexplained weight loss or gain and, accordingly, decreased appetite or increased cravings
- Sleep disturbance, either insomnia or excessive sleeping
- Irritability or angry outbursts
- Agitation, restlessness or anxiety
- Fatigue and loss of energy
- Poor concentration, indecisiveness and distractibility
- Feelings of low self-esteem
- Thoughts of death or suicide

Depression affects each person in a different way, so the symptoms will vary. For some people, depression symptoms are so severe that it's obvious something isn't right. Other people feel generally miserable or unhappy without really knowing why.

It's extremely important to see your doctor if you become concerned about any changes. The symptoms may not get better on their own — and depression may get worse if it isn't treated. Even if the symptoms aren't associated with depression, it's important to identify underlying reasons for distress.

Depression is the most common condition that accompanies dementia. Although brief periods of discouragement and apathy may be expected when someone is dealing with a diagnosis of Alzheimer's, prolonged despondency should not go untreated. When dementia is present, the negative impact of depression on emotions and intellect can be even more extreme.

Delirium

Delirium is a state of mental confusion and clouded consciousness. Individuals with delirium go through a range of extreme emotions.

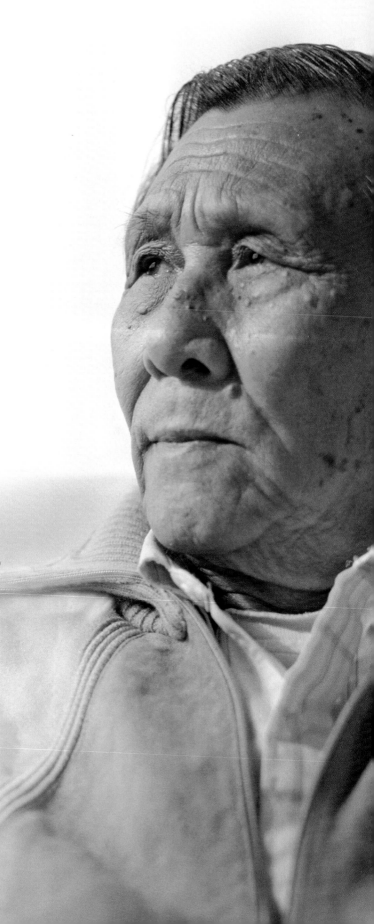

Symptoms of delirium may include:

- Wandering attention or inability to stay focused
- Poor memory, particularly of recent events
- Rambling or nonsense speech
- Disorientation
- Agitation, irritability or combative behavior
- Hallucinations
- Sleep disturbance

Though the signs and symptoms of delirium may be mistaken for those of dementia, there are important differences. One difference is that the signs and symptoms of delirium usually appear over a short period of time, from a few hours to a few days. And the symptoms may fluctuate throughout that time.

Another difference is that delirium is often caused by a treatable condition. In such cases, emergency medical treatment of delirium is critical because the underlying cause may be a serious infection such as bacterial meningitis.

Delirium may occur in older adults who have lung or heart disease, long-term infections, poor nutrition, or hormone disorders. Delirium may also result from medication interactions, alcohol or drug abuse, or emotional stress. Someone with dementia can develop delirium, often due to another medical condition such as a urinary tract infection.

Whether depression or delirium occurs alone or in combination with dementia, both are treatable conditions. That's a reason to see your doctor if you or a loved one exhibits symptoms of cognitive impairment. The sooner the condition can be diagnosed, the sooner you can find relief and start to feel better.

Chapter 3

Diagnosing abnormal signs and symptoms

Sarah is a 68-year-old woman who hasn't felt her normal self in months. In addition to increasing forgetfulness, Sarah has frequent moments of confusion and anxiety. She needs more help around the house but gets defensive and snaps at friends and neighbors when they try to help her — something she never did before.

Her daughter is urging Sarah to see a doctor, but she is reluctant. She claims that if the family can just be patient for a little longer, she'll work things out and "shake" the symptoms on her own. If she were being honest, however, Sarah might admit that she's afraid of going in for medical tests.

Like many other people, Sarah hopes that what she doesn't know won't hurt her. Her daughter assures her that seeing a doctor is the right thing to do. The truth is that whatever the result — good news or bad news — the doctor will find ways to make Sarah's life easier and ease everyone's concerns. The sooner that Sarah makes an appointment, the better are her chances for getting help.

People often don't recognize a serious medical problem when the signs and symptoms first appear. They may pass them off as "getting old." Or they may view the forgetfulness, confusion and mood swings as separate problems and don't draw connections between them. Some people may be aware that something's going on but are reluctant to dig deeper. Like Sarah, they're afraid of what they might learn — they'd just as soon not know whether or not they have a serious condition.

It's true that if Sarah is experiencing memory loss, confusion and extreme mood swings, a doctor will very likely consider dementia as a possible diagnosis. But a neurodegenerative disease isn't the only cause of these symptoms.

It's also possible she has a potentially reversible condition, such as a thyroid disorder, depression or drug interaction. The earlier Sarah makes an appointment, undergoes the evaluation and receives a diagnosis, the more

New guidelines for neurocognitive disorders

The Diagnostic and Statistical Manual of Mental Disorders (DSM) is used by medical specialists for the diagnosis of more than 300 mental health conditions, including neurocognitive disorders. The criteria often guide treatment decisions and also are used to determine health insurance coverage and benefits and to reimburse health care providers. In 2013, the fifth edition of this authoritative handbook, commonly referred to as DSM-5, was published by the American Psychiatric Association.

The DSM-5 outlines three main categories of neurocognitive disorder: mild neurocognitive disorder (NCD), major NCD and delirium. In making a diagnosis, one of the categories will be paired with the condition considered responsible for the symptoms — for example, a person may be diagnosed with mild NCD due to Alzheimer's disease. This reflects the two-step diagnostic process: First, determine the level of cognitive impairment and its effect on a person's ability to function in everyday life, and, second, determine the cause of the impairment.

While the classifications in the fifth edition differ from previous editions of DSM, there may be little change in how clinicians actually diagnose Alzheimer's disease. The new terminology of mild NCD and major NCD, which will be used by psychiatrists, corresponds closely to the constructs of mild cognitive impairment due to Alzheimer's disease and dementia due to Alzheimer's disease that are used in this book.

options she'll likely have that may improve her symptoms and better her life.

For example, the doctor may find that Sarah's problems with memory and doing household chores are age-related. What about her confusion and moodiness? Those could be a result of drug interactions from new medications that were prescribed last month. By changing her prescriptions, Sarah could feel her life rapidly returning to normal.

On the other hand, the doctor may perform tests that exclude treatable causes, pointing the diagnosis toward dementia. Though such a diagnosis may be difficult to hear, there are advantages to receiving the news early. Sarah can use the time to establish a support system, organize affairs and arrange for care in the months ahead. The earlier the diagnosis, the better you can:

Prepare for the changes ahead. Extra time allows you to learn more about the disease, which may lessen anxiety and fear. It also allows family members to prepare adequately for new living arrangements and day-to-day care.

Explore all of the treatment options. Although no drug can stop or reverse the disorder, some drugs can help treat the early-stage symptoms of dementia and greatly improve quality of life. Perhaps a new drug that's still in clinical trials may be the one that's able to slow progress of the disease.

Treat coexisting conditions. You may experience depression, anxiety or a sleep disorder in addition to dementia. Often, treating these conditions results in improved general health and potentially better cognition.

Arrange medical, legal and financial care. Early diagnosis may allow you to actively participate with your family in critical long-term decisions, particularly decisions that relate to your care in later stages of the disease.

Common tests and evaluations

Although a physician may be your primary contact, a whole team of medical professionals may be involved in diagnosing a neurodegenerative disorder, including specialists such as a neurologist and psychiatrist. The basic evaluation includes a medical history, a physical examination, a neurological evaluation, and cognitive and neuropsychological tests.

Some of the tests are used to assess a person's current level of cognition (memory, reason, judgment, attention) and whether or not brain function has been altered. Other tests are used to identify or eliminate medical conditions other than dementia that could be a cause of the symptoms.

Some tests may help determine the specific type of dementia, if that's what the symptoms are pointing to. The medical team will use all of the test results to find ways to ease the impact of symptoms and improve quality of life.

The following are tests and procedures that you can expect during a diagnostic evaluation of the symptoms.

Medical history

To compile a medical history, the doctor will typically begin by interviewing the person who is exhibiting the signs and symptoms. The doctor will often include insights in the interview from someone that the person spends a lot of time with.

Interviewing a spouse, partner, family member or friend is important because it's often difficult for an individual to remember every detail. It allows the doctor to get another perspective on what is often one person's subjective account of what happened, influenced by emotions and preconceptions.

The purpose of the interview is to establish a chronology of events, identify signs and symptoms that could be associated with dementia, and determine the degree to which they impact the person's life. The doctor will want to record personality and mood changes, and assess how the person performs tasks now in comparison with his or her previous level of competence — including household chores, mental computations and social interactions.

Interview questions may include:

- What's your daily routine like?
- What were the first symptoms and when did you notice them?
- Have the symptoms gotten worse or remained relatively constant?
- Are the symptoms severe enough to interfere with daily activities?

The doctor may also ask questions about past or ongoing medical concerns, any over-the-counter or prescription medications being taken, a family history of dementia and other diseases, and the social and cultural background of the family.

Preparing for an appointment

A medical history is an integral part of the diagnostic process. It's a good idea to have the following information prepared before your appointment:

- Primary concern that made you seek an evaluation in the first place
- Changes you've noticed in daily routines or in your performance of common tasks
- Any signs and symptoms that you feel are particular problems, including when they began, how frequently they recur and how they affect activities in daily life
- General outlook on life
- Current and past medical problems, including when they were diagnosed and what treatments were prescribed
- Family history of medical problems, including relationships and ages of the individuals when the problems were diagnosed
- Medications currently being taken, including both prescription and nonprescription medications — and don't forget about herbal and dietary supplements

Physical examination

Assessing the current status of the person's physical health is another critical element of the diagnostic process. Any number of factors, such as congestive heart failure, hypothyroidism, or vision and hearing problems, may affect cognitive functions. This part of the diagnostic process may include:

- **General physical.** Reveals medical conditions that may be contributing to cognitive impairment as well as to other symptoms.
- **Electrocardiogram.** Records heartbeat patterns that may help identify various heart conditions.
- **Chest X-ray.** Produces internal images to help assess general health as well as identify factors that may be contributing to symptoms.
- **Nutritional assessment.** Checks nutritional health and weight status, both of which are reflective of overall physical health.

Neurological evaluation

This series of tests focuses on the function of the brain, spinal cord and peripheral nervous system, evaluating balance, sensation, reflexes and other neurological elements. The tests can help assess muscle strength, nerve function and the ability to feel different sensations. A neurological exam may identify signs of Parkinson's disease, strokes, tumors or other medical conditions that can impair cognition as well as physical function.

Mental status evaluation

These tests help determine which cognitive functions may be impaired. The assessment may include interviews and written tests to evaluate:

- Recent memory
- Remote memory
- Attention span
- Awareness of time and place
- Word comprehension, especially in relation to reading and writing
- Ability to perform daily activities

Common neuropsychological tests

To test ...	The doctor may ask a person ...
Recent memory	To learn a list of words and repeat them, then recall them after a delay of several minutes, and after that, identify them from a longer list of words
Remote memory	To relate facts from personal history — such as childhood recollections, where the person lived, worked or went to school, or when he or she got married
Language skills	To name common objects in the room, such as a desk, light switch or curtain; to follow commands, such as repeating a simple phrase or pointing at different items in succession
Motor skills	To stack blocks, arrange pencils in a specific design or demonstrate how he or she brushes teeth
Executive skills	To count to 10, point out the similarities and differences in related words, or list words that begin with a certain letter

Additional evaluations may include doing simple calculations, language exercises (such as spelling words backward) and drawing simple designs.

Neuropsychological tests

This battery of tests helps determine the nature and severity of cognitive impairment. The tests are designed to evaluate memory, language competency, judgment, reasoning and problem-solving. They can also assess the level of coordination between a person's vision and muscular movement.

Test results indicate a person's ability to handle a variety of common but complex tasks, such as following recipes and managing finances. They also help decide whether it's safe for that person to be living alone, or to what degree he or she should have assistance at home.

These tests may be critical for differentiating between dementia and another condition, such as depression, that's existing at the same time, especially in the early stages of dementia. The tests may also help distinguish between different dementia types that have similar signs and symptoms, such as Alzheimer's disease, dementia with Lewy bodies and frontotemporal degeneration.

Other diagnostic procedures

If a doctor has conducted the common diagnostic tests but is still looking for answers, he or she may recommend other procedures. These tests may eliminate a potential cause unrelated to dementia or reveal more about a particular symptom.

Laboratory blood tests and urine tests can help pinpoint a treatable cause, such as thyroid problems, anemia, infections, and medication or vitamin levels. For example, a routine test can measure vitamin B levels in the bloodstream as well as liver and thyroid functions. A urine test may detect certain drugs or uncover a urinary tract infection, which can cause confusion or impair cognition in some older adults.

A psychiatric assessment may be recommended as well. This helps determine if the person has depression or another condition that mimics dementia. This assessment may reveal certain cognitive patterns that are clues to the underlying condition.

A doctor may recommend imaging tests, using sophisticated, noninvasive technology, to get a better picture of what's going on inside your brain. Brain imaging can't replace standard diagnostic procedures, but may provide clues or confirm suspicions that help identify the cause of the symptoms.

The different kinds of brain imaging are often categorized as either structural or functional. Which category is selected by the medical team will depend on what kinds of information may be of greatest help to the diagnosis.

Structural imaging

Structural imaging provides pictures showing size, shape and location of the internal structures of your brain. It may be used to help detect strokes, tumors, brain injury, hydrocephalus or other structural abnormalities. The procedure can also reveal shrinkage (atrophy) of brain tissue.

Computerized tomography (CT). Computerized tomography is an imaging technology that's used extensively in diagnostic evaluations of the brain. For the test, you lie on a table inside a doughnut-shaped machine. A scanner inside the machine rotates around you, emitting a series of X-ray beams. A computer collects and processes these scans, combining them into a single, detailed, image. A CT scan makes internal structures visible that are difficult to see on an ordinary X-ray.

Magnetic resonance imaging (MRI). Rather than X-rays, magnetic resonance imaging uses magnetic fields and radio waves to produce the image. For the test, you lie on a table inside a long, tube-like machine that produces a magnetic field. The magnetic field aligns atomic particles in your cells. When radio waves are broadcast in their direction, the particles produce signals that vary according to the type of tissue. Images produced with MRI may show different tissues and more detail than those of a CT scan.

Functional imaging

Functional imaging shows brain activity rather than brain structure. It does so by detecting changes in the chemical composition of brain tissue, such as glucose or oxygen, or in blood flow in the brain. The images help associate mental function, such as listening to a conversation or recalling a memory, with different regions of the brain. Based on the observable changes, a doctor may be able to identify brain activity associated with Alzheimer's disease, for example, rather than frontotemporal degeneration.

Structural imaging

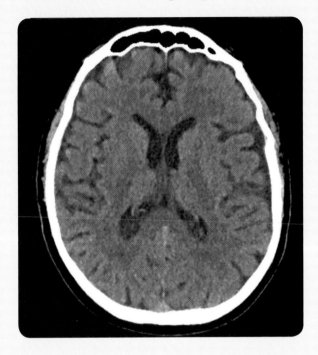

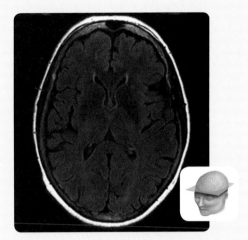

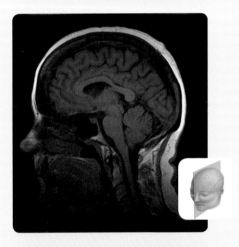

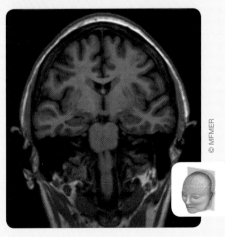

Structural imaging reveals the size and shape of internal structures of the brain. The image above is a computerized tomography (CT) scan of a normal brain showing the cerebral cortex. This view is an axial perspective, meaning from directly above or below the subject.

The column on the right contains magnetic resonance imagining (MRI) scans, a type of structural imaging that provides slightly more detail than does a CT scan. The image at the top of the column is from the axial perspective. Other imaging perspectives include sagittal (middle), which is a view taken from either the left or right side of the subject, and coronal (lower), which is taken from either the front or back of a subject. The different perspectives may be critical to a diagnosis because each perspective can provide different details about a neurological disorder such as Alzheimer's disease.

© MFMER

Normal	Severe AD

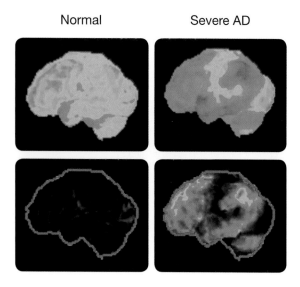

These PET images use a radiotracer to show the conversion (metabolism) of glucose into energy (known as FDG-PET). The top images reveal glucose metabolism in a normal brain (left) and in a brain with severe Alzheimer's (right). Warm colors indicate high metabolism while cool colors indicate low metabolism, and low metabolism means low activity. The bottom images compare these same scans to a statistical norm. Now the color scale is reversed, with cool colors indicating areas of normal activity — making a normal brain appear practically black — and warm colors indicating areas of low activity.

Types of functional imaging include:

Positron emission tomography (PET). This technology detects emissions from a small amount of radioactive material (tracer) injected into your body. PET technology is able to reveal the way in which various tissues in the brain actually use energy.

Single-photon emission computerized tomography (SPECT). Similar to PET technology, a SPECT scan uses a radioactive tracer. A camera that detects the tracer rotates around your head to create 3-D images.

Functional magnetic resonance imaging (fMRI). Similar to an MRI, an fMRI uses magnetism — in this case, the magnetic properties of blood — to record activity in different areas of the brain and to detect changes in this activity over short periods of time. The fMRI technology is used primarily for research and not for diagnosis.

Imaging molecular pathways. Using radioactive tracers (radiotracers) with PET or MRI technology allows researchers to detect biological processes in the brain at the molecular level. When introduced into the brain, these biomarkers trigger chemical changes that are detected by the imaging technology.

A critical development in molecular imaging is the ability to detect amyloid plaques in the living brain. Before this breakthrough, the only way to determine the existence of plaques in the brain was through autopsy.

Amyloid imaging is currently used for research purposes. At this point, the technique cannot predict the development of dementia due to Alzheimer's nor can it replace other diagnostic tests. But amyloid imaging can be a valuable tool for tracking progress of the disease and the effects of medication therapy.

In 2012, the Food and Drug Administration approved the use of the biomarker florbetapir F 18 (Amyvid) with PET imaging to detect amyloid plaques. Pittsburgh compound B (PiB) is another biomarker developed for the same purpose.

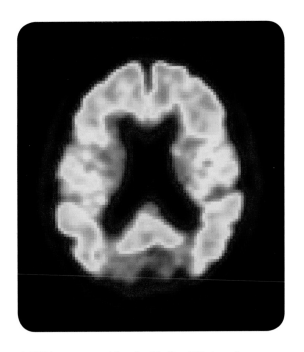

A PET scan combined with the Pittsburgh compound B (PiB) radiotracer reveals how much amyloid-beta is in the brain. Bright yellow and orange colors show areas where the radiotracer has been retained, indicating the presence of plaques.

When symptoms signal dementia

The official criteria most often used to diagnose dementia are established by the American Psychiatric Association and described in a handbook called the Diagnostic and Statistical Manual of Mental Disorders (DSM). The fifth edition (referred to as DSM-5) was published in 2013.

Typically, the following criteria must be met in order for a physician to diagnose dementia due to Alzheimer's:

Problems with at least two cognitive functions. The test results from a thorough evaluation indicate severe impairment in learning and memory, as well as difficulty in one other area of cognition, such as language skills, basic motor functions, recognizing familiar objects or abstract reasoning.

Disruption of daily living. Cognitive impairment is severe enough to disrupt daily activities and personal relationships. The changes represent a serious decline from previous levels of function and independence.

Symptoms aren't linked to depression or delirium. Cognitive changes can't be explained by the presence of a major psychiatric disorder, such as depression. And they don't occur exclusively during a period of delirium — a state of mental confusion and broken concentration and attention that's sometimes mistaken for dementia.

The doctor may look for evidence of uncharacteristic behavior, such as apathy, anxiety, irritability, and inappropriate actions or language. Although these may not be considered cognitive decline, they're common indicators of dementia — and often some of the earliest signs noticed by family and friends that something may be wrong.

People with dementia may repeat questions or conversations over and over again. They may misplace personal items, forget important events or appointments, or get lost on familiar routes. They may have difficulty remembering common words or make speech and writing errors. Often, people with dementia have trouble recognizing familiar faces or objects, and may have difficulty operating simple tools, such as a scissors or fork and knife.

Lack of insight — of understanding what's happening — is common in the early stages of dementia. Those affected by dementia may be unaware of memory loss or other cognitive problems. They may make plans that are unrealistic. For example, a person may insist on investing a lot of money into a business in which he or she has never shown any previous interest. Or, someone with serious balance problems may announce that he or she is going on a vigorous wilderness hike.

People affected by dementia may not observe accepted mores and conventions. They may tell inappropriate or off-color jokes in public and disregard social rules, such as being polite, maintaining personal space and keeping one's voice down. They may act overly friendly with complete strangers. And they may neglect basic hygiene, such as bathing, brushing teeth and wearing clean clothes.

All of these signs and symptoms may be caused by conditions other than dementia in a variety of circumstances. For that reason, it's important not to jump to conclusions if you or a loved one experiences them — especially if just one of these symptoms appears. Remember that dementia is a syndrome, or a collection of symptoms.

It's also important not to self-diagnose, either by checking a symptoms list or taking a screening test — the kind found online or at the drugstore. Such tests are inaccurate and the results can be easily misinterpreted, causing either undue worry from a low score or a false sense of security from a high score. It bears repeating that no single test can unequivocally determine whether you have dementia due to Alzheimer's.

It's more important that you work with your doctor and the other specialists recommended to you. They have the skill, experience and resources to accurately assess the symptoms, make a diagnosis and offer appropriate plans for treatment.

Ruling out other conditions

In addition to ruling out other causes of dementia that may be treatable, such as a metabolic imbalance or substance abuse, your doctor will want to make sure your symptoms are not caused by certain factors or conditions that aren't dementia but are capable of producing the symptoms of dementia. These factors or conditions include:

Delirium. Delirium affects attention and concentration and may cause fluctuations in your consciousness, making it seem as if you may have dementia. But the condition usually comes on suddenly, as opposed to the gradual and more insidious nature of dementia. Be aware that delirium and dementia can occur simultaneously, and they're not always easy to distinguish from each other.

Age-associated impairment. As you get older, your ability to learn and retain new information may decrease a bit, and you may not process information as quickly as you once did. But overall, your cognitive functions are still intact and you have only minor difficulties navigating your daily routine.

Mild cognitive impairment. Some people have problems with memory loss but their difficulties aren't enough to disrupt daily living. Their test results indicate some cognitive impairment but don't meet the criteria for dementia. These people may have mild cognitive impairment, a condition that is not as severe as dementia but of greater concern than the memory changes associated with typical aging.

Mild cognitive impairment increases the risk of developing dementia in the future, so your doctor may conduct regular tests to check for further cognitive changes.

Depression. Depression can produce symptoms similar to dementia, such as unresponsiveness, lack of concentration and confusion. People with depression are generally more aware of cognitive difficulties than are people with dementia, whose family and friends are usually the first ones to notice a problem.

Identifying the cause

The various tests and procedures described in this chapter may help a doctor reach a diagnosis of dementia. But that's not the end of the examination. The doctor must consider an even more complex question: What process or condition is causing these signs and symptoms of dementia?

As described earlier in Chapter 2, many conditions — from vitamin deficiencies to Alzheimer's disease — can cause dementia. And although the different types of dementia have signs and symptoms in common, each type develops in a characteristic pattern with variations that are often subtle.

For example, memory loss is a primary symptom of both Alzheimer's disease and frontotemporal degeneration (FTD). But in Alzheimer's, memory loss is often one of the first symptoms to develop and is very obvious. In FTD, emotional problems typically develop first, with memory loss occurring in later stages of the disease.

So how do doctors go about identifying a cause of dementia? In the same way they diagnose the presence of dementia in the first place — through a systematic process of evaluation, testing, analysis and comparison.

Once again, doctors must consider the various signs and symptoms collectively in order to narrow the field of potential causes. If the person hasn't exhibited any emotional problems to this point and a brain scan shows no damage to the frontal or temporal lobes, for example, frontotemporal degeneration isn't likely to be the culprit. It can be moved down the list of possible causes.

Sometimes determining a type of dementia may be easier than at other times. For example, if strokes are part of the medical history and the doctor establishes that cognitive decline started shortly after a stroke, that's a good indication of vascular cognitive impairment.

Other times, additional testing and lab work may be required to determine the cause of dementia. Memory loss and cognitive decline may clearly suggest dementia, for example, but it may not be until Parkinson's, HIV, brain tumors and myriad other causes have been ruled out — and crucial brain scans studied — that the doctor may diagnose the cause as Alzheimer's disease.

Sometimes, even after completion of all the tests, the type of dementia still cannot be determined. For example, several characteristic symptoms of dementia with Lewy bodies are the same as those of Alzheimer's disease. The same may be said of common cognitive symptoms of vascular cognitive impairment and of Alzheimer's.

Adding to the challenge, these different causes can coexist — a single person can be affected by more than one type of dementia at the same time.

Even if the medical team is unable to determine the exact cause of dementia, that doesn't change the level of care that a person will receive. He or she can still be well supported and cared for, can still plan for the future and, when appropriate, can still receive treatment for his or her symptoms that will greatly improve quality of life.

After the diagnosis

Being diagnosed with a progressive form of dementia or having a loved one diagnosed with dementia can be a very frightening experience. You'll need to give yourself plenty of time to work through a broad range of feelings and to adjust emotionally.

Don't be afraid to ask family members, friends and colleagues for help. A doctor, nurse or psychologist can work with you and your family to develop strategies to manage the symptoms as they progress. He or she can help you determine the right time and manner in which to tell others about the diagnosis. There may be resources in your community that could provide valuable assistance, such as local chapters of the National Association of Area Agencies on Aging or Alzheimer's Association.

If you've been diagnosed with a specific disease, take advantage of this time to learn more about it. Many neurodegenerative diseases, including Alzheimer's disease, frontotemporal degeneration, and dementia with Lewy bodies, as well as vascular cognitive impairment and more, are explored in depth in later chapters.

Types of cognitive and functional decline

Dementia is a syndrome involving various forms of cognitive decline. Sometimes, these forms can have confusing, often similar-sounding names, for example, aphasia, agnosia and apraxia. Here are easy-to-understand explanations of these common symptoms of dementia.

Memory loss

Sometimes known as amnesia — though this term sounds outdated now — memory loss is the one symptom that's essential to a diagnosis of dementia. This common symptom of cognitive decline is marked by an inability to recall past events, either partially or in full. Problems with recent memory are often the earliest and most noticeable signs of this decline.

Difficulties with language use

Aphasia is the deterioration of your ability to use and understand language. For example, those affected may have trouble coming up with the names of familiar people, places and objects. Their speech is often nonsensical, repetitive, and peppered with nonspecific words such as *thing* and *it*. They may have difficulty understanding spoken and written language.

Difficulties understanding spatial relationships

The term *visuospatial* combines the root words visual and spatial. It follows that people with visuospatial decline are easily disoriented and have difficulty moving about, for example, judging the height of a step or the distance around an obstacle in their path. They may have trouble finding their way to the bathroom in a house where they have lived for 30 years.

Difficulties managing time and effort

Executive functioning refers to decision-making and the ability to carry out those decisions. People with an impairment of executive functioning will have trouble with organizing, prioritizing and thinking abstractly, so they tend to avoid situations that require processing new information. Managing finances, outlining a report, organizing a family vacation or throwing a large party would prove too difficult for people with this form of cognitive decline.

Inability to recognize familiar objects

Agnosia describes the failure to recognize or identify objects despite being able to see, hear and feel them normally. For example, a person walks into a classroom and is not able to recognize the chairs and desks in that room. Or the person cannot identify the shapes of different eating utensils at the table. As dementia progresses, those affected with agnosia may have difficulty recognizing their children or spouses and partners — or even their own reflections in the mirror.

Inability to carry out routine movements

Apraxia is a problem with your ability to carry out many learned movements — even though you're aware, and your senses and motor skills are in working order. For example, someone with apraxia may be unable to wave to a neighbor, although he or she sees the neighbor waving in greeting and understands what is expected in response. Apraxia may make tasks such as feeding and dressing yourself impossible. There's also a form of apraxia that affects speech.

Attention deficit

People experiencing this form of cognitive decline will find it difficult to concentrate on words being spoken to them or on tasks they're attempting to accomplish. They feel scatterbrained and highly distractible and are able to focus on one thing for only brief periods of time.

Loss of muscle coordination

Ataxia is a lack of coordination while performing voluntary movements — those movements that you make a conscious decision to perform. People with ataxia may appear clumsy or unstable while walking, climbing stairs or picking up objects because their movements are often jerky and disjointed.

Future trends

Most of the tests that are currently performed to diagnose dementia are primarily used to exclude potential causes, a process of narrowing the list down to the one or two most likely problems. A definitive diagnosis of Alzheimer's generally can't be made until autopsy, when examination of brain tissue yields direct evidence of the abnormalities characteristic of the disease.

Ideally, a test or range of tests would be available that identifies which disease process is taking place in the brain while the person is still alive, without having to wait for an autopsy report.

Researchers are attempting to reach this goal. Clinical trials, for example, indicate that samples of cerebrospinal fluid contain certain biomarkers indicating the presence of disease-specific abnormalities. Tests such as these would help achieve greater certainty in diagnosis much sooner.

If a loved one has received a diagnosis of Alzheimer's and you want to learn more about the disease, this book is also for you. Becoming familiar with the type of dementia affecting your loved one will help you anticipate changes and prepare for the experiences ahead. Learning how to cope with a diagnosis of dementia can be found in the Action Guide for Caregivers, located at the back of this book.

Part 2

Alzheimer's disease

Chapter 4

The basics of Alzheimer's disease

Alzheimer's disease (AD) is the most common cause of dementia among adults age 65 and older. Family members and friends see the poignant impact of the disease in loved ones — a gradual loss of intellect and memory, impairment of good judgment, changes in personality, and the inability to perform routine tasks of daily living.

Alzheimer's is a neurodegenerative disease. As the brain's nerve cells degenerate and communication pathways break down, cognition becomes more impaired. People with Alzheimer's ultimately lose some or all of their ability to communicate, recognize familiar objects, control behavior and satisfy basic physical urges, such as the need to eat or to urinate. In the final stages of Alzheimer's disease, they are bedridden and dependent on others for care.

The course that Alzheimer's disease may take is variable. It may run from two to 20 years after the first signs and symptoms appear. The disease is terminal, and death generally occurs from the complications of being immobile and unable to eat and drink properly — which can include pneumonia and other infections, malnutrition, dehydration, and circulatory problems.

This is the first of several chapters in Part 2 devoted to Alzheimer's disease. This chapter describes the biology of the disease and introduces two of the most characteristic features of Alzheimer's: amyloid plaques and neurofibrillary tangles.

Subsequent chapters in Part 2 describe different stages that the disease may take as it develops, but they're presented in reverse order. In Chapter 5, the fully developed disease is presented — the stage that experts have studied the most and that most people want to know about.

Chapter 6 describes mild cognitive impairment (MCI), a possible precursor to Alzheimer's. The next chapter introduces a newly identified stage known as preclinical Alzheimer's disease — when the earliest indications of change occur in the brain, before any symptoms appear (asymptomatic), putting a person at higher risk of the disease.

the interior of the brain. The hippocampus acts as the central switchboard of your memory system. That's why memory loss is closely associated with the dementia caused by Alzheimer's. There also may be disorientation and the loss of visuospatial function — the perception of where objects or places are located in relation to each other.

In addition to the hippocampus, Alzheimer's disease attacks other parts of the limbic system, including the amygdala. And the disease spreads from there to the frontal, parietal and

Pattern of degeneration

Alzheimer's disease affects the brain by destroying its most basic components — the nerve cells (neurons) that relay messages within the brain and between the brain and the rest of the body. This neurodegenerative disease also wreaks havoc with the communication points (synapses) between neurons, further impairing communication.

Neuron loss due to Alzheimer's disease occurs first in the hippocampus, a part of the limbic system located in

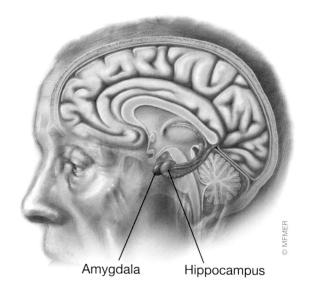

Amygdala   Hippocampus

© MFMER

The hippocampus, a key component of the memory, is affected at the onset of Alzheimer's disease. The disease spreads to amygdala and other parts of the limbic system, and from there, to the cerebral cortex.

temporal lobes of the cerebral cortex. As neuron communication is damaged or destroyed in these areas, other cognitive functions become impaired, such as language skills and executive skills such as decision-making.

Gradually, the disease robs people of their ability to perform routine self-care and undertake household tasks that they may have done for many years. Since the limbic system is the part of the brain that influences instincts and emotions, neuron loss in this area also may explain the aggressive behavior and paranoia that people with Alzheimer's often exhibit.

In addition, Alzheimer's disease destroys neurons at a location deep within the brain called the basal nucleus of Meynert. This area is rich in a chemical called acetylcholine (as-uh-teel-KOH-leen), and damage to the structure causes a sharp drop in acetylcholine levels. Acetylcholine is a neurotransmitter that plays an important role in the formation and retrieval of memories, which compounds the memory loss due to the disease's impact on the hippocampus.

Alzheimer's disease decreases levels of other neurotransmitters in the brain, such as dopamine, glutamate, norepinephrine and serotonin. The chart below indicates other cognitive functions that may be impaired or lost when levels of these neurotransmitters are reduced. As Alzheimer's spreads through the brain and more nerve cells die, the size of the brain shrinks (atrophies), a feature that can be seen on brain imaging.

Neurotransmitters affected by Alzheimer's

Neurotransmitter	Primary function
Acetylcholine	Attention, learning and memory
Dopamine	Movement
Glutamate	Learning and remote memory
Norepinephrine	Emotional response
Serotonin	Mood and anxiety

Proteins gone awry

Two abnormal structures in the brain are characteristic of Alzheimer's disease — amyloid plaques and neurofibrillary tangles. In 1907, Dr. Alois Alzheimer published an account of a woman exhibiting severe memory loss and paranoia. An examination of brain tissue after her death revealed heavy accumulations of both structures, which he described in his report.

Plaques and tangles aren't unique to Alzheimer's. They've been observed in other forms of dementia. In fact, they can develop in people who show no symptoms of dementia at all. But in people with Alzheimer's, plaques and tangles occur in far greater numbers.

Plaques

Plaques are large, undissolvable (insoluble) clumps of tissue found between and around living nerve cells. These plaques

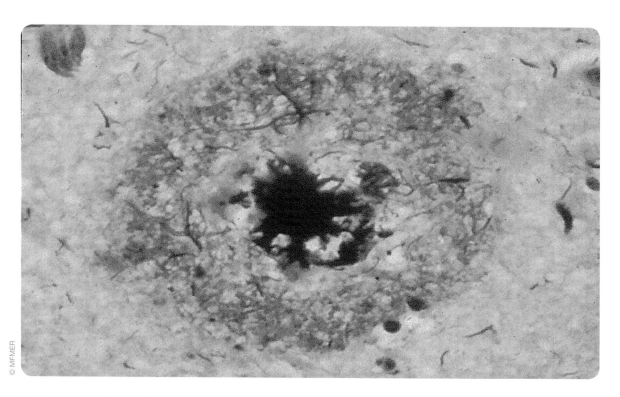

© MFMER

The dark, irregular spot in this microphotograph is the dense core of an amyloid plaque in brain tissue. The discoloration surrounding the core indicates the presence of inflammation.

consist mainly of a protein called amyloid-beta, mixed with bits of cellular material and other protein fragments.

Amyloid-beta is, in fact, a protein fragment cut off, or snipped, by enzymes from the amyloid precursor protein (APP). The normal function of APP is uncertain, but studies indicate that the protein plays a role in neuron growth and maintenance.

APP becomes lodged in a cell like a pin stuck in a cushion — partly inside and partly outside the membrane, the thin outer covering of a cell. In this position, APP is snipped off outside the membrane by the enzymes.

Various kinds of protein fragments are snipped from APP, but the amyloid-beta fragments appear to be longer and stickier than the others. "Stickier" in this regard means a tendency of the protein fragments to collect together, form into a clump, and harden into plaques — unlike other protein fragments that dissolve easily and are removed as waste from the brain.

The prevailing theory among scientists is that amyloid-beta somehow acts as a catalyst for much of the neuron damage that occurs in Alzheimer's. A significant clue, for example, is that rare, inherited forms of Alzheimer's are almost always associated with an increase in the level of amyloid-beta in the brain.

The abnormal processing and buildup of amyloid-beta seems to occur early in the disease process. Imaging techniques that allow doctors to observe structures and functions deep inside the living brain indicate that amyloid deposits may develop many years before any signs or symptoms of cognitive impairment appear.

Scientists have begun referring to this initial stage, which includes other physiological markers of Alzheimer's but no outwardly noticeable symptoms, as preclinical Alzheimer's disease.

Stages of toxicity. Amyloid-beta fragments pass through several stages before forming a plaque. A growing body of research suggests that the fragments may be more toxic in some stages of plaque formation than in other stages.

At first, a few amyloid-beta fragments clump together and yet are still fairly easy to dissolve and remove from the brain. In this stage they're called oligomers (OL-ih-go-murz). When several oligomers join together, the clumps become larger and stickier, forming

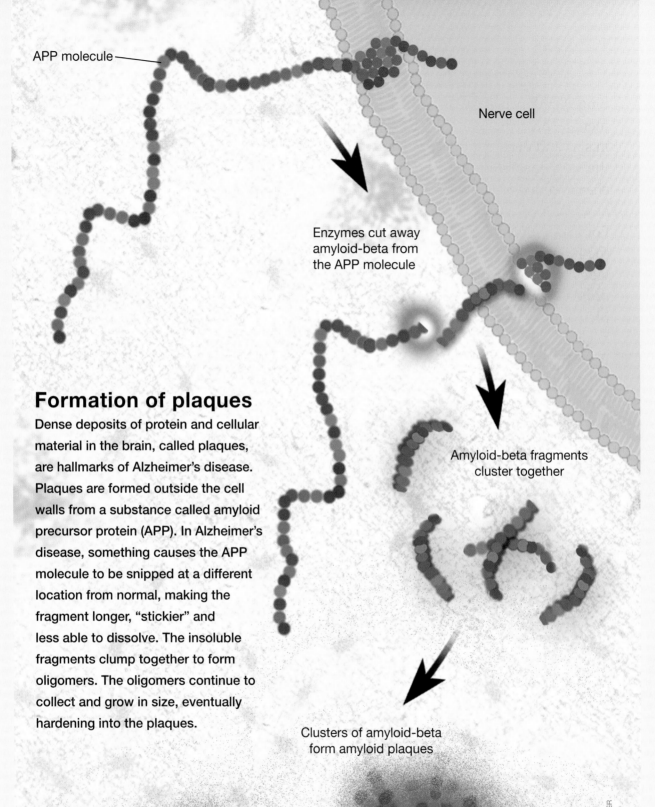

APP molecule

Nerve cell

Enzymes cut away amyloid-beta from the APP molecule

Formation of plaques

Dense deposits of protein and cellular material in the brain, called plaques, are hallmarks of Alzheimer's disease. Plaques are formed outside the cell walls from a substance called amyloid precursor protein (APP). In Alzheimer's disease, something causes the APP molecule to be snipped at a different location from normal, making the fragment longer, "stickier" and less able to dissolve. The insoluble fragments clump together to form oligomers. The oligomers continue to collect and grow in size, eventually hardening into the plaques.

Amyloid-beta fragments cluster together

Clusters of amyloid-beta form amyloid plaques

© MFMER

long, slender chains of amyloid fragments. These chains continue to grow in size and density until they form the hard, insoluble plaques that are so characteristic of Alzheimer's.

For a long time, scientists believed that the fully developed amyloid plaques were responsible for neuron death. But as more evidence is uncovered about plaque formation, some scientists are beginning to reconsider this position. They argue that the time when amyloid-beta is most toxic to neurons is during the earlier oligomer stage, before the plaques have formed.

The researchers believe that oligomers attack and destroy the brain's synapses — the narrow spaces that neurons must bridge in order to communicate with one another — resulting in memory loss and other cognitive impairments.

According to this theory, by the time large plaques have formed, the amyloid-beta fragments may have already lost their toxicity and the insoluble clumps are merely inactive masses, or "litter" of the disease process.

Not by amyloid-beta alone? Even as research continues to expand and refine basic understanding of the mechanisms that cause Alzheimer's, aspects of the disease still refuse to fit neatly into a logical, coherent pattern.

On one hand, tests reveal that some people have a large amount of amyloid-beta in their brains but suffer little damage to the neurons — and these individuals remain cognitively sound until death. On the other hand, tests show that some people may have normal levels of amyloid-beta in their brains but still show measurable damage to the neurons.

This evidence prompts a series of questions. Can neuron destruction still occur without abnormal levels of amyloid-beta in the brain? Are other processes required for neuron damage and the subsequent development of dementia to take place? Are some people more resistant to damage from amyloid-beta than are others, enabling them to live longer without noticeable cognitive impairment?

Researchers suspect that people who have cognitive impairment but show little evidence of amyloid-beta accumulation may, in fact, be on a non-Alzheimer's disease pathway.

These are questions that scientists hope to resolve before a clear outline of the disease process can be established.

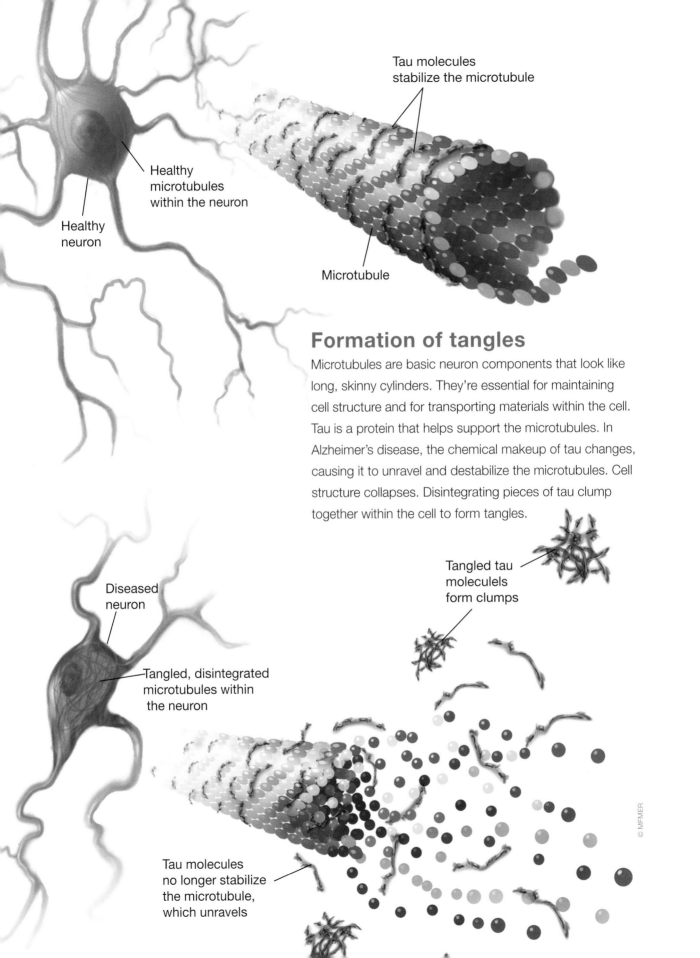

Tau molecules
stabilize the microtubule

Healthy
microtubules
within the neuron

Healthy
neuron

Microtubule

Formation of tangles

Microtubules are basic neuron components that look like long, skinny cylinders. They're essential for maintaining cell structure and for transporting materials within the cell. Tau is a protein that helps support the microtubules. In Alzheimer's disease, the chemical makeup of tau changes, causing it to unravel and destabilize the microtubules. Cell structure collapses. Disintegrating pieces of tau clump together within the cell to form tangles.

Tangled tau
moleculels
form clumps

Diseased
neuron

Tangled, disintegrated
microtubules within
the neuron

Tau molecules
no longer stabilize
the microtubule,
which unravels

Tangles

Neurofibrillary tangles are the other characteristic structure of AD. Tangles occur inside a cell body, caused by the breakdown of a protein called tau (pronounced tou). Tau helps uphold cell structure. But as AD develops, the protein undergoes chemical changes that cause it to malfunction. Instead of stabilizing cell structure, strands of tau unravel and clump together, forming tangled masses inside the cell.

The development of tangles has a devastating effect on a neuron. Internal cell structures called microtubules collapse, which disrupts the transportation of nutrients and the transmission of electric impulses within the cell body. This leads to a breakdown of vital cell functions.

Tangles and plaques appear firmly intertwined in the disease process, but scientists are still trying to determine exactly what role they play. For example, the

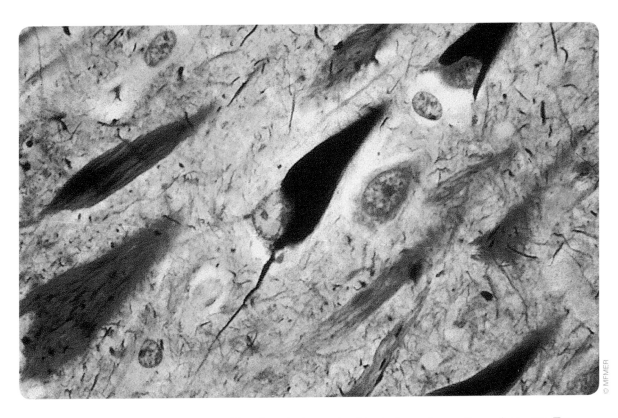

The dark, solid mass at the center of this microphotograph of brain tissue is a collapsed neuron. Tau protein within the cell has twisted, loosened and formed into tangles, undoing the structure of the cell.

What about genetic screening?

Screening kits are available for presenilin 1 (PSEN1) mutations associated with the early-onset form of AD, and for the APOE e4 allele associated with the late-onset form, but specialists don't routinely recommend genetic testing.

If someone is exhibiting early symptoms of dementia and another close family member has already been diagnosed with the early-onset form, then screening for the PSEN1 mutation may be useful for a diagnosis.

But screening for the APOE e4 allele has little predictive value. That's because having the allele doesn't mean you'll get AD, and not having the allele doesn't mean you won't get the disease.

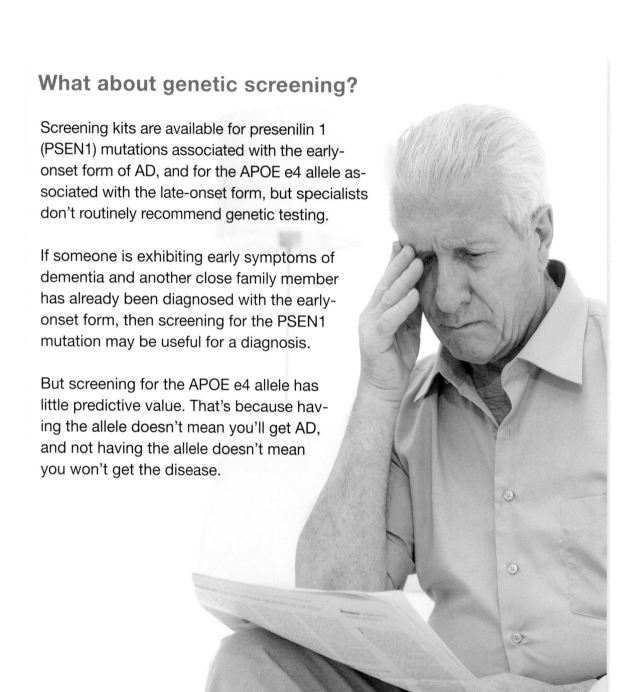

number of tangles in the brain seems to correlate more closely with the timing and severity of dementia symptoms than does the number of plaques.

Studies also indicate that tau is key to how toxic amyloid-beta is to neurons. In particular, a specific type of tau appears to strengthen amyloid-beta's effect. Normally, tau has a certain number of phosphate molecules attached to it. In AD, however, certain tau strands carry an unusually large number of phosphate molecules. These strands are referred to as hyperphosphorylated tau (p-tau). Evidence suggests that without elevated levels of p-tau, amyloid-beta deposits appear to have little effect on cognitive decline.

Contributing factors

Although plaques and tangles are the prominent features of Alzheimer's — and the most extensively studied ones — many scientists feel that research on the disease is only beginning. Recent studies involving therapies designed to clear amyloid-beta from the brain have so far failed to produce a corresponding improvement in cognitive signs and symptoms. This implies that amyloid-beta is not the only factor at play in the disease process.

The hypothesis that seems increasingly likely is that Alzheimer's, like many other diseases, is a result of multiple factors, as varied as your genes, your lifestyle, and your body's resilience to age-related changes and to other diseases. Following are factors that may contribute to or are somehow associated with Alzheimer's disease.

Genetics

Some genetic mutations, or defects, are known to cause a small number of inherited forms of Alzheimer's disease. These genes include the amyloid precursor protein (APP) gene and two presenilin genes, presenilin 1 (PSEN1) and presenilin 2 (PSEN2). People who inherit one of these rare mutations usually experience symptoms before the age of 65 — a condition known as early-onset Alzheimer's disease.

Symptoms of the inherited form of Alzheimer's are generally no different from the noninherited form — they just occur at an earlier age. A parent who has one of the known mutations has a high chance of passing it on to his or her child — each child has a 50 percent chance of inheriting the abnormal gene and developing the disease.

Something all genetic mutations known to cause Alzheimer's have in common is the abnormal processing of APP and the excessive production of amyloid-beta fragments. It's based on this knowledge that many scientists have hypothesized the central role of amyloid-beta in the disease process, even in the more common, late-onset form. However, it's possible that although early-onset and late-onset Alzheimer's have symptoms in common, early-onset may develop in one way and late-onset in another way.

Apolipoprotein E

In addition to genetic mutations, scientists have identified a normal gene, the apolipoprotein E (APOE) gene, that may increase your risk of the late-onset form of AD, which occurs after age 65. Before being linked to Alzheimer's disease, the APOE gene was known in the medical community for its role in carrying blood cholesterol through the body.

There are three variants, or alleles, of APOE — named e2, e3 and e4. Unlike mutations associated with early-onset

Alzheimer's, it's a naturally occurring variant of APOE — the e4 allele — that plays a role in the disease process. While inheriting one of the APP, PSEN1 and PSEN2 mutations is certain to lead to early-onset Alzheimer's, inheriting the APOE e4 allele doesn't mean a person develops the late-onset form.

But having the e4 allele greatly increases your risk of the disease. This risk appears to peak around 70 years of age and levels off in later years. Having the e4 allele may also lower the age that the disease begins — usually several years earlier than forms of Alzheimer's in which the e4 allele is not involved.

Research indicates that the APOE e4 allele is associated with increased levels of amyloid-beta in the brain, but exactly how this happens is under debate. Some researchers suspect that unlike the other alleles, the e4 allele is simply ineffective at dissolving amyloid-beta.

Surprisingly, another of the APOE alleles — the e2 allele — may have a protective effect against Alzheimer's disease. This is suggested by the fact that people who carry a mutated APP gene — a known cause of early-onset Alzheimer's — as well as the APOE e2 allele have failed to develop dementia, as would be expected.

Oxidative stress

Oxidative stress happens after damage to certain structures within the cell body called mitochondria — these structures are cellular energy factories. Damaged mitochondria tend to overproduce highly reactive molecules called free radicals.

Free radicals at normal levels perform a number of useful tasks, but too many free radicals become a problem. They overwhelm and damage the cell, resulting in tissue breakdown and damage to DNA.

What causes oxidative stress? Normal aging may cause a buildup of free radicals, as can various disease-related factors. Evidence also suggests that the formation of amyloid plaques and possibly inflammation play roles.

Signs of oxidative stress have been observed in the brains of people with Alzheimer's disease, particularly in later stages when plaques and tangles are plentiful.

There are also indications of oxidative stress in the earliest stages of the disease. This has led some researchers to question whether stress may lead to the formation of plaques and tangles. Some even argue that plaques and tangles may form as protective measures against the stress.

Other researchers contend that a chronic state of low-level oxidative stress, combined with other factors, may be sufficient to trigger damage to the brain's neurons.

Regardless of whether oxidative stress initiates or results from neuron damage, most researchers agree that it plays a part in the disease process.

Inflammatory response

Inflammation is your body's natural protective response to injury. It may involve pain, swelling, heat and redness of the inflamed region. Various studies have observed that some inflammation develops in the brain tissue of people with Alzheimer's disease.

What causes this phenomenon? Even as amyloid plaques develop between neurons, immune cells (microglia) go about their work of clearing dead cells and other waste products from brain tissue. Scientists speculate that the microglia identify plaques as foreign substances and try to destroy them, triggering inflammatory response.

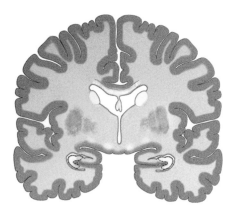

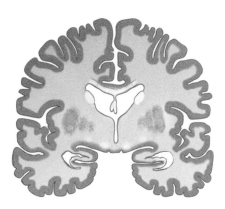

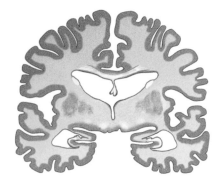

© MFMER

This sequence illustrates another characteristic feature of AD, showing a normal brain (top), a brain with MCI (middle) and a brain with Alzheimer's disease (bottom). With extensive neuron damage taking place as the disease progresses, the brain gradually shrinks in size.

The microglia may also be trying to remove damaged neurons. Or they may be activating compounds that cause inflammation — examples include the protein interleukin-1, the enzyme COX-2 and another group of proteins that take action against cells marked by microglia for removal.

Although scientists believe the inflammation develops before plaques have fully formed, they aren't sure how this relates to the disease process. There's also debate about whether inflammation damages the neurons or is in any way beneficial for clearing away the plaques.

Vascular brain injury

As one of the largest, busiest organs in the body, the brain depends on a vast network of blood vessels to feed it the oxygen and nutrients necessary to operate successfully. The brain also relies heavily on the heart's capacity to pump enough blood for its needs.

Over time, the brain's vascular system begins to resemble that of the rest of an aging body — arteries in the brain become more narrow and less elastic, some become clogged with fatty deposits, and new capillary growth — offshoots from the main arteries — slows down. The heart may not pump with its previous efficiency. As a result, the brain receives an insufficient amount of blood, and the blood that does arrive may not flow as well as it once did.

The wear and tear of age on the cerebrovascular system can result in microscopic injuries and bleeding, inflammation and oxidative stress. In addition, the presence of other conditions such as high blood pressure, atherosclerosis or head trauma can further aggravate these effects.

It's possible that a faulty, aging vascular system in the brain may create an environment for neuron destruction to occur. Various studies have linked cardiovascular risk factors in midlife — such as high blood pressure, high cholesterol and obesity — to later cognitive impairment and dementia.

Alzheimer's disease and cerebrovascular disease — such as stroke or ministrokes, which in themselves can cause brain injury and dementia — frequently occur together in the same individual. Almost all people with severe cerebrovascular disease also have an abundance of amyloid-beta in their brain tissue. And many people with Alzheimer's disease also have severe cerebrovascular disease.

Exactly how one condition affects the other is unclear. One emerging theory is that amyloid-beta deposits are initially produced as protective agents rather than toxic ones. This theory views amyloid deposits as sturdy, insoluble patches that work to seal off leaky blood vessels in the brain.

A problem arises when chronic vascular injury — whether due to cardiovascular disease or traumatic injury — leads to an overabundance of amyloid deposits, which choke out small blood vessels and leave behind free-floating amyloid fragments. It's at this stage, some scientists argue, that amyloid deposits become harmful.

If this is true, it may explain why immunization therapy trials designed to eliminate amyloid-beta have led to microscopic bleeding in the brains of some participants, insomuch as the therapy may have removed active amyloid "scabs" from injured blood vessels.

Unraveling the link between vascular disease and dementia remains elusive. For example, evidence that anti-high-blood pressure and anti-cholesterol drugs have a preventive effect against dementia is relatively thin. Trials focusing on specific age groups may help to illuminate the association.

Insulin resistance

Diabetes and Alzheimer's disease are connected in ways that aren't completely understood, but a number of studies indicate that people with diabetes — especially type 2 diabetes — are at higher risk of developing AD.

Because diabetes damages blood vessels, it has long been recognized as a risk factor for vascular dementia and may be a risk factor for Alzheimer's in similar ways as high blood pressure and high cholesterol (see previous section on vascular brain injury).

But there may also be a link between insulin and dementia, as a result of the complex ways that type 2 diabetes affects the ability of the brain and other tissues in the body to use sugar (glucose) and respond to insulin.

Insulin is a hormone produced by the pancreas that helps regulate your body's use of glucose. With type 2 diabetes, either your pancreas doesn't produce enough insulin or your body becomes resistant to the effects of insulin. As a result, too much glucose accumulates in your bloodstream.

Glucose is the brain's main source of energy. The disruption of insulin's role in regulating glucose can affect the brain in a variety of ways, but in general, it decreases energy metabolism while increasing inflammation and oxidative stress.

Chronic high blood glucose also can trigger the production of toxic molecules (advanced glycation end products) in the brain. Combined, these conditions have damaging effects on neuron generation and repair.

In the context of Alzheimer's disease, imbalanced levels of insulin may affect the clearance of amyloid-beta and increase the amount of tau with an abnormal number of phosphate molecules (hyperphosphorylation).

As with other contributing factors, scientists are exploring whether the disruption of insulin regulation is a causative factor in Alzheimer's disease or whether Alzheimer's disease is what causes insulin defects.

Protective factors

An increasing amount of research suggests that while there are many factors that appear to increase your risk of Alzheimer's disease, there are also many factors that may protect against AD.

Various studies indicate that a number of lifestyle habits — such as exercising, eating a diet rich in fruits and vegetables, engaging in mentally stimulating activities, and staying socially connected — may reduce your risk of developing Alzheimer's disease.

Whether these daily habits act against the basic disease mechanisms of Alzheimer's or whether they build up a reserve of brain capacity that can be accessed when other areas of the brain become damaged is still under study.

Response to a growing crisis

The social burden of Alzheimer's disease is staggering, and the crisis is only getting worse. According to the Alzheimer's Association, more than 5 million Americans are living with the disease, and that number may triple to over 13 million by 2025. As the sixth leading cause of death in the United States, approximately one in three older adults dies from Alzheimer's or from another disorder causing dementia.

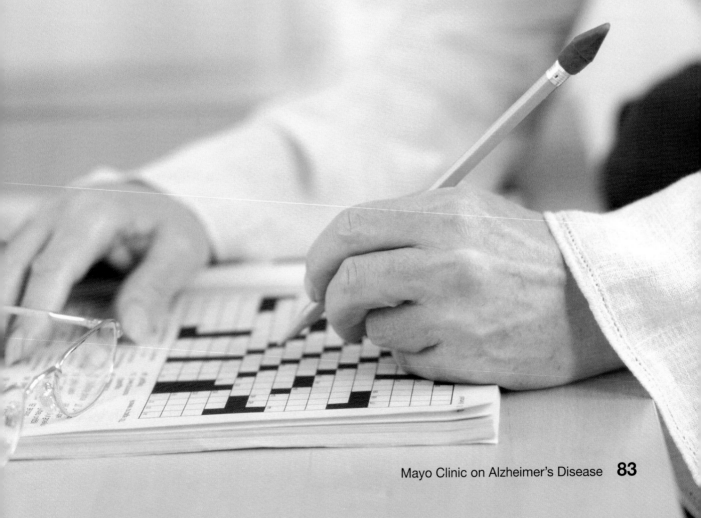

It's estimated that taking care of loved ones with dementia involves more than 15 million caregivers, providing more than 17 billion hours of unpaid care. More than 60 percent of these caregivers rated the emotional stress they've experienced as high or very high, and more than one-third reported symptoms of depression. In 2013, the direct costs of Alzheimer's care to Americans are an estimated $203 billion. These costs are expected to reach as high as $1.2 trillion by 2050.

In 2012, the U.S. government enacted the National Plan to Address Alzheimer's Disease, in full recognition of this growing health crisis and the unsustainable costs it will incur on American citizens if the disease is not stopped. The Plan reflects input from literally thousands of specialists and organizations across the country.

The National Plan is directed by the Department of Health and Human Services, with assistance from the Advisory Council on Research, Care and Services and solidly backed by federal agencies. It outlines specific goals for meeting some of the most burdensome challenges associated with Alzheimer's disease. The National Plan will guide the country's fight against Alzheimer's disease for the next 15 years.

The five primary goals of the National Plan include:

- Being able to prevent and effectively treat Alzheimer's disease by 2025
- Training health care providers and developing new approaches to improve the quality of care
- Expanding services and support for caregivers, and developing a better system to assess caregiver needs
- Undertaking a nationwide public awareness campaign to educate Americans about Alzheimer's
- Improving the collection of data to monitor the progress of research

The National Plan is an ambitious attempt to deal with the health crisis from both a research and care perspective, and builds a solid framework on which to accomplish the goals.

For more information about the National Plan and the progress being made, visit the website maintained by the Department of Health and Human Services: *www.alzheimers.gov.*

Chapter 5

Dementia due to Alzheimer's disease

As previously described, dementia is not a disease but a syndrome — a collection of signs and symptoms that often indicates the underlying cause. When a person is diagnosed with dementia due to Alzheimer's disease, he or she shows a specific set of signs and symptoms that a specialist attributes to Alzheimer's and to the exclusion of other conditions that cause dementia.

People who develop this form of dementia may experience Alzheimer's differently — for example, age of onset and severity. These differences can be influenced by many factors, including age, physical health, family history, and cultural and ethnic backgrounds.

Nevertheless, there are certain patterns in the disease process that are common in almost everyone who has dementia due to Alzheimer's. Using these patterns as benchmarks, physicians typically describe the development of Alzheimer's in stages ranging from mild to severe. What distinguishes one stage from another is the appearance of or a change in various indicators, in terms of cognition (how a person thinks), behavior (how a person acts) and function (how a person performs basic tasks).

In this book, three stages are used to characterize dementia due to Alzheimer's: mild, moderate and severe. Keep in mind that these stages are relatively general in nature, and may not fit individual circumstances exactly. Some signs and symptoms may appear throughout the disease process and are not restricted to one stage. Others may simply never develop for some people.

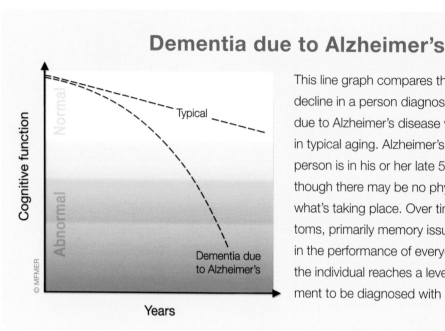

Dementia due to Alzheimer's

This line graph compares the sharp cognitive decline in a person diagnosed with dementia due to Alzheimer's disease with what may occur in typical aging. Alzheimer's may start when a person is in his or her late 50s or early 60s, even though there may be no physical indication of what's taking place. Over time, signs and symptoms, primarily memory issues, start to interfere in the performance of everyday tasks. Eventually, the individual reaches a level of cognitive impairment to be diagnosed with dementia.

Once the signs and symptoms of dementia appear, the time frame in which this unrelenting disease runs its course can be highly variable. If a person is older than 80 when he or she is diagnosed with dementia due to Alzheimer's, the disease may take its toll in just a few years. If, on the other hand, a person is still fairly young at the time of diagnosis, he or she may live with the disease for 10 years or more.

Death caused by dementia due to Alzheimer's often results from a breakdown of the immune system and from the complications of being immobile and unable to eat or drink — complications that may include pneumonia, malnutrition and dehydration.

Diagnosing Alzheimer's disease

To determine if certain signs and symptoms of dementia are caused by Alzheimer's disease, a physician must decide whether this evidence clearly meets criteria that have been established to make a diagnosis. Different professional and governmental organizations have worked together to create standards for diagnosing Alzheimer's disease, including the American Psychiatric Association and the National Institute on Aging in conjunction with the Alzheimer's Association.

Essentially, the criteria attempt to outline a distinctive pattern of signs and symptoms that's typical of Alzheimer's and that rule out other possible causes of dementia.

Doctors can't diagnose Alzheimer's with 100 percent accuracy — something that's currently possible only at autopsy. But studies show that a majority of the Alzheimer's diagnoses are later confirmed by autopsy results. Because of this, the established criteria are considered fairly reliable in making a diagnosis of "probable" Alzheimer's.

In general, what doctors look for to satisfy the diagnostic criteria for dementia due to Alzheimer's include:

- The presence of certain signs and symptoms of dementia
- A gradual onset of the signs and symptoms
- Indications that the signs and symptoms are clearly getting worse

The earliest, most prominent signs and symptoms are ones that fit the pattern considered typical of Alzheimer's disease, such as memory loss, language difficulties, problems in recognizing familiar objects, places or faces, and impairment of reasoning, judgment and executive functions.

The examination should make clear that another condition is not a cause of the dementia, such as stroke, a different type of neurodegenerative disease, use of brain-affecting medications or another disease that might affect cognition.

In some cases, where there is still some degree of uncertainty, a doctor may qualify the diagnosis as "possible" Alzheimer's. This may occur if a person's signs and symptoms fit the criteria for Alzheimer's dementia but have come on suddenly or the person has just had something like a stroke, which might explain some of the symptoms.

While autopsies remain the gold standard for a definitive diagnosis of Alzheimer's, it's possible that doctors may soon begin using imaging and lab tests to help confirm the diagnosis. These tests are already being conducted in research settings.

For example, analyzing positron emission tomography (PET) scans with a radioactive tracer or samples of cerebrospinal fluid can highlight the existence of amyloid plaques and neurofibrillary tangles in the brain. Doctors with access to these forms of testing may use them in practice, but so far, the methods are too new to be recommended for the general public.

Warning signs of Alzheimer's

Some of the earliest signs and symptoms of dementia due to Alzheimer's may include:

- Memory loss that disrupts daily life, often of recent events
- Difficulty performing familiar tasks, such as following recipes or using appliances
- Problems with language, for example, calling objects by the wrong name or not being able to find the right word in conversations
- Disorientation to time and place, for example, becoming lost in familiar places and unable to find a way home
- Poor judgment, for example, spending money unwisely or dressing inappropriately for the weather or the season
- Problems with abstract thought, such as struggles with problem-solving or calculating numbers
- Misplacing personal items, often in unusual places
- Changes in mood and behavior, for example, undergoing extreme mood swings for no apparent reason
- Changes in personality, for example, becoming more suspicious, irritable or paranoid
- Loss of initiative, for example, becoming more passive and withdrawn

These are certainly not all of the signs and symptoms of dementia due to Alzheimer's. At the same time, most individuals with the disease will not experience everything listed.

And just because you may have one or more of these symptoms does not mean you have Alzheimer's — they may be a result of another, treatable cause or even of normal aging. Whenever you notice that a symptom is new or that it has changed, that's the best time to discuss these concerns with your doctor.

Mild Alzheimer's

Increased forgetfulness is the most common complaint in the early stages of dementia due to Alzheimer's disease. At first, the person may have difficulty with recent memory — new information such as names or appointments — while remote memory remains intact. Usually, the memory loss presents itself as a new, more intense pattern of forgetfulness that persists.

Still, the early signs of Alzheimer's dementia are often hidden and subtle, making it difficult to recognize that something is actually wrong. There may be slight problems with communication. There may be uncharacteristic changes in personality. It may be easier for the person to become disoriented or confused while performing tasks in his or her daily routine.

Even if people sense there are problems, they may not associate the changes with an illness. Many people in the early stages seem to be less aware and less concerned about their problems than are their family and friends — this lack of awareness may itself be an early indication of the disease.

Stages of Alzheimer's

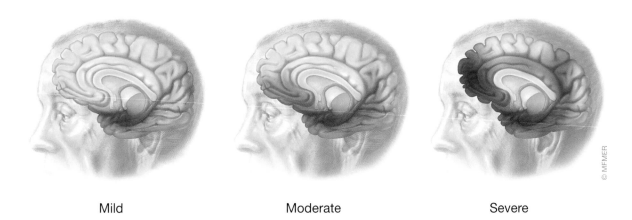

| Mild | Moderate | Severe |

© MFMER

Alzheimer's destroys the brain's most basic component, the nerve cell (neuron). In its mild stage, neuron loss occurs in the area of the hippocampus and spreads to the amygdala (see purple shading). In its moderate stage, the disease spreads into the cerebral cortex. In its severe stage, most of the brain is affected, except for the occipital lobe at the back of the brain.

Some of the signs and symptoms in the mild stage of Alzheimer's include:

- Not remembering recent events
- Asking the same question repeatedly
- Getting lost in conversation and unable to find the right word
- Not being able to complete familiar tasks, for example, someone who loves to cook having difficulties with a recipe
- Having problems with abstract thought, for example, using a credit card for financial transactions
- Misplacing items in inappropriate places, such as putting a watch, wallet or handbag in the refrigerator
- Undergoing sudden, intense changes in mood or behavior
- Showing an inability to concentrate for more than just a few minutes or to take the initiative to follow through and complete projects
- Showing less interest in what's going on in the surroundings
- Showing an indifference toward personal appearance, for example, being unwashed, disheveled and poorly dressed
- Not observing normal courtesies to others, for example, ignoring greetings and simple questions
- Feeling disoriented about time and place, for example, uncertainty about the locations of familiar stores in town
- Becoming lost while driving on familiar streets

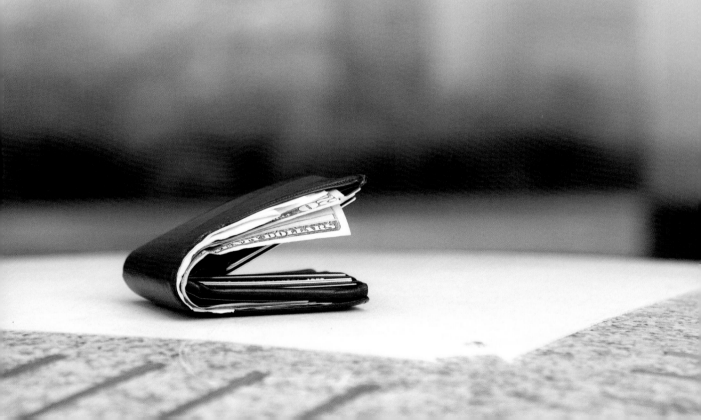

What does it feel like to have Alzheimer's?

This was a question asked by members of Mayo Clinic's Alzheimer's Disease Research Center to a group of people who had received a diagnosis in the mild stage of Alzheimer's. How they responded was revealing. While some interviewees were philosophical about their condition, others were more pragmatic.

"Loss of independence. It doesn't feel right to become more dependent on others by letting them get the idea that you can't do anything. I give in and let others take over completely. You lose out when you let others take over. We need to slow down so I can stay involved."

"Fear. You hear it's so debilitating and that gets you down."

"When they hear Alzheimer's, people back up like you've got a 'disease.' Almost like you should be ashamed. Like they are wondering if it's catchy or if maybe she's going to die soon."

"Expectations others have for me are often too high or too low. I can't keep up with my spouse. It's quicker and easier to let my spouse take over."

"I need to be reminded of tasks or activities."

"I don't recognize places when we go for drives. That scares me."

"It takes me much longer to remember why I went into a room."

"I need to work at a slower pace. People around me seem like they are on a merry-go-round — going faster and faster. I can't keep up. I want to stay active, but I need to take more time to do things."

Even as the mild stage of Alzheimer's develops, the person may still be employed and trying to go about business as usual. Difficulties at work may be passed off as stress, lack of sleep, fatigue or simply getting older.

The person may try to compensate for problems with memory by sticking to places and routines that are familiar while avoiding new or strange situations. The growing awareness of memory loss may lead to feelings of anger, frustration and helplessness.

It's not unusual for a person to take strong emotions out on others. Depression also is common at the mild stage. Having depression is a serious development that should be evaluated and treated as soon as possible.

Moderate Alzheimer's

At the moderate stage of dementia due to Alzheimer's disease, warning signs that before had seemed out-of-place occurrences have now become obvious problems. The person may not only be experiencing memory loss but also may be having difficulty thinking clearly

and exercising good judgment. He or she likely needs help with many day-to-day activities, including personal care. Moods may change literally from one moment to another.

Generally, these developments have alerted family members, friends and neighbors that something is definitely wrong. If there had been any reluctance previously to seeing a doctor, these new concerns may prompt a doctor visit now. Signs and symptoms of the moderate stage may include:

- Forgetting to turn off appliances such as the iron and stove.
- Consistently forgetting to take medications even with constant reminders.
- Having difficulty with tasks involving calculation and planning, such as balancing a bank account, paying bills, counting out change, going grocery shopping, preparing dinner and scheduling appointments.
- Having difficulty with tasks that require skilled movements such as tying shoelaces and using utensils.
- Losing the ability to communicate and interact with others, including reading and writing.
- Exhibiting extreme behaviors, such as aggressiveness, withdrawal and outbursts of anger.

Example of dementia due to Alzheimer's

A man brought his 67-year-old wife to the doctor because of serious concerns about memory loss. His wife was well educated and an entrepreneur who had owned her own business for many years. Now, increasingly, she was unable to remember appointments, easily confused her orders and needed constant help with finances. She could no longer go on business trips for fear of muddling her itinerary, getting lost and forgetting purchases. Outside of work, she had withdrawn from social activities that she long enjoyed. And recently, she left food cooking on the stove unattended, resulting in a small kitchen fire.

The woman had no serious medical problems, took no medications and passed an initial physical examination, which showed nothing significantly wrong. Mental status testing, however, revealed mild problems with naming common objects and a disorientation to the exact calendar date. Further testing indicated short-term memory impairment and problems with language and calculations. A diagnosis was made of Alzheimer's disease.

- Beginning to have problems recognizing familiar faces, sometimes confusing one friend with another.
- Behaving inappropriately in public, for example, talking loudly, interrupting conversations and engaging complete strangers.
- Feeling increasingly agitated and restless, particularly at night
- Sleeping for excessively long periods of time or hardly sleeping at all. Some people may sleep 10 to 12 hours at night and still nap during the day, while others may sleep only two to four hours at night and stay awake throughout the day.
- Having false beliefs (delusions) or seeing or hearing something that's not really there (hallucinations).

The progression of a loved one into the moderate stage of Alzheimer's can be a trying time for someone thrust into the unanticipated role of caregiver. As both the caregiver and the person with dementia grapple with the changes, it takes time to develop a new perspective on the evolving relationship.

Severe Alzheimer's

In the severe stage of Alzheimer's, the disease has progressed to a point where the person is no longer able to think or reason. Self-awareness seems to have disappeared completely.

The essential tasks of living, such as bathing, dressing, eating and going to the bathroom, require a caregiver's full assistance. The person's personality may have changed completely.

Motor activities have deteriorated to the point where the person can no longer walk, sit up or communicate. In fact, the person seems unmotivated to move at all without prompts from other people.

Signs and symptoms at the severe stage of Alzheimer's include:

- Having little or no memory, be it recent or remote
- Having difficulty with speaking and understanding words
- Showing little or no emotion
- Grasping objects or people and not letting go
- Having difficulty recognizing family members and friends, including a spouse — perhaps not even recognizing himself or herself when looking in a mirror
- Needing assistance with all forms of personal care, including using the toilet, bathing, dressing, eating and moving around
- Experiencing frequent incontinence due to the lack of bladder and bowel control
- Feeling increasingly weak and sleeping more
- Being highly susceptible to infections due to a weakened immune system
- Having difficulty chewing and swallowing, and because of these problems, losing weight

A person in the final stage of Alzheimer's has become bedridden. His or her body systems are severely weakened, which increases the risk of developing other health problems. And because of the weakened body systems, these complications are frequently more severe in someone with Alzheimer's than in a person without the disease.

The most frequent cause of death in people with dementia due to Alzheimer's disease is called aspiration pneumonia. It occurs when a person can't swallow properly and instead inhales food or liquid into the lungs, which causes a deadly infection.

Where is my wife?

This haunting question was asked of a wife, caring for her husband with Alzheimer's disease. She describes the changes that occurred in their relationship in this way:

It is heartbreaking for your spouse not to know you. But I have learned not to let it get to me. I tell my husband that his wife will soon be back or, if he persists, that she has gone to visit family. At times, he tells me that his wife has gone to visit family, and I should sleep in the guest room. Well, I tell him that this bed is just like mine and I would sleep better in it. He will get in bed and sleep at the farthest edge. But before he goes to sleep, he reaches over and holds my hand and kisses me good night.

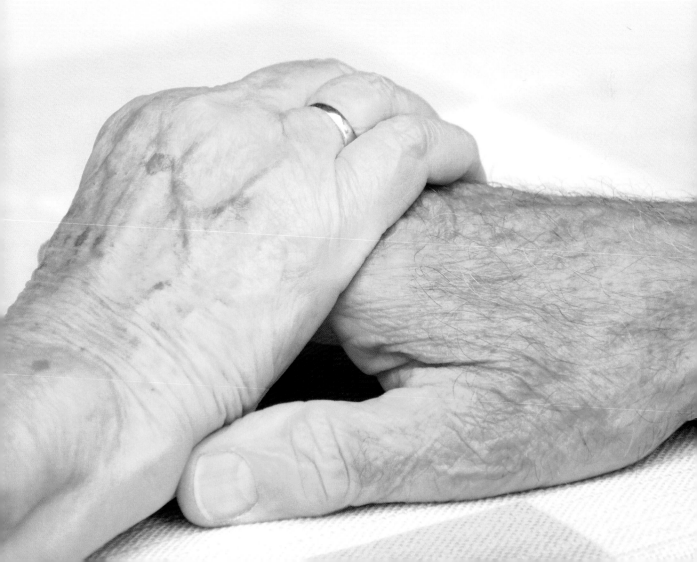

Concurrent conditions

Certain conditions may develop at the same time that Alzheimer's does. The signs and symptoms of these conditions can obscure or complicate a diagnosis. They may also hasten or increase the severity of cognitive decline. The fact that many of these conditions are treatable emphasizes the importance of getting an early diagnosis. Conditions that commonly coexist with Alzheimer's include depression, anxiety and sleep disorders.

Depression

According to the Alzheimer's Association, up to 40 percent of people with Alzheimer's experience significant depression at some point during the course of the disease. It's especially common during the early stages when social isolation, diminishing mental and physical abilities, and loss of independence occurs. Brief periods of discouragement and apathy may be natural in such circumstances, but prolonged despondency is not.

Although coexistence is common, scientists aren't sure of the exact relationship between depression and dementia due to Alzheimer's. Studies indicate that chronic feelings of sadness or worthlessness may be linked to the awareness of mental decline — despite the fact that many people with Alzheimer's lose insight into their behavior early in the disease process.

Other research has found that the biological changes caused by Alzheimer's may increase a person's genetic predisposition to depression. Some studies suggest that the symptoms of depression, such as apathy and lack of motivation, may be among the earliest signs of Alzheimer's. Other studies indicate that the presence of depression may increase your risk of Alzheimer's.

What's clear is that depression will strongly impact the quality of life for a person with Alzheimer's disease as well as for his or her caregiver. In addition to the emotional problems, depression can lead to weight loss and physical frailty.

Depression is associated with earlier placement in assisted living and nursing homes, greater disability in the performance of daily living skills, and more physical aggression toward caregivers. Also, depression in a person with Alzheimer's increases the chances of depression in caregivers.

Diagnosing depression in a person with Alzheimer's can be especially challenging due, in part, to the person's growing inability to describe how he or she feels. Experts encourage caregivers or anyone else involved in the daily life of the person to take part in doctor visits to provide a more complete picture of the person's moods.

Counseling and nondrug therapy can be helpful, especially for people with mild depression. A professional therapist can help a person with Alzheimer's develop daily routines and find enjoyable activities. The therapist can help caregivers learn problem-solving and coping skills. Sometimes, making use of eldercare services can provide a needed break for both the person with Alzheimer's and his or her caregiver. Antidepressants can help relieve more severe symptoms of depression.

Anxiety

The symptoms of anxiety — fearfulness, agitation, apprehension, fidgeting or pacing, excessive worry, restlessness and even anger — are common among people with Alzheimer's. In addition, anxiety and depression often occur together at the same time. It's not hard to imagine how someone whose memory — of the past, of how to do routine tasks, of familiar faces and places — is failing would frequently feel anxious and insecure.

Anxiety is associated with some of the challenging behaviors that may occur in someone with Alzheimer's. These include agitation, wandering, inappropriate behavior, hallucinations, verbal threats and physical abuse. These behaviors are frequently the reasons for placing a loved one in a nursing home. Treating the anxiety may improve these symptoms and, in turn, reduce the stress and fatigue on the caregiver.

Treatment for anxiety generally employs strategies to manage the behavior. A common method for managing excess worry, irritability or restlessness is to identify the behavior that's causing concern, find out what may be causing it, and adapt the person's environment to minimize his or her discomfort. See chapter 8 for more on behavioral strategies.

If anxiety symptoms are severely disruptive, the doctor may prescribe short-term doses of medications that may ease some of these symptoms. These medications include anxiolytics, selective serotonin reuptake inhibitors or antipsychotics.

The primary side effect of medication is sedation, but some medications may worsen memory and cognition and cause other side effects. Therefore, medication should be used with caution.

In addition, antipsychotics are associated with an increased risk of death when used to treat behavioral disturbances in older adults who have dementia. This is usually as a result of a heart-related event, such as heart failure, or as a result of infections, such as pneumonia.

Sleep disorders

Disturbed sleep patterns are common among people with Alzheimer's, particularly in later stages of the disease. These disturbances take many forms. Some people may sleep more than they ever did before — up to 16 hours a day. Others may sleep less, perhaps only two to four hours at night. Furthermore, the cycle of sleep and wakefulness may be reversed between night and day. Restlessness and nighttime wandering are common symptoms.

Factors that may contribute to excessive sleeping include medication side effects, metabolic problems and boredom. On the other hand, anxiety and depression can contribute to insomnia, as can lack of daytime physical activity, too much napping, certain medications and the excessive intake of stimulants such as caffeine.

Keeping a person with Alzheimer's occupied and engaged during the day, monitoring napping and caffeine intake, increasing physical activity, and maintaining a reasonable bedtime (not too early) may improve sleep patterns.

Other sleep disorders that commonly affect people with Alzheimer's include sleep apnea, restless legs syndrome and periodic limb movements during sleep. Some people may "act out" their dreams. People with Alzheimer's may snore loudly and experience episodes of snorting or gasping, a creepy-crawly sensation in their legs (especially at night), or nightmares.

These signs and symptoms should be discussed with a doctor. Most sleep disorders are treatable, and successful treatment can improve cognition, mood and quality of life.

The sleep disturbances often affect the caregiver's sleep patterns as well. If this happens, the caregiver should find alternate ways to get rest, so he or she doesn't become sleep deprived.

Concurrent causes of dementia

Alzheimer's disease sometimes occurs at the same time as other dementia-causing disorders. This presents a challenge to the doctor attempting to make a diagnosis. Because treatment options may vary, your doctor will carefully study all of the signs and symptoms and perform various tests in hopes of distinguishing between Alzheimer's and another cause of dementia.

Vascular cognitive impairment

Based on autopsy reports, up to half of people with Alzheimer's disease also have signs and symptoms of vascular cognitive impairment (vascular dementia). Vascular cognitive impairment typically is a result of interrupted blood flow to the brain, either because of blocked arteries or because of a series of strokes. A person's cognitive abilities deteriorate step by step with each additional stroke.

Not surprisingly, a major risk factor is a history of strokes. Other risk factors include high blood pressure and high cholesterol levels. Paralysis, vision loss, and difficulty with speaking and using language are commonly found in people who have vascular cognitive impairment. Often, the onset of this disorder is sudden and abrupt, but occasionally the disease progresses more slowly, making it difficult to distinguish from Alzheimer's.

It may be that Alzheimer's and vascular cognitive impairment are more closely intertwined than thought. For example, some studies suggest that dementia due to Alzheimer's is more likely to occur in someone who has had a stroke than in someone who has not.

The combination of vascular injury and Alzheimer's features, such as plaques and tangles, may make it easier for neuron damage to occur in the brain, ultimately leading to dementia. You can read more about vascular cognitive impairment in Chapter 12.

Dementia with Lewy bodies and Parkinson's disease

The hallmark features of Alzheimer's dementia — amyloid plaques and neurofibrillary tangles — can exist in combination with other brain disorders, including dementia with Lewy bodies and Parkinson's disease.

Lewy bodies are abnormal protein deposits in the brain that progressively destroy neurons and disrupt cell communication. When these protein deposits are widespread throughout the brain, a person with dementia with Lewy bodies may first experience problems with concentration and other cognitive symptoms.

Later in the course of the disease, stiffness and slowness of movement occur. The person also may experience visual hallucinations. In people who have both Alzheimer's disease and dementia with Lewy bodies, memory loss occurs along with these symptoms. For more information on dementia with Lewy bodies, see Chapter 11.

Some people with Alzheimer's also develop Parkinson's disease. Parkinson's is a crippling illness affecting nerve cells in parts of the brain that control muscle movements. It's characterized by limb stiffness, tremors, difficulty with walking and speech impairment.

Lewy body structures often appear in the brain tissue of people with Parkinson's disease, as well as in the brain tissue of some people with Alzheimer's disease. This suggests a close but still undetermined relationship among all three disorders.

Advancing our understanding

Scientists describe dementia due to Alzheimer's disease in stages according to changing signs and symptoms as the disease spreads through different parts of the brain. Scientists have also identified conditions, including other causes of dementia, which may exist concurrently with Alzheimer's.

This knowledge helps determine the treatment for various cognitive and behavioral symptoms of Alzheimer's disease, greatly improving the quality of life for the person with dementia and reducing the workload stress for the caregiver. For more practical information on the handling of Alzheimer's symptoms, turn to the Action Guide for Caregivers in this book.

Chapter 6

Mild cognitive impairment

Neurologists emphasize that a neurodegenerative disorder such as Alzheimer's typically doesn't begin in the manner of a virulent, aggressive disease — one month your cognition appears fine and the next month you're struggling with memory loss and extreme mood swings.

Rather, the onset of a neurodegenerative disorder tends to be gradual, with milder symptoms developing into more severe ones throughout the course of the disease. As mentioned in Chapter 2, researchers describe this transition in terms of a cognitive spectrum.

The word *spectrum* can mean "a range or a continuous whole" — in this case, it refers to a person's history of cognitive change in relation to aging and disease; a collection of signs and symptoms from their onset to a point where they have produced the extreme changes associated with dementia.

For many years, scientists' attention focused on the severe end of this spectrum, due to the immediate and extensive care that a person with dementia is in need of. More recently, much research has switched to the milder end of the spectrum. Investigators are intrigued by the concept of a "pre-dementia" stage, when symptoms are more severe than typical aging but aren't severe enough to be dementia.

The common term for this stage is mild cognitive impairment (MCI). Depending on the underlying cause, a person could be diagnosed with MCI due to Alzheimer's disease or due to another neurodegenerative disorder.

Mild cognitive impairment due to Alzheimer's

Cognitive function — Normal / Abnormal

Typical

MCI due to Alzheimer's

Dementia due to Alzheimer's

© MFMER

Years

This line graph places mild cognitive impairment (MCI) along the trajectory of cognitive decline leading to dementia due to Alzheimer's disease. It should be pointed out that just because a person is diagnosed with MCI due to Alzheimer's does not mean the inevitable transition to dementia is just around the corner. For some people diagnosed with MCI, the symptoms get no worse, and, in fact, sometimes they improve. Scientists are attempting to discover mechanisms that may trigger or obstruct the process.

What is MCI?

Mild cognitive impairment is characterized by a person having subtle difficulties with certain cognitive skills even while most other aspects of cognition remain relatively normal.

A person with MCI may experience new, mildly deteriorating patterns of forgetfulness, yet still be able to live independently, handle his or her finances, perform household tasks capably, and drive a car with few problems. This person may have developed memory loss greater than what occurs in typical aging but not so severe as to be classified as dementia.

Of significance is the fact that not everyone with mild cognitive impairment goes on to develop dementia. For sure, the presence of MCI signals higher risk, but some individuals remain at this stage while others revert back to a normal cognitive status. In other words, dementia is not an inevitable future after a diagnosis of MCI.

Nevertheless, as research reveals more about the process of cognitive decline, a greater understanding of MCI will no doubt contribute clues to the way in which dementia develops. And this understanding may expand the options for treating conditions that cause dementia such as Alzheimer's.

Subcategories of MCI

Mild cognitive impairment is a term that encompasses a wide range of experience. At present, two broad categories of mild cognitive impairment have been identified, based on their predominant signs and symptoms: amnestic MCI and nonamnestic MCI.

Amnestic MCI. Stemming from the word *amnesia*, amnestic MCI is characterized primarily by memory loss. Impairment in other cognitive functions, such as attention and language use, may exist but is usually mild. The person is likely to be living independently and functioning fully within his or her community. Worry about forgetfulness, either new or worsening, is the most likely reason for someone with this condition to want to see a doctor.

When memory is tested, the person doesn't perform as well as others of similar age and education, but the impairment doesn't meet the criteria for dementia due to Alzheimer's disease.

Amnestic MCI is divided into subcategories. If only memory loss is present, then the condition is classified as amnestic MCI-single domain. If other areas of cognitive impairment are detected in addition to memory loss, then the classification is amnestic MCI-multiple domain. For example, a person having difficulty with concentration and in performing household tasks in addition to forgetfulness may be classified as amnestic MCI-multiple domain.

Amnestic MCI is the most common form of mild cognitive impairment and is also the most studied in medical literature. Some but not all studies indicate that this form is more common in men than in women. Generally, amnestic MCI is believed to be a precursor to Alzheimer's.

Nonamnestic MCI. This subcategory of MCI applies to a person who experiences difficulty in a cognitive area other than memory, such as reasoning, judgment, language and communication skills, or visuospatial skills.

Researchers hypothesize that a mild yet persistent problem with executive skills, such as decision-making and prioritizing, may represent the early stages of a non-Alzheimer's type of dementia, such as frontotemporal degeneration. They also believe that mild language difficulties may be linked to several types of dementia. Mild problems with executive skills or visuospatial skills often precede the dementia with Lewy bodies.

As with amnestic MCI, one cognitive skill (nonamnestic MCI-single domain) or multiple skills (nonamnestic MCI-multiple domain) may be affected.

Causes

For either amnestic or nonamnestic MCI, there may be one or more underlying causes. The causes are grouped into the following categories:

Neurodegenerative. A progressive disorder that destroys neurons in the brain (for example, Alzheimer's disease, dementia with Lewy bodies or frontotemporal degeneration)

Vascular. A disorder that affects blood vessels of the brain, limiting blood supply and causing cell damage and death (vascular cognitive impairment)

Psychiatric. Certain conditions that affect memory, concentration and mood (for example, depression)

Medications. Certain drugs that cause side effects affecting brain function

Sleep disturbances. Inadequate sleep, due to insomnia, sleep apnea or other problems, may affect cognition in a manner characteristic of MCI

Metabolic disturbances. Disruption of body metabolism, such as vitamin B-12 deficiency and hypothyroidism, may cause mild cognitive problems

If you notice mild changes in cognitive function, a thorough medical evaluation may help determine whether they have a treatable or untreatable cause.

Diagnosis

The criteria that are proposed for making a diagnosis of mild cognitive impairment include:

- Evidence of modest cognitive decline — often involving memory loss but possibly problems with concentration, decision-making, language, and visuospatial, motor or social skills — preferably confirmed by family or friends, or by neuropsychological testing
- Generally normal participation in the activities of daily living, including household tasks, work responsibilities and social functions
- Symptoms that aren't the result of delirium or another mental disorder, such as depression or schizophrenia
- Symptoms that are not severe enough to be dementia

In practice, a diagnosis of MCI can be challenging. A memory complaint is often subjective, based on how much a person feels it impacts his or her life, and that assessment can vary considerably. Furthermore, the person must be aware of the memory problems in order to make the complaint — and people with memory loss often lack that awareness. In this regard, a description of the incidents involving memory loss from someone who knows the person well can be helpful.

Usually, the complaint regards a new pattern of forgetfulness, such as asking the same question repeatedly or difficulty with remembering dates and names that once were easy to remember. Occasionally forgetting appointments is fairly normal, but regular slips in the routine may be signs of a serious underlying condition.

The doctor will conduct an extensive interview to gather information about the events and about the person's history. The doctor will also conduct a mental status evaluation to assess any evidence of cognitive decline. If there appears to be greater change than is warranted for someone of that age and educational status, but still not reaching the level of dementia, the doctor may suspect mild cognitive impairment.

Neuropsychological testing can help determine whether the person's memory and other cognitive functions are impaired by comparing them to other people in his or her age group. A series of evaluations over time is best, as they capture the signs of decline.

Still, a diagnosis of MCI is partly dependent on the doctor's judgment, within the context of each individual case. In general, an experienced physician will rely on a combination of personal interviews, medical history and clinical test results to identify and measure cognitive change when making a diagnosis.

Depending on the signs and symptoms, a diagnosis may be made for amnestic- or nonamnestic-MCI and designated either a single-domain or multiple-domain category.

Brain imaging tests

Sophisticated imaging technology may be called upon to clarify and refine a diagnosis of MCI. For example, to exclude possible structural causes of cognitive impairment, such as a tumor or the effects of physical trauma, doctors often request magnetic resonance imaging (MRI) of the brain. MRI can also be used to assess the health of blood vessels and the extent of any cerebrovascular disease in the brain.

In addition, detecting small changes in brain volume (brain mass) can provide diagnostic clues to MCI. Imaging allows scientists to gather data about the hippocampus — a structure in the brain important for memory.

Studies indicate that the volume of the hippocampus is frequently smaller in the people who progress from MCI to dementia than in the people who don't move from MCI to dementia. In light of this knowledge, refined measurements of the hippocampus may, at some time, be used as a tool for predicting the risk of dementia in people who have been diagnosed with MCI.

Scientists are studying other forms of imaging that may prove helpful in diagnosing mild cognitive impairment and in identifying individuals who are at higher risk of moving to dementia. For example, functional imaging — imaging that evaluates brain activity rather than physical structure — indicates that certain changes in activity may accompany the onset of mild cognitive impairment. These changes may potentially serve as markers for an increased risk of Alzheimer's.

Molecular imaging may be another valuable diagnostic tool, for example, positron emission tomography (PET) scans using tracers that readily stick to amyloid-beta in the living brain. The stain pattern of these tracers may allow doctors to monitor the development of amyloid plaques, potentially helping confirm a diagnosis of MCI.

When preventive treatments for Alzheimer's are discovered and become readily available, it will be important to identify people with MCI who are at higher risk of developing dementia, as they will be the ones most likely to benefit from treatment.

Outcome

Long-term studies indicate that people with mild cognitive impairment, particularly amnestic MCI, have a higher risk of Alzheimer's disease — they tend to develop dementia due to Alzheimer's at a much higher rate than do people who don't have MCI. Exactly how many people with MCI go on to develop Alzheimer's, and the rate at which this occurs, is the subject of ongoing research. The numbers vary from study to study, at least in part due to varying criteria for identifying MCI.

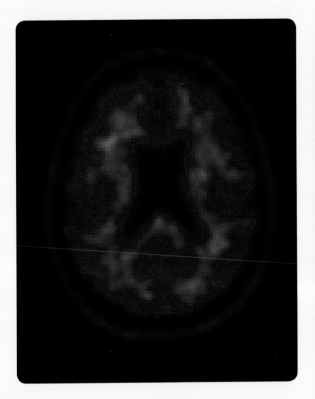

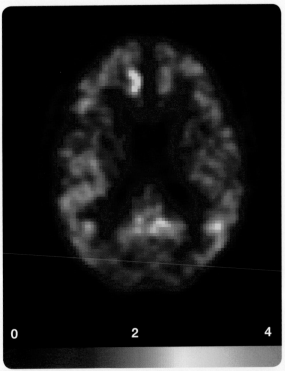

0   2   4

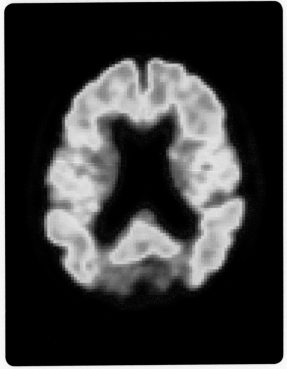

These PET scans using the Pittsburgh Compound B (PiB) radiotracer demonstrate the
progressive buildup of amyloid-beta in the living
brain. As the color bar indicates, cooler colors
such as blue and green indicate lower levels of
amyloid-beta, while warmer colors such as yellow and orange indicate higher levels. The upper
left image is a brain that is cognitively normal
— and with normal levels of amyloid-beta. The
upper right image is a brain with mild cognitive impairment, showing a pervasive buildup of
amyloid-beta. The lower right image is a brain
diagnosed with Alzheimer's disease indicating areas with abnormally high levels of amyloid-beta.

A long-term study of Catholic clergy yielded some information about the course and outcomes of mild cognitive impairment over a follow-up period of four and one-half years. For the study, the clergy had agreed to annual cognitive evaluations as well as postmortem brain donation.

From among nearly 800 participants, more than 200 were diagnosed with mild cognitive impairment at the start of the study. The study results showed that those with MCI were three times more likely to develop Alzheimer's than were those with no MCI.

But there was great variability in the study. Some participants remained at the same level of mild impairment while others reverted back to a normal cognitive state. Still others shifted from MCI to normal and then shifted back to MCI again. The more severe the cognitive symptoms were, the more likely a study participant was to progress to dementia.

In a study of more than 1,200 older adults who had no dementia on enrollment, approximately 3 to 4 percent developed amnestic MCI over the course of the study. All participants were evaluated every two years for a period of 10 years. Among the participants with amnestic MCI:

- Between 10 and 17 percent of this subgroup progressed to Alzheimer's disease every two years. This study found that people with MCI had four times the risk of developing Alzheimer's disease as did people with no MCI.
- Up to 5 percent progressed to a non-Alzheimer's form of dementia.
- Between 10 and 20 percent remained stable with MCI — with cognitive functions getting neither better nor worse.
- Between one-third and one-half of participants either improved or reverted to normal, worsened but didn't become demented, or had mixed results.

Other studies report variations of these figures, but, in general, most confirm the concept of mild cognitive impairment as a distinct stage that puts you at higher risk of dementia, but not on an inevitable path to developing the syndrome. Those who do develop dementia tend to do so within two to three years of being diagnosed with MCI.

Shift from MCI to dementia

Researchers are working to identify the factors that could contribute to a person's risk of moving from MCI to dementia. Some of the factors under question include genetics, such as the e4 variant of the apolipoprotein E (APOE) gene, as well as vascular factors, such as high blood pressure and diabetes. You can learn more about these factors in Chapter 4.

Scientists are also examining whether the presence of biomarkers — such as abnormally high levels of certain proteins in your cerebrospinal fluid or blood, or the subtle loss of brain mass — may help diagnose MCI and pinpoint the people who are more likely to develop dementia.

For example, several studies suggest that measuring the levels of specific forms of amyloid-beta and tau in cerebrospinal fluid can help identify the people with MCI who are most likely undergoing pathological (disease-related) changes that are characteristic of a neurodegenerative disorder such as Alzheimer's disease.

It's likely that a combination of risk factors will be more predictive of dementia than any single factor. By discovering which elements indicate the early signs of a neurodegenerative process, doctors hope to identify people most likely to benefit from monitoring or from participating in clinical trials.

Inside the MCI brain

Scientists are investigating the pathological changes that may occur in a person with MCI. What impact do these changes have on brain function? Answering this question is a step toward understanding the earliest stages of dementia and possibly providing new opportunities for treatment.

What researchers have discovered is that the brain of a person with MCI doesn't show the heavy load of amyloid plaques and neurofibrillary tangles that are present in the Alzheimer's brain. However, certain disease-related changes are underway, particularly in sections of the temporal lobes — areas of the brain vital to memory and learning.

Several findings cast an interesting light on the subject, but the manner in which this knowledge fits within the big picture is not yet understood.

- Autopsies performed on people diagnosed with MCI reveal a strong association between neurofibrillary tangles and cognitive impairment — the distribution of the tangles correlates well with how severely cognition is impaired.

- When a similar analysis is made of amyloid plaques, the MCI brain appears to more closely resemble a normal brain than an Alzheimer's brain — meaning many fewer plaques are present.
- There's evidence of non-Alzheimer's neurodegenerative disorders in the MCI brain, including a strong presence of vascular disease.

These findings suggest that at the MCI stage, pathologically, Alzheimer's disease or any other neurodegenerative disorder has not yet fully developed in the brain. This opens up the possibility of intervening early in the disease process and preventing a disorder from progressing more.

Treatment

Most research suggests that by the time a person is diagnosed with Alzheimer's disease, it's too late to stop the disorder or reverse neuron damage that has occurred. Research focused on MCI may lead to strategies that help prevent development or delay progress of AD. Several studies have been conducted to evaluate the effects of different compounds introduced to the MCI brain during the transition to Alzheimer's.

As a starting point, researchers examined drugs and other compounds that have already shown some effect on Alzheimer's disease. One of the primary research targets has been cholinesterase inhibitors. These drugs can help stabilize cognitive function in the disease's early stages by increasing levels of the neurotransmitter acetylcholine in the brain. Acetylcholine is a chemical that typically decreases during the development of Alzheimer's.

Cholinesterase inhibitors include donepezil (Aricept), rivastigmine (Exelon) and galantamine (Razadyne, formerly known as Reminyl). For more information on these medications and how they work, see Chapter 8.

Other therapies for AD that have been studied in relation to MCI include:

- **Antioxidants.** Substances such as vitamin E, ginkgo and selegiline may protect neurons from oxidative stress that appears to play a role in the development of AD.
- **Anti-inflammatory agents.** Medications such as nonsteroidal anti-inflammatory drugs (NSAIDs) may help reduce brain inflammation.
- **Drugs that regulate brain chemicals.** Dopamine agonists and glutamate receptor antagonists may

help normalize levels of other neurotransmitters reduced by the disease process.

- **Treatment of atherosclerosis.** Since vascular disease can damage blood vessels in the brain and often coexists with dementia, doctors speculate that controlling high blood pressure, diabetes and other vascular risk factors also may help prevent dementia.
- **Management of sleep disorders.** While more research needs to be done, there is preliminary evidence that the treatment of sleep apnea and insomnia, and less napping during the day, may decrease the risk of dementia.
- **Healthy lifestyle.** Increasing evidence suggests that eating a healthy diet and staying physically active may help reduce the risk of cognitive decline and dementia.

Unfortunately, no research has provided definitive results in terms of postponing or preventing the progression of MCI to dementia. But medical investigators are hopeful that a greater understanding of the disease process and more-powerful tools for identifying those at risk will enable the better design of research studies and eventually the discovery of more-effective treatments, especially preventive ones.

Vitamin E and donepezil

Years ago, results were published from a large study comparing the effects of vitamin E, a cholinesterase inhibitor (donepezil) and a placebo (inactive pill) on people with amnestic MCI over a period of three years. The study enrolled over 700 participants and of these, more than 200 developed Alzheimer's during the course of the trial.

In the study, vitamin E appeared to have no benefit in slowing the progression to AD. On the other hand, people who received donepezil progressed at a slower rate than did those in the other groups for the first 12 months. By the end of trial, however, this effect had disappeared, and there was no significant difference in the total number of people in each group who had developed AD.

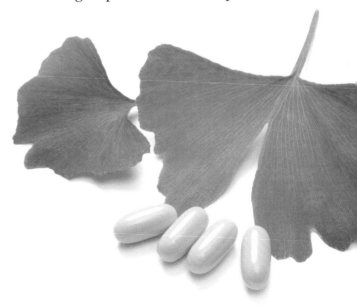

Researchers still aren't certain why donepezil worked only for a short time. They speculate that the drug's effects simply wore off after a period of time or that the burden of the disease gradually overtook the modest effects of the drug. Nonetheless, the fact that donepezil temporarily delayed the progression to AD is an incentive to pursue further studies in treating mild cognitive impairment.

The study revealed other results that scientists are still sorting through. For example, the study confirmed previous findings that the APOE e4 variant was a genetic risk factor for Alzheimer's — three-quarters of the people who progressed from MCI to Alzheimer's were APOE e4 carriers. The effects of donepezil, however, appeared to last the longest among this group, reducing their risk of Alzheimer's by about a third for most of the study.

Not enough is known about this aspect of Alzheimer's to recommend that people be tested for the APOE e4 variant, but it does provide material for future study. It may be that treatments can be designed according to a person's genetic profile, not unlike other diseases where a particular gene represents increased risk, such as the BRCA gene in breast cancer.

Making progress

Most scientists are certain that preventive treatment for Alzheimer's will be developed in the next few decades. It stands to reason that identifying those at high risk of the disease, such as people with mild cognitive impairment or even at an earlier, pre-MCI stage, will be important for getting the maximum benefit from treatment.

The challenge facing scientists who study MCI is twofold: One direction lies in refining the parameters for diagnosing the condition and identifying those individuals with MCI who will go on to develop dementia. The other direction lies in identifying and developing treatments that prevent MCI from progressing into dementia.

Chapter 7

Preclinical Alzheimer's disease

What if the signs and symptoms of dementia signaled a later stage of Alzheimer's disease (AD) and not a beginning one? More and more, scientists are coming to believe that the earliest pathological changes in the brain start long before there's any clear evidence of disease. By the time people become aware of the signs and symptoms of dementia, Alzheimer's disease is already well established.

For individuals who have developed dementia due to Alzheimer's, scientists have identified a prolonged early period when the disease is present but no signs and symptoms are perceptible. They refer to this stage as preclinical Alzheimer's disease.

During this stage, very subtle changes are taking place in the tissues and in

the chemical composition of the brain that lay the foundation for Alzheimer's and increase your risk of getting it. But these changes don't typically register in the conventional tests and evaluations that are performed during a medical visit to measure your cognitive and intellectual decline.

One way to understand the preclinical concept of AD would be to compare it to the early phase of heart disease when arteries start to narrow from the buildup of fat and cholesterol (atherosclerosis). While you may not feel different or notice any changes, these deposits gradually accumulate until they block blood flow to your heart. The blockage can cause a heart attack, with obvious signs and symptoms. But when you experience the attack, you're usually caught off guard by the event.

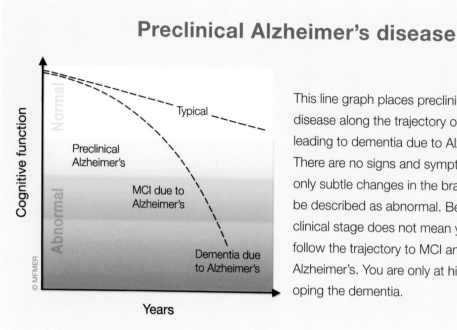

Preclinical Alzheimer's disease

Cognitive function

Normal

Abstract

Typical

Preclinical
Alzheimer's

MCI due to
Alzheimer's

Dementia due
to Alzheimer's

© MFMER

Years

This line graph places preclinical Alzheimer's disease along the trajectory of cognitive decline leading to dementia due to Alzheimer's disease. There are no signs and symptoms at this stage, only subtle changes in the brain that still cannot be described as abnormal. Being in the preclinical stage does not mean you will inevitably follow the trajectory to MCI and dementia due to Alzheimer's. You are only at higher risk of developing the dementia.

In similar fashion, gradual changes in the brain proceed at an almost undetectable pace. But at a certain point, these changes reach a level that causes irreparable damage to the brain, resulting in the loss of cognitive skills and an inability to function without assistance.

A critical difference between a neurodegenerative condition such as Alzheimer's and a cardiovascular condition such as atherosclerosis is that a buildup of fat and cholesterol in the arteries is detectable and measurable. During regular checkups, your doctor can conduct tests to make sure your arteries are functioning and healthy. If you have signs of atherosclerosis, the doctor can make recommendations to treat your arteries and reduce your risk of a heart attack.

Early changes in the brain that may signal a higher risk of Alzheimer's disease are only now being identified and studied. Researchers are searching for ways to accurately detect and measure these changes and to determine when intervention may be most effective.

The hope is that therapeutic measures, similar to the medications and lifestyle changes for atherosclerosis, can be established for the preclinical phase of Alzheimer's that dramatically reduce the risk of ever reaching dementia.

Early changes in the brain

What takes place during preclinical Alzheimer's disease? When are these "silent" changes in the brain detectable? Studies based primarily on brain imaging and cerebrospinal fluid samples provide some of the answers.

Based on these results, scientists have built a hypothetical model describing the sequence of events that define the preclinical stage. These events precede mild cognitive impairment (MCI) due to AD. The sequence includes a buildup of amyloid-beta protein in the brain, neuron damage, loss of brain mass and subtle cognitive changes.

Amyloid-beta buildup

Many scientists believe that accumulation of amyloid-beta, the material that forms amyloid plaques, may be the earliest measurable feature of Alzheimer's. This change occurs before other known physiological changes in the brain. What scientists aren't sure of is how long it takes for signs and symptoms to appear once the accumulation begins. Available evidence suggests it may be a decade or more.

There are currently two ways that scientists determine how much amyloid-beta is accumulating in the brain. One is by measuring the concentration of a specific type of amyloid-beta protein (amyloid-beta 42) in a person's cerebrospinal fluid. A low concentration in the sample suggests that amyloid waste isn't being cleared from the brain efficiently and is building up in the brain.

Another way of gauging amyloid-beta accumulation is by scanning the brain using positron emission tomography (PET) and radiotracers that seek out and attach to plaques. These radiotracers light up on the PET scan, indicating the location and volume of plaques.

Test results showing low levels of amyloid-beta 42 in cerebrospinal fluid or high amounts of amyloid-beta in a PET scan correspond well to a pattern of development that will eventually lead to Alzheimer's disease.

A drawback of these tests is that they may not be as specific as researchers would like. For example, the tests may show how much amyloid-beta is deposited as hardened plaques, but reveal little about how much exists in the form of oligomers, the still-soluble protein fragments that may be more toxic to neurons than are plaques.

Markers of disease-related change due to Alzheimer's

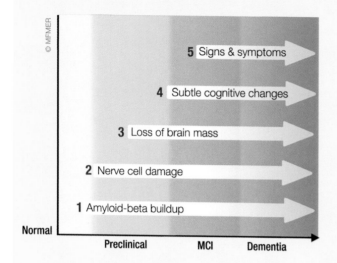

© MFMER

5 Signs & symptoms

4 Subtle cognitive changes

3 Loss of brain mass

2 Nerve cell damage

1 Amyloid-beta buildup

Normal

Preclinical   MCI   Dementia

The buildup of amyloid-beta in the brain is thought to precede signs and symptoms of dementia by several years, even decades. Nerve cell (neuron) damage happens next, fostered by neurofibrillary tangles. The loss of brain mass and subtle cognitive changes become evident late in the preclinical stage. Functional changes become apparent midway through the MCI stage.

In addition, people who test positive for amyloid-beta buildup in the brain don't always score poorly on neuropsychological tests. So, just because a person may have all the physiological characteristics of preclinical Alzheimer's doesn't mean he or she will later exhibit signs of cognitive change.

It's possible that simply having amyloid plaques in the brain isn't enough to produce the signs and symptoms of cognitive decline. More likely, dementia results from a combination of amyloid-beta buildup and other common features, such as a buildup of neurofibrillary tangles as well as nerve cell damage (neuron injury).

Nerve cell damage

As amyloid plaques build up in the brain, signs of nerve cell damage also begin to appear. To get an indication of neuron injury, researchers measure the level of tau protein in cerebrospinal fluid. Tau helps uphold neuron structure but as Alzheimer's develops, tau disengages from the structure, causing cell collapse. Loose tau filaments clump together inside the cell, forming tangles and disrupting cell activity. Some loose tau is released into cerebrospinal fluid.

Measures of tau in cerebrospinal fluid samples from people with Alzheimer's disease correlate well with the amount of tangles recorded in their autopsy reports. This suggests that cerebrospinal-fluid concentrations of tau may be good real-time predictors of tangle formation and, as a result, of the level of dysfunctional or collapsed neurons in the brain.

Brain imaging that detects neuron damage is called an 18-F fluorodeoxyglucose (FDG)-PET. This test uses a PET scan with the FDG tracer to measure synaptic activity — how well neurons communicate across the spaces (synapses) that separate cells. Where communication is disrupted, the scan shows less activity (the brain is not using glucose as expected). With Alzheimer's, this decreased uptake appears in a distinct pattern.

This imaging test is an indirect measure of nerve cell function, and the loss of function isn't specifically related to Alzheimer's. But investigators believe the results may help identify the preclinical stage: The FDG-PET shows decreased synaptic activity, but individuals still aren't showing cognitive decline. Scientists point out that in studies of cognitively normal, older adults, FDG-PET results typically corroborate findings of the two proposed Alzheimer's biomarkers found in cerebrospinal fluid: low levels of amyloid-beta 42 and high tau concentrations.

Loss of brain mass

Over time, accumulation of amyloid-beta protein and increased cell damage are thought to cause a substantial loss of neurons. This causes actual shrinkage (atrophy) in specific areas of the brain. In dementia due to Alzheimer's, magnetic resonance imaging (MRI) often shows significant atrophy in the area of the hippocampus. But researchers believe that loss of brain mass may begin earlier, as part of the preclinical stage.

Several studies using MRI have noted brain atrophy in individuals who have a genetic mutation for early-onset Alzheimer's but still haven't developed the symptoms of dementia. Researchers developed a composite measure of brain atrophy over time as the disease progresses — a specific pattern known as the "AD signature." They decided to test brain atrophy as a biomarker of Alzheimer's in cognitively normal adults with no known genetic mutations.

Based on MRI, the investigators classified study participants according to each person's AD signature. They hypothesized that individuals with the more-prominent signatures were at higher risk of preclinical Alzheimer's and would experience greater cognitive decline in the follow-up period than would those

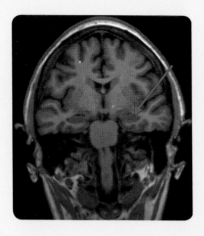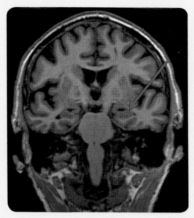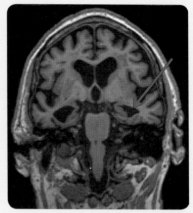

This series of coronal MRIs represent the pattern of brain atrophy known as the "AD signature" in three 70-year-old individuals. The left image is the brain of a person who is still cognitively normal, the center image is a person diagnosed with MCI, and the right image is a person diagnosed with Alzheimer's. In addition to the loss of overall brain mass — for example, the widening central cavity of the brain — the red arrows highlight shrinkage of the hippocampus. The hippocampus, which is associated with memory processing and retrieval, is one of the earliest brain structures affected by Alzheimer's.

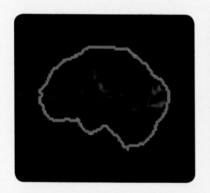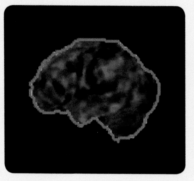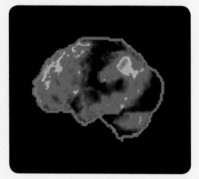

These sagittal PET scans show the progression of hypometabulism from a brain that is cognitively normal (left) to a brain with MCI (center) and to a brain with Alzheimer's disease (right). Hypometabolism means that certain chemical processes in the brain have slowed down — in this case, it's the uptake of glucose, and less uptake means less brain activity. A scan that is primarily black and blue means metabolism is relatively normal. Colors that range from green to yellow, orange and red indicate metabolism levels that are progressively lower. The changes of this sort may become evident only at the end of the preclinical stage, when subtle cognitive changes are only beginning to develop.

who were at average or low risk. Their hypothesis proved correct. In addition, more than half the high-risk participants also had low levels of amyloid-beta 42 in cerebrospinal fluid samples.

Studies such as these suggest that detecting subtle decreases in brain mass may support other indications of preclinical Alzheimer's disease.

Subtle cognitive change

Although much of the evidence for preclinical Alzheimer's is focused on physiological changes in the brain, there's evidence suggesting that subtle cognitive changes may occur before dementia sets in.

Studies assessing cognitive function in people prior to the appearance of signs and symptoms of dementia indicate a long, gradual decline in memory and nonmemory-related functions — up to a decade before the onset of dementia. Some studies also show a period of more accelerated decline that may begin years before the onset of mild cognitive impairment.

Scientists are working to develop sophisticated neuropsychological tests that are more sensitive to even small changes in cognitive function. Tests such as these, in addition to the presence of other Alzheimer's biomarkers, could help confirm a diagnosis of preclinical Alzheimer's.

Diagnostic guidelines

Based on these newly defined biomarkers, researchers have developed a set of potential guidelines for the diagnosis of preclinical Alzheimer's. At present, these guidelines are used for research purposes only — primarily as a way to identify people who may be at high risk of Alzheimer's and might benefit from participating in clinical trials.

Scientists recognize that not everyone who has the biomarkers for preclinical Alzheimer's — heavy amyloid-beta accumulation in the brain, evidence of tau in cerebrospinal fluid, indications of brain atrophy or subtle cognitive decline — is destined to develop dementia or even to develop mild cognitive impairment. Researchers have yet to identify the specific factors that contribute to a particular person moving along the trajectory from preclinical changes to MCI to dementia.

These biomarkers are, at best, indirect measures of the actual disease process. There may be other, as yet undiscovered, mechanisms critical to the development of Alzheimer's disease.

Additional factors may influence the process, such as cardiovascular disease or brain diseases other than Alzheimer's. Head trauma, depression, apathy and chronic stress have been linked to a higher risk of MCI and dementia. Certain factors may have a protective effect, as well, such as a larger cognitive reserve capacity, genetic factors or environmental influences.

In light of current understanding, scientists are proposing that three stages constitute the development of preclinical Alzheimer's disease.

Stage 1: Amyloid-beta buildup

In the opening phase, amyloid-beta starts accumulating in the brain, even as the person shows no signs or symptoms of cognitive impairment. Whenever amyloid-beta builds up, the condition is called amyloidosis. Evidence of this accumulation in the brain is obtained through PET scans and samples of cerebrospinal fluid that show

low levels of amyloid-beta 42. By the time symptoms of dementia do appear, amyloid-beta accumulation is no longer increasing in the brain and has largely leveled off.

Stage 2: Amyloidosis plus neuron injury

Next in the preclinical sequence, signs of neuron damage accompany the amyloid-beta buildup in the brain. This stage is marked by a higher concentration of tau proteins in cerebrospinal fluid samples. FDG-PET scans show areas of low brain metabolism, indicating that neurons are losing proper function. Neurodegeneration and the AD-signature pattern of brain atrophy become apparent on MRIs.

Stage 3: Amyloidosis plus neuron injury plus cognitive decline

In the final stage of the preclinical sequence, subtle signs of cognitive decline start to appear. Sometimes, these signs indicate a slight decline from the previous performance of a baseline test, even if the test results still fall within the "normal" range. Or challenging memory tests may detect subtle cognitive change. A person in this third phase is on the border of meeting the criteria for mild cognitive impairment.

Shortly after these research guidelines were published, a team of Mayo Clinic researchers tested the criteria on a group of 450 adults between the ages of 70 and 89 who had undergone neuropsychological evaluation and were deemed cognitively normal. On these adults, the researchers conducted PET scans to gauge the level of amyloid-beta deposition in the brain and FDG-PET and MRI scans to gauge the presence of neurodegeneration.

Out of this group, 43 percent had no signs of amyloid-beta accumulation, neuron injury or subtle cognitive changes, which meant they were aging normally. About 30 percent were classified as either stage 1, 2 or 3 of preclinical Alzheimer's. Incidentally, almost a quarter of the participants showed no sign of amyloid-beta buildup but did show signs of neuron injury. These people may be in the preclinical stages of a different, non-Alzheimer's disease process.

Experts have noted that not everyone progresses through the complete sequence from stage 1 to stage 2 to stage 3 to MCI. A longer follow-up study might reveal additional information that illuminates the reasons why certain individuals move through the complete sequence while others stop along the way.

What's next?

Now with a basic framework developed to detect preclinical Alzheimer's, researchers must resolve several important challenges in order to make such a diagnosis useful:

- Standardize the techniques for measuring biomarkers so that all researchers and physicians are using the same guidelines.
- Agree on very specific thresholds in biomarker testing that separates the three stages or distinguishes normal aging from preclinical Alzheimer's. For example, what amount of amyloid-beta accumulation in PET scans or increase of tau protein in cerebrospinal fluid constitutes stage 1 or stage 2?
- Refine the techniques for biomarker testing in order to gain more specific information. For example, current biomarkers can provide evidence of amyloid accumulation, but a more useful test might be one that identifies the more-toxic oligomer forms of amyloid-beta.

- Develop and refine neuropsychological tests that are more sensitive to very subtle changes in cognition and behavior.
- Identify the factors that represent the biggest risk for a person who has preclinical Alzheimer's to develop dementia due to Alzheimer's.
- Identify treatments that may best prevent further damage and destruction of neurons in the brain.

Various trials are already underway that are attempting to accomplish these goals and more.

Earlier treatment, better results?

The ultimate goal of research is to arrest Alzeheimer's disease in its preclinical stage, before irreversible brain damage can happen and dementia sets in.

Identifying the individuals who are in the preclinical stage is a critical first step toward accomplishing this goal. And the biomarkers described in this chapter can be used not only to determine people who might be at risk of Alzheimer's but also to monitor their response to different therapies.

It's possible that drugs that have failed to help individuals in the MCI and dementia stages of Alzheimer's disease may be more effective in the preclinical stage. Also, experts are interested in testing whether therapies that alter the production of amyloid-beta — the earliest biomarker of Alzheimer's disease — or modify its clearance from the brain might be effective means of preventing neurodegeneration and blocking the path to dementia.

For example, many studies are focused on immunizing the body against amyloid-beta buildup, either by administering amyloid antibodies directly or by activating the body's immune system to produce its own antibodies. Although human trials of an amyloid vaccine have been unsuccessful so far, researchers are hoping to still find safe, effective ways to use this approach in the preclinical phase.

You can read more about potential new treatments in Chapter 9. Chapters 14 and 15 contain information on lifestyle measures, such as ways to keep your mind sharp and expand your "brain power" (cognitive reserve), that may help ward off dementia.

Chapter 8

Treatment of Alzheimer's disease

Scientists are searching intently to find a cure for Alzheimer's disease — developing and testing new approaches and methods that may stop or slow its progress, or possibly even prevent the disease. But for now, no treatment is available that can halt Alzheimer's or check its course.

Treatment strategies currently in use are focused instead on easing the signs and symptoms of dementia and alleviating associated problems. "But if treatment doesn't offer a cure, what's the point of taking it?" you may ask yourself. In fact, there's much good that can be accomplished.

Treatment can reduce the severity of your symptoms, at least in the early stages of the disease, and have a positive impact on your quality of life throughout its course. Treatment can help maintain memories, reduce anxieties, raise spirits, relieve health concerns, encourage alertness during the day, and foster quality sleep at night. That's a lot to offer.

Treatment strategies for Alzheimer's disease most often involve a combination of medications, behavior adaptations and personal assistance. Some medications have been designed to treat the cognitive symptoms of Alzheimer's, while others are used more generally for mental health.

Caregivers and medical specialists rely on a variety of behavioral, social and personal care strategies to help people with Alzheimer's live to their fullest capacity and maintain independence for as long as possible.

Treatment goals

Living with Alzheimer's disease can challenge the courage, fortitude, patience, creativity and adaptive skills of everyone involved. Whether it's the person with Alzheimer's, other family members or the primary caregiver, the level of stress is intense and the demands are challenging. Coping with the disease requires trust and honesty to deal with a host of complex issues.

The one constant you can depend on is change. The symptoms are going to change or intensify as the disease progresses. In response, treatment and care must be adapted or refined to meet changing goals. What worked in the milder stages of Alzheimer's may no longer be as effective for more moderate and severe stages.

Just as important as setting a treatment strategy is acknowledging the need for team effort. You don't have to face this challenge alone. The most effective approach coordinates care among a group of people, which may include the primary caregiver, physicians, nurses, social workers, clinicians, friends, family and, most important, the person with Alzheimer's. Adequate resources, guidance and support can be provided at every step along your path.

Navigating the treatment process

If you or someone you know has received a diagnosis of Alzheimer's, here are three key guidelines to remember as you explore your options and begin the treatment process.

Know your resources. To make use of available resources, you need to know where you can find them. The Alzheimer's Association is a trusted source of information and may be able to refer you to additional resources close to home.

With chapters throughout the United States, the Alzheimer's Association can help you find specialists, support groups, in-home services, respite care, financial planners and assisted living facilities. At the back of this book, you'll find a list of organizations, including the Alzheimer's Association, which may be helpful to contact.

Ask for help. Many people dealing with cognitive impairment, whether it's the person with the condition or the caregiver, find it difficult to ask for help. You may feel like you should be able to handle the pressures on your own. Unfortunately, this mindset often makes the problems worse.

For a person with early-stage Alzheimer's, it can be frightening to admit that you have the disease. But at this emotionally fragile time, while you're coming to terms with your condition, it's important to remain connected to family and friends for crucial support.

If you're the caregiver, wearing yourself out to the point of exhaustion won't help you or your loved one. To care for others, you must first care for yourself. Enlist the help of family members and friends, seek advice from experts, and take advantage of resources.

Don't give up. Just because there's no cure for Alzheimer's right now doesn't mean it's a waste of time to seek out treatment for the disease. There's a lot that can be done to ease symptoms, build up emotional resilience and improve quality of life. But it takes commitment and persistence.

Undoubtedly, Alzheimer's disease will bring dramatic changes to your life. But along with bad moments, you'll also have good moments and even humorous moments. When possible, step back from the immediate demands of coping. Focus on something else — enjoy a morning cup of coffee or watch a favorite movie. Giving yourself time to breathe helps keep you going.

Following these simple guidelines can help you actively participate with your health care team in accessing the full arsenal of therapies that are available to help you manage the disease, for a time at least. Becoming well informed about Alzheimer's disease will help you and your loved one face the challenges of the disease with dignity and grace.

Medications for cognition

The medications commonly prescribed for Alzheimer's disease can help with memory loss, confusion, poor judgment, lack of concentration and many other cognitive symptoms. But these drugs don't work for everyone, and they may not be as useful in later stages, as the dementia worsens.

The Food and Drug Administration (FDA) has approved two types of medications to treat the cognitive symptoms of Alzheimer's disease. These medictations will be described in the following sections. Neither type of medication treats the underlying causes of the disease. Rather, these drugs help keep the brain's communication network working as well as it can.

Acetylcholine: The thoughtful messenger

Acetylcholine is one of the body's primary chemical messengers (neurotransmitters), functioning in both your central and peripheral nervous systems. It controls muscle contractions and hormone secretion and also plays a key role in thinking and memory skills.

In the 1970s, neuroscientists became aware of a dramatic drop in the level of acetylcholine that occurs in people with Alzheimer's disease. Since then, scientists have learned that the level of acetylcholine in the brain relates directly to the severity of dementia — the lower the level, the more severe the symptoms. This evidence has led to the development of medications designed to increase acetylcholine levels, or at least to prevent a reduction of the neurotransmitter.

Although scientists are still not sure of the exact role acetylcholine plays in thinking and memory, most agree that it's involved in what's called selective attention. This term refers to the way your brain filters incoming information and processes some messages while ignoring others — essential tasks at the start of the memory process. Some researchers speculate that a shortage of acetylcholine may affect conscious awareness as well as memory retrieval.

Cholinesterase inhibitors

In people with Alzheimer's, the sharp drop in levels of the brain chemical acetylcholine is caused at least in part by an enzyme known as acetylcholinesterase (as-uh-teel-koh-lih-NES-tuh-rays). Drugs that block, or inhibit, this enzyme from acting on acetylcholine are called cholinesterase (koe-lin-ES-tur-ays) inhibitors. They help maintain acetylcholine levels by slowing the chemical's breakdown. Most of the medications currently approved by the FDA for treating cognitive symptoms work in this manner.

Available cholinesterase inhibitors are donepezil (Aricept), rivastigmine (Exelon) and galantamine (Razadyne).

Tacrine (Cognex) is an older cholinesterase inhibitor that's no longer used because of severe side effects.

Cholinesterase inhibitors play a valuable role in managing the disease during the mild to moderate stages of Alzheimer's. They not only can stabilize memory, judgment and attention, but also seemingly improve behavior.

As the disease progresses into advanced stages, however, the benefit of taking one of these drugs may decline as memory and thinking problems worsen — although for some people, continuing use of these drugs may be beneficial. Whether or not to use this medication in advanced stages is a decision to discuss with your doctor.

Although these medications are generally well tolerated, gastrointestinal problems, such as nausea, diarrhea, stomach pain, loss of appetite and vomiting, are common. These problems often go away with time. Other side effects include bad dreams and muscle cramps.

Donepezil. The most commonly prescribed cholinesterase inhibitor, donepezil (Aricept) comes in tablet form and is taken once a day. The doctor may start a person with a dose of 5 milligrams (mg) and then increase the dose to 10 mg if the drug is well tolerated. A 23-mg dose is available but not recommended because it increases side effects without added benefit.

In clinical trials, people with Alzheimer's who took donepezil did better on cognitive assessments than did those who were given an inactive substance (placebo). Another benefit of donepezil is that, in smaller doses, its side effects are generally mild.

Rivastigmine. This drug is similar to donepezil in its action. Rivastigmine (Exelon) can be taken as a tablet twice a day, in doses ranging from 3 to 12 mg. Higher doses of rivastigmine may be more effective than lower doses but also cause more-severe side effects.

This medication is also available as a patch that's worn on the chest, back or upper arm. The patch is easier for most people to tolerate than is the capsule, and it's useful for people who don't like taking pills. Taking the capsule form of rivastigmine with food may help minimize side effects.

Galantamine. Galantamine (Razadyne) improves both cognition and behavior. The medication comes in tablet form, and the dosage is increased gradually, to no more than 12 mg twice a day. A once-a-day formulation is also available. Side effects are usually mild, similar to those of donepezil.

People taking a cholinesterase inhibitor often wonder if the medication is doing any good. They're tempted to stop taking it if they don't see immediate benefits. These drugs are designed to maintain cognitive functions, which are not always easy to self-check and assess. Some people who stop taking an inhibitor will experience a sudden, dramatic drop in functional ability.

How long treatment with cholinesterase inhibitors should continue is uncertain. At least one of these drugs — donepezil — has been studied long enough to show that its effects persist even into the advanced stages of Alzheimer's disease. Usually, treatment lasts for about three to five years until the symptoms of dementia become severe enough to offset any benefit from taking the medication.

Currently, there's no evidence to suggest that one cholinesterase inhibitor is any better than another one. Based on personal preference, a doctor might switch prescriptions at some point if the person has an allergic reaction to one of the drugs or can't tolerate a drug's side effects.

Scientists are testing whether such drugs are helpful for mild cognitive impairment. A large study of the use of donepezil among people with MCI found that it did slow progression to dementia — but only temporarily.

Preliminary studies of galantamine in people with MCI showed no real cognitive benefits. Unfortunately, the researchers observed a higher number of deaths among the people receiving galantamine as opposed to participants receiving a placebo. Additional research on the effectiveness of cholinesterase inhibitors for MCI is ongoing.

NMDA antagonists

Memantine (Namenda) is the first drug of its type to be approved for treating Alzheimer's disease in the United States. It's officially classified as an N-methyl-d-aspartate (NMDA) receptor antagonist. It regulates the interactions of glutamate — a neurotransmitter involved in memory and learning — and NMDA neuron receptors.

A receptor is the part of a neuron that receives the impulse during cellular communication. The impulse triggers the release of neurotransmitters from a neuron into the space separating it from an adjoining neuron. The neurotransmitters bind to specific receptors on the neighboring cell, allowing the impulse to be passed on (for more on cell communication, see Chapter 1).

Normally, glutamate binds to NMDA receptors to help with memory storage. But too much glutamate overstimulates the receptors. This may be one cause of neuron degeneration. Memantine works by blocking NMDA receptors so glutamate can't bind to them. This reduces excess glutamate and helps regulate glutamate activity.

Memantine is used to treat moderate to severe Alzheimer's disease. It can help people maintain their ability to handle daily tasks. The drug is usually started at a low dose and increased to 20 mg a day (10 mg twice a day). An extended-release capsule of 28 mg is also available that can be taken once a day. Memantine is usually well tolerated, but occasional side effects may include headache, constipation, confusion, dizziness and seizures.

Because cholinesterase inhibitors and memantine differ markedly in their actions, they may be used together. But little or no evidence shows that the combination is any more effective than using either type of medication alone.

Nutritional supplements

A growing number of herbal mixtures, vitamins and dietary supplements are promoted for cognitive health. Unfortunately, these over-the-counter remedies offer more hype than hope.

Of the many vitamins and supplements that have been tested in clinical trials, none has shown any benefit for thinking and memory. These include vitamin-B6, vitamin-B12, vitamin E, folic acid, ginkgo and huperzine A — a moss extract used in Chinese medicine.

Other supplements marketed for memory improvement or dementia prevention also lack scientific backing. Some examples are beta carotene, caprylic acid, coenzyme Q10 and coral.

Some research has suggested that a Mediterranean diet — one rich in fruits, vegetables, olive oil, legumes, whole grains and fish — may prevent or slow the progress of cognitive decline. Foods containing high levels of antioxidants or the spice turmeric also may be helpful. Although study results indicate that the Mediterranean diet can have a positive impact on heart health, no clinical trials have directly tested its potential benefit on the brain. For more information, see Chapter 15.

Before taking any herbal medicines, nutritional supplements or vitamins, talk to your doctor. The supplements promoted for cognitive health can interact with medications that have been prescribed for Alzheimer's disease or other health conditions. Claims about the safety and effectiveness of supplements aren't based on the rigorous scientific research required by the FDA. Work closely with your health care team to create a treatment strategy that's right for you or your loved one.

Strategies for behaviors

As Alzheimer's disease progresses into the later stages, extreme changes in mood and behavior become more common. This may be a result of cell communication breakdown, particularly in the limbic system, the part of the brain associated with emotions and memories. Challenging behaviors associated with Alzheimer's include aggres-

Nonmedication therapy for cognitive symptoms

Aside from medications, memory aids can help a person with Alzheimer's disease cope with cognitive loss and maintain a degree of independence. You can do this by writing down information and keeping it in visible places, along with well-placed clocks and calendars. Create a list of the day's activities, including specific instructions for accomplishing tasks such as getting dressed and preparing food. Make a list of important phone numbers. Label drawers with their contents and label the doorways to different rooms (for example, "bathroom" and "bedroom"). For more memory retention tips, see Chapter 14.

For a caregiver, reassurance may be the most important thing you can provide as your loved one's disease progresses. If your loved one becomes worried about a family member who is no longer living, for example, it's often more comforting to reassure him or her that everything is OK rather than to insist on the person accepting reality. You'll find more information about all aspects of caregiving in the Action Guide for Caregivers.

sion, agitation, delusions, hallucinations, resisting help, sleep disturbances, paranoia and wandering.

Be aware that people with Alzheimer's are gradually losing their ability to communicate. The behaviors often described as challenging may be their only way to express discomfort, stress and frustration. Even if speech remains intact, there may be difficulties in expressing thoughts correctly. The behaviors may be an attempt to communicate urgent feelings and needs.

Try to avoid labeling a behavior or the person who displays that behavior as "bad" or a "problem." Troublesome behaviors rarely occur on purpose. They're part of the disease process. Also, these labels create the expectation of "good" behavior that the person may be unable to meet. Unfulfilled expectations may lead to a sense of futility or anger.

The following strategies may be helpful in dealing with challenging behaviors.

Identify secondary causes

Behavioral problems aren't always a direct result of Alzheimer's. They may occur from other causes. A wide range of physical, emotional, environmental and social factors can have profound effects on a person with dementia. If these problems can be identified, the care team can focus on eliminating, modifying or preventing them.

Distinguishing between the symptoms caused by Alzheimer's and those from a secondary source can be challenging. You may look for a nondementia-related cause for behavior if you notice a:

- Behavior that's brand new
- Sudden, noticeable decline in functional ability
- Conspicuous worsening of confusion and disorientation

If you observe one of these indicators, consult your doctor. Treating a secondary problem often improves behavioral issues, even though the improvement may be temporary.

Health problems. Physical discomfort generally brings out complaints from anyone. A person with Alzheimer's disease is no exception. But behaviors may be the only way to indicate that something's wrong.

Challenging behaviors can arise from pain, hunger, fatigue, drug side effects, dehydration, constipation, illness, infection and impaired hearing or vision.

If you suspect an underlying health problem may be prompting your loved one's behavior, talk to your doctor about ways to manage the problem.

Emotional issues. Anxiety and depression are common conditions among people with Alzheimer's disease. They may show excessive concern over upcoming events or begin to wander, scream or act aggressively. Feelings of anxiety can be caused by any number of factors, including illness, abuse, loss or frustration.

Feelings of depression may translate into tearfulness and a pervading sense of worthlessness. Depression may also come across as a worsening of cognition and lead to social withdrawal, weight loss and disruptive behavior.

Fortunately, both anxiety and depression are treatable. For caregivers, the diagnosis of a loved one can lead to more realistic expectations of what can be accomplished and how to better communicate and provide support.

People in early stages of Alzheimer's who are depressed but still communicating well can benefit from support groups and professional counseling. Physical exercise and planned activities also may help alleviate anxiety or depression by providing a sense of purpose and self-worth.

Environmental factors. A person's surroundings can have a significant impact on his or her behavior. Both understimulation and overstimulation may pose problems. With nothing to do, a person with Alzheimer's may become bored or restless and resort to wandering. But multiple or unnecessary distractions may only confuse and overwhelm the person.

Television shows may be misunderstood or mistaken for reality, resulting in frightened or angry reactions. Disembodied voices coming from radios, paging systems or people conversing out of sight also may contribute to confusion, paranoia, agitation, hallucinations and delusions.

Changed surroundings can confuse the person. For example, moving to a new residence or admission to a hospital can trigger behavior change. Introducing a new caregiver, rearranging furniture, or even asking the person to change clothes can be disruptive.

Creating a serene, constant and predictable environment provides a greater sense of familiarity and comfort and reduces the risk of disruptive behavior. Avoiding excess stimulation and hubbub may help achieve this.

Social isolation. Although people with Alzheimer's progressively lose their ability to communicate, they still retain basic desires to belong, be loved and feel useful. Social isolation can lead to depression, anxiety, agitation, delusions, aggression and wandering. Encouraging social interaction that is stimulating but not overwhelming can help prevent the feeling of isolation.

Stay engaged

One approach that may improve the quality of life for people with Alzheimer's is to encourage them to take part in the routine tasks of daily living. This helps them feel more involved in the normal rhythms of life.

At the same time, it's important to respect the ways in which your loved one can feel comfortable and achieve success. What someone with dementia is able to accomplish day to day may vary. Tasks, such as getting dressed, may sometimes present little problem and at other times seem overwhelming.

Try these suggestions to help engage your loved one in daily activities.

Break each task into simple steps. Limit choices and allow extra time for your loved one to accomplish the chore. Rushing the process may only cause frustration and panic.

Avoid confrontation. Argument and accusation will usually be counter-productive. Raising your voice will only make your loved one more upset. Speak in a soft voice, focusing on the positive, to diffuse a tense situation.

Allow your loved one to do as much as possible. This reinforces existing skills and helps maintain a greater sense of independence. Rather than doing everything yourself, you can allow your loved one to participate in getting dressed. Provide clothing with elastic waistbands, sweaters with easy-to-pull zippers instead of buttons, and shoes that don't need to be tied.

Encourage involvement in recreational activities. Enjoyable pastimes may include listening to music, painting, playing board games, walking or reading. How the activity is performed is less important than how much fulfillment and social interaction it provides. For example, the joy of paging through a morning newspaper together may be far greater than being able to discuss or remember its content.

Join, validate, distract

As the disease progresses, people with Alzheimer's tend to lose their comprehension of the present and revert to a past reality, such as when they were a child or young adult. In their minds, their parents may still be alive and their children may still be toddlers.

If loved ones are confronted with present reality, they may respond with anger, aggression and withdrawal, and be even more determined to pursue a particular course of action.

In such circumstances, it may be more constructive to *join* the person's reality, *validate* how the person is feeling, and find a way to *distract* the person with another thought or activity. Generally, it's best to respond as though you believe what the person has said is true. Then, give an explanation that makes sense in that context.

For example, you might tell your mother that her long-deceased parents aren't home because they've gone to visit relatives, or that there's no need for her to go to school today because it's Saturday. It's more important to comfort your mother than to make sure she's factually correct. Frame your response in a way that will reassure her.

Keep in mind that the emotions your loved one is expressing are very real to him or her, even if the reasons behind them aren't logical. Don't pass them off as misplaced or nonsensical. Show that you're paying attention and listening. Make eye contact and give feedback. Empathize and acknowledge that you recognize the concerns being expressed.

Find activities that can distract your loved one's attention away from these emotions. If your mother becomes upset because she thinks she needs to go home and care for her young children, for example, you can join her reality and acknowledge how upset she is without making light of her distress.

Provide an explanation for the absence of the children that makes sense to her — for example, say that the children are at a birthday party and having a great time. They won't be home for several hours. Then distract her with an activity such as baking cookies or listening to favorite music as you "wait."

Anticipate problems

Heading off problems before they occur is an effective way for a caregiver to manage behavior. This is sometimes called the ABC method — A stands for

The personal connection

Helping people with Alzheimer's stay socially connected can be particularly effective for behavioral symptoms. Even when people are cognitively impaired, they remain remarkably attuned to interactions with others. They respond to interpersonal cues and emotional support, and they still want to feel a sense of identity, especially within their families.

As a caregiver, you can reinforce your loved one's role as a mother, father, aunt or uncle by sharing family stories and pictures. Spend time together talking — even if the person doesn't understand everything being said, he or she probably still enjoys the interaction.

Another proven strategy for social connections is to use activity and support groups, elder care programs and counseling services.

antecedent (cause), B for behavior and C for consequence. Most behaviors have an antecedent. And behaviors generally have a consequence. Consequences that are negative can be much more difficult to resolve than ones that are positive.

As a caregiver, you may be tempted to concentrate on the consequences of a behavior because they tend to be things that demand your immediate attention and cause the greatest harm. But using forethought goes a long way toward resolving the problem. By addressing the antecedent, you may be able to avert both the behavior and the consequence.

For example, seeing a car parked in the driveway may provoke outbursts of anger in a person with Alzheimer's — the person may be reminded that he or she can no longer drive. If you're able to drive, the anger may be directed at you.

Your attempts to soothe your loved one may be futile. His or her attention remains focused on the car, parked in full view outside the window.

The ABC approach can guide your response to this behavior. Identify the antecedent (parked car), the behavior (anger) and the consequence (hours of distress). You might decide that from now on, you'll park the car out of sight. By addressing the antecedent, you've eliminated the cause of the outburst and the needless frustration and anger.

Not all behaviors have such apparent antecedents. But whether the antecedent is clear or not, being adaptable is an important part of caregiving. With wandering, for example, you may simply go along with the behavior. If the wandering is relatively harmless and can be done safely, it may be an appropriate outlet for feelings.

Be creative. See what works and what doesn't work. And go easy on yourself. If an approach isn't successful some days, keep in mind that you're doing the best you can. Simply try something else the next day.

Medications for behaviors

Sometimes, behavioral therapy and social interaction aren't enough to the soothe challenging behaviors of a loved one or alleviate symptoms of anxiety and depression. To help, your doctor may prescribe medications that can improve behavioral symptoms.

Unfortunately, no single medication can treat all of the behavioral symptoms associated with Alzheimer's disease. And, although medications may be of some benefit, they're generally a second line of defense. That's because these drugs can intensify cognitive impairment and their side effects may be more severe in older adults.

As a result, it's important to discuss this strategy with your doctor, weighing the risks and benefits of a drug before taking it. In general, these medications are best when used only when necessary and for a short period of time.

Cholinesterase inhibitors may improve behavioral as well as cognitive symptoms. If a person with Alzheimer's isn't already taking a cholinesterase inhibitor, a doctor may recommend one before prescribing any of the medications that follow.

Anti-anxiety drugs. Anxiety may be relieved with a class of drugs known as anxiolytics (ang-zee-o-LIT-iks). These medications are generally recommended for occasional or short-term use.

Anxiolytics work best for stressful events that can be predicted, such as visiting the dentist or taking a weekly bath. Taking a low dose of the medication one hour before the dental visit or bath can help ease the anxiety of this situation.

Side effects include sleepiness, decreased learning and memory, dizziness and loss of coordination. There is also a risk of generating even more agitation. Anxiolytics include lorazepam (Ativan), oxazepam and buspirone.

Antidepressants. If a person with Alzheimer's is also diagnosed with depression, drug therapy is often recommended. The most commonly prescribed antidepressants are selective serotonin reuptake inhibitors (SSRIs). These have proved effective while causing relatively few side effects. SSRIs act primarily by blocking the receptors for the neurotransmitter serotonin while leaving acetylcholine receptors undisturbed.

Some SSRIs can cause anxiety and agitation, so they should be used with caution in people who already have these symptoms. Other side effects may include insomnia, tremor, nausea, diarrhea, headache, decreased appetite, dizziness, sweating and dry mouth.

Your doctor will start the medications at a low dose, then gradually increase the dose while monitoring closely for side effects.

Commonly prescribed antidepressants include citalopram (Celexa), paroxetine (Paxil), sertraline (Zoloft), fluoxetine (Prozac, Sarafem), escitalopram (Lexapro) and mirtazapine (Remeron).

Antipsychotics. These medications may be prescribed for people with dangerous or extremely challenging behaviors, such as aggression, delusions and hallucinations. Antipsychotics are divided into two major groups: conventional and atypical. Both groups work by blocking certain neurotransmitter receptors, particularly dopamine, in hopes of regulating the emotions.

Conventional antipsychotics are limited in use for Alzheimer's because their side effects — muscle spasms, rigidity, tremor, gait disturbance and sedation — tend to be severe and typically outweigh any benefits they may provide.

Atypical antipsychotics may be used to treat agitation or psychosis. They generally have fewer side effects than conventional antipsychotics.

The decision to use an antipsychotic medication must be considered cautiously. Older adults with dementia who are treated with antipsychotic drugs for behavioral problems face an increased risk of death. The FDA requires these medications to carry a warning label about the risks, as well as a reminder that they're not approved for treating dementia symptoms.

In addition, atypical antipsychotics can raise blood glucose levels to abnormally high levels, which can lead to diabetes. Some experts recommend regular screening for diabetes in people who take atypical antipsychotics.

Antipsychotics also block acetylcholine receptors, which are already in short supply due to Alzheimer's. This action tends to speed cognitive decline.

Commonly prescribed antipsychotic drugs include olanzapine (Zyprexa), risperidone (Risperdal) and quetiapine (Seroquel).

Mood stabilizers. Although not as commonly prescribed as atypical antipsychotics, mood stabilizers (or anticonvulsants) may also be used to treat hostility or aggression. They're not often recommended, however, as there's not much evidence to support their effectiveness for Alzheimer's, and side effects such as sedation can be severe. These drugs include divalproex (Depakote), carbamazepine (Carbatrol, Tegretol) and lamotrigine (Lamictal).

A good perspective

Alzheimer's disease may be incurable, but it's not untreatable. Many studies have shown that actively managing Alzheimer's and other conditions that cause dementia can significantly improve quality of life, both for the person with the neurodegenerative condition and for his or her caregiver.

This means taking advantage of all the treatment options — social and behavioral strategies as well as medications — addressing any coexisting health conditions, and working with a team of health care professionals and personal caregivers.

Even as symptoms of Alzheimer's progressively worsen, therapies to improve cognition, stabilize emotions and ease challenging behaviors can greatly enhance the quality of life for people with Alzheimer's and for their caregivers. A focus on a person's strengths as well as needs remains the strongest weapon against this unrelenting disease.

Chapter 9

Research trends in treatment and care

A massive effort is currently underway to find effective treatments for Alzheimer's disease (AD) and other conditions that cause dementia. Initiatives also have been launched that address the financial burden of Alzheimer's on society, as prevalence of the disease is expected to triple in the coming decades.

Guiding this common effort is the National Plan to Address Alzheimer's Disease, released by the Department of Health and Human Services in 2012. This ambitious plan intends to establish an effective means of treating Alzheimer's by 2025. In addition, the plan has established goals to enhance the quality of care, expand support to people with AD and their families, enhance public awareness, and improve data collection to track research.

To make the plan a national priority, specialists joined together to propose specific steps for achieving these goals. An advisory council was created to evaluate the implementation and progress of the plan. Millions of federal dollars were set aside for research.

Scientists are pursuing the plan on many fronts, such as identifying risk factors, developing new imaging technology and therapeutic approaches, and evaluating the impact of environment and lifestyle on the disease process. This diverse body of knowledge is growing rapidly, in hopes of finding success by 2025.

This chapter highlights some of the key research trends. Each new effort brings more hope for finding ways to prevent and treat Alzheimer's.

Causes

Based on current research, it appears likely that the late-onset form of Alzheimer's disease, which develops after age 65, is caused by the interaction of a variety of genetic and environmental factors. The thinking is that no single factor by itself will cause a neurodegenerative disorder, but in combination with other risk factors, the likelihood of Alzheimer's is greater.

Scientists have identified several of the risk factors that play a part in this disease process. They're also attempting to unlock secrets to the pathological mechanisms that cause the interactions. Following are some of the latest research efforts that may reveal the potential causes of Alzheimer's disease.

Genetic risk factors

Researchers are studying genetic factors associated with the increased risk of Alzheimer's. A strong genetic link is supported by studies involving twins. The results showed that an estimated 60 to 80 percent of the risk of Alzheimer's disease among the study participants was genetic — although environmental factors also appeared to play important roles.

The search for genetic links to Alzheimer's has accelerated recently with use of an approach called genome-wide association studies (GWAS). This technology involves rapidly scanning a complete set of human DNA (genome) to find the variations associated with a particular disease.

Through this and other means, researchers have identified several genes that may increase the risk of Alzheimer's. Some genes, such as APP and presenilin, are linked to the early-onset form of the disease. But the gene that has received the most attention is a variant of apolipoprotein E (APOE), and linked to the late-onset form.

APOE e4. One of three common variants (alleles) of the APOE gene is APOE e4. Evidence confirms that this variant is a risk factor for mild cognitive impairment and Alzheimer's disease. The APOE gene has several responsibilities in the brain, including neuron repair and helping reorganize neuron connections (plasticity). Impairing either function would make a person more susceptible to dementia.

The APOE e4 allele, in particular, is more likely to be defective or produce toxic effects in the brain than are the other alleles, although the reasons for this are not clear. For example, people with the APOE e4 allele typically have more amyloid-beta deposits in their brains — a hallmark of Alzheimer's disease — than do people with other APOE variants.

Other genes. With the advent of GWAS studies, researchers are discovering other genetic variants that may increase the risk of late-onset Alzheimer's. These variants are thought to affect a variety of cell functions. While individual variants may only be weakly linked to Alzheimer's, the impact of multiple variants in combination may be significant on this risk.

SORL1, a gene that normally helps transport amyloid precursor protein (APP) within cells, has been connected to Alzheimer's. Some variants of the gene appear to increase production of "sticky" amyloid-beta fragments, which clump together to form plaques.

A variant of the GAB2 gene is also thought to increase risk. A normal GAB2 gene may help prevent the formation of neurofibrillary tangles, so a change in this gene could leave a person more susceptible to tangles.

Other genes that may be linked to Alzheimer's include:

- CLU. This gene helps regulate the clearance of amyloid-beta.
- CR1. This gene helps regulate inflammation in the brain.
- PICALM. This gene is linked to neuron communication.
- TREM2. This gene helps regulate inflammation in the brain.

Similar to APOE, these genes may increase risk but are not a direct cause of Alzheimer's disease. As technology advances, even more genes linked to the disease may be identified.

Aging and family history

Two risk factors for Alzheimer's disease are aging and family history. In general, your risk increases as you grow older, especially after age 65. And risk increases if you have close relatives who have Alzheimer's, even more so if they developed the disease at an early age.

Some scientists speculate that, in fact, everyone is susceptible to Alzheimer's, the only difference being the age of onset — a factor that might be influenced by genetics. For example, if your father developed Alzheimer's at age 70, then you will likely have the tendency to develop Alzheimer's at around the same age.

To test this theory, scientists collected the family histories of people with Alzheimer's and of people without dementia. Their findings suggest that if you have a close relative with AD, your inherited risk increases with age but appears to peak close to the age at which the relative developed the disease. After that time, surprisingly, your risk declines to a point where it's about the same as that of someone with no family history of dementia.

Another interesting result of this study: The older a person is when he or she develops Alzheimer's, the lower the risk for his or her relatives to get the disease. In other words, as the age of onset increases, the risk to others decreases.

What this may imply is that as you age, genetic risk factors tend to diminish while environmental factors tend to become more influential.

Vascular risk factors

Mounting evidence draws connections between heart health and brain health. Factors such as chronic high blood pressure, high cholesterol, and a history of heart disease, heart attack or heart failure may increase your risk of Alzheimer's disease.

Researchers have observed similarities between the risk factors for stroke and for vascular cognitive impairment. High blood pressure can damage blood vessels in the brain, leading to blocked vessels and insufficient blood flow. Without nutrients from the bloodstream, neurons suffer damage and die. Vascular cognitive impairment — a form of dementia caused by damaged blood vessels — often develops at the same time as does Alzheimer's.

The APOE e4 allele is a risk factor for both cardiovascular disease and Alzheimer's disease. It's possible that the role of APOE for processing cholesterol in the body may also affect the onset of Alzheimer's in the brain.

If the risk factors for cardiovascular disease also influence the risk of dementia, this may offer a potential avenue for prevention. You may be able to improve brain health by managing cardiovascular health through diet, exercise and medications.

Underlying biological mechanisms

Scientists are attempting to clarify the processes taking place in the brain that ultimately lead to the destruction of neurons. Two areas of research are prominent: amyloid plaques and neurofibrillary tangles.

Amyloid plaque formation. As discussed in Chapter 4, amyloid plaques are the end result of a sequence of events taking place in the brain. Amyloid-beta fragments trimmed from the cell surface collect and form into long chains called amyloid fibrils. The fibrils combine with other substances to form oligomers that eventually harden into plaques. Amyloid plaques appear in disproportionate numbers in the brains of people with Alzheimer's disease.

Scientists are investigating the role that plaque development may play in dementia. For example, the structure of amyloid fibrils resembles a molecular "zipper." In order for fibrils to form, the amyloid fragments must be aligned just right. When that happens, the fibrils zip up so tightly that it's difficult to undo them. This may help explain why plaques are so hard to dissolve. So, finding ways to disrupt fibril formation could potentially prevent the accumulation of plaques.

Other research involves the oligomers, toxic compounds that lead directly to plaques. Oligomers attack synapses — the spaces that cells must bridge in order to communicate with other cells. The loss of synapses disrupts communication and causes memory loss. Scientists have learned that oligomer levels are high in people who have Alzheimer's.

Some researchers believe oligomers may be a missing puzzle piece that clarifies the relationship between plaques and Alzheimer's disease. In studies, mice genetically programmed to develop plaques were vaccinated with antibodies to fight the plaques. Although the mice retained the same number of plaques after vaccination, they showed improved cognition, including rapid reversal of memory loss. The vaccine may have actually targeted oligomers instead of the intended plaques.

Neurofibrillary tangles. Another subject of intensive research is the role that neurofibrillary tangles play in the development of dementia. Tangles — abnormal masses of tau protein inside neurons — are characteristic of several neurodegenerative disorders, including Alzheimer's and frontotemporal degeneration with parkinsonism.

Are the tangles a cause of disease or a byproduct of it? To answer this question, scientists are studying mice that exhibit tau abnormalities. By administering different medications to the mice that may

Plaques without dementia

Although people with Alzheimer's have a high number of plaques in their brain tissue, many people without dementia were found to have plaques when their brains were examined during autopsy. Interestingly, the people with plaques but no dementia also have the APOE e4 allele, putting them at higher risk of Alzheimer's disease. This raises a number of questions. Were these individuals in an early stage of Alzheimer's but died before the disease progressed to a symptomatic stage? Or did some factor prevent them from developing full-blown Alzheimer's? Research continues to try solving these unanswered questions.

prevent or eliminate the tangles, the scientists are hoping to discover a therapy that is also helpful to humans.

Several aspects of neurofibrillary tangles are worth noting. Scientists have discovered that in certain disorders, the tangles are distributed in distinct patterns in the brain. Also, the basic building blocks of tau (amino acids) have a different genetic sequence in different dementias. Scientists are hoping to use the distribution patterns and distinctive biochemical makeup of tau as "bar codes" to distinguish between different dementing disorders.

Research on the tau protein may shed more light on how Alzheimer's progresses through the brain. Scientists have learned that tangle formation can spread from neuron to neuron, suggesting that strands of tau from a diseased neuron may be released into synapses and taken up by adjoining cells that are healthy. Within a new cellular environment, the diseased strands may affect healthy tau, resulting in the breakdown and death of the neuron.

Early diagnosis

A promising area of research is focused on detecting neurodegenerative conditions in their earliest stages. Researchers believe that new medications may be most effective if they can be given early in the disease process, before a condition such as Alzheimer's has caused irreparable harm. Early detection also would allow people to benefit more from preventive therapies or treatments that may keep dementia symptoms from becoming more severe.

As researchers work to identify early signs and symptoms, they're also developing criteria that can help diagnose Alzheimer's at a preclinical stage. Some tests look for early cognitive or biological signs (biomarkers) of change. For example, a new test has been developed that can detect oligomers in cerebrospinal fluid. Imaging techniques are also being explored for this purpose.

Precursor stages of Alzheimer's

A new, exciting area of research explores early recognition of the disease-related (pathological) changes in the brain. One of these precursor stages, known as preclinical Alzheimer's disease, is a new diagnostic category that's discussed in Chapter 7. Researchers are looking to identify the subtle changes that occur during this stage, which may happen many years before any signs and symptoms of dementia appear.

As discussed in Chapter 6, the transitional stage following preclinical Alzheimer's in the disease spectrum

is mild cognitive impairment (MCI). People with MCI will not necessarily get Alzheimer's disease but are at a higher risk to develop it.

It's challenging, even for a specialist, to examine an older adult and try to distinguish preclinical Alzheimer's and MCI from the forgetfulness of typical aging. Scientists are working to precisely define and specify diagnostic criteria for both stages. Establishing these standards will assist doctors in diagnosing varying symptoms accurately.

Cognitive tests

Doctors use a variety of interview-type tests to assess a person's cognitive abilities. In these tests, the person responds to a set of questions or completes a series of simple tasks. Researchers are working to develop new tests that may help identify the earliest stages of memory impairment or accurately predict a person's risk of dementia.

This effort may involve simply modifying existing resources. For example, in a modified version of a standard cognitive test, a person views a list of common words and is later asked to recall as many words from memory as possible. Rather than using the same score for all recalled words, researchers have weighted the scoring in hopes of gleaning more information and improving their ability to detect MCI and early-stage dementia.

Researchers have developed testing to predict a person's 10-year risk of Alzheimer's with 70 percent accuracy. When this test was combined with two other tests, results were able to predict a person's five-year risk of Alzheimer's with more than 80 percent accuracy. And researchers have developed a simple equation factoring in test results with age and education to determine a person's probability of developing Alzheimer's within five or 10 years.

Biomarkers and imaging techniques

A biomarker, or biological marker, is a measurable substance in the body that can indicate a normal biological process, the presence of disease or a response to therapy. This substance may be naturally occurring or be introduced into the body. Finding a biomarker for Alzheimer's disease would greatly help scientists' ability to identify people at high risk or in the earliest stages of the disease and enable these people to receive prompt treatment.

Some features of disease, such as the plaques and tangles of Alzheimer's, are generally studied during autopsy. Imaging techniques under investigation will allow scientists to study the living brain to detect and monitor biomarkers that may reflect the disease process. This imaging can also help monitor the brain's response to treatment.

Cerebrospinal fluid (CSF) biomarkers. Research is focused on measuring substances in CSF samples that accurately detect the development of Alzheimer's disease. One study concludes that amyloid-beta 42, which is the predominant form of amyloid-beta in plaques, may be a sensitive biomarker in samples and help predict the transition from mild cognitive impairment to Alzheimer's.

The characteristic Alzheimer's "signature" in a CSF sample is a low level of amyloid-beta 42 along with high levels of total tau and phosphorylated tau. A problem with using this test for diagnosis is the wide variability between results from various laboratories.

Blood plasma biomarkers. Researchers at Mayo Clinic recently published study results in which they measured the chemical fingerprints of cellular activity that can be detected in blood plasma. This includes changes in substances such as sugars, lipids and amino acids. The researchers found that these changes closely matched the CSF biomarkers that they were also monitoring. This suggests that blood may become a reliable means to diagnose, monitor and evaluate Alzheimer's, with large-scale clinical applications.

Imaging amyloid plaques. Several radioactive tracers (radiotracers) have been developed to show amyloid plaques in the living brain. These compounds, administered as an intravenous drug, readily stick to the plaques, which "light up" during positron emission tomography (PET) imaging. Previously, amyloid plaques could only be detected during an autopsy.

One of these radiotracers, florbetapir F 18 (Amyvid), has been approved by the Food and Drug Administration to detect amyloid plaques in Alzheimer's disease. More study is needed to test reliability before this technique can be used regularly for diagnosis.

Monitoring the hippocampus.
The hippocampus is part of the brain that's essential for memory. And the hippocampus is usually one of the first structures affected by Alzheimer's — it shrinks as the disease progresses. To

confirm a diagnosis of Alzheimer's, doctors often use magnetic resonance imaging (MRI) to check for a smaller than normal hippocampus.

MRI monitoring of the hippocampus is useful for other purposes, for example, detecting progression from cognitively normal to MCI to Alzheimer's (see this progression in Chapter 7). Imaging can also monitor the rate of progression or the effect of experimental treatment, and detect other causes of hippocampus atrophy, including head injury, sleep apnea and cardiac arrest.

Other forms of MRI are being explored as monitoring tools. Magnetic resonance spectroscopy is a test that measures the amounts of certain metabolic substances (metabolites) in the body. Some studies have found that abnormal levels of certain metabolites may indicate the progress of Alzheimer's.

Diffusion-weighted MRI is a way to measure hippocampus atrophy in the earliest stages. The test measures minor structural change, for example, revealing how much space water molecules in the brain have to move around in. If the hippocampus is even microscopically smaller than normal, the test reveals that extra space is available for the molecules.

Imaging tau protein. Radiotracers have recently been developed that show the presence of tau protein in the living brain with the help of PET imaging technology. This development is important for evaluating the impact of neurofibrillary tangles on the Alzheimer's disease process.

Measuring brain activity

Another way to compare a normal brain with a cognitively impaired brain is by measuring brain activity. All brain cells use glucose for energy during normal cellular operations. PET scans can measure the chemical processing of glucose (metabolism) as well as other vital functions, such as blood flow and oxygen use. PET imaging of people with Alzheimer's and MCI reveals areas of reduced glucose metabolism.

A similar form of imaging called single-photon emission computerized tomography (SPECT) measures blood flow in the brain and shows which areas are more active or less active. The imaging technique has indicated reduced brain activity in people with dementia that correlates well with the results of cognitive tests, suggesting that the changes captured on the SPECT images reflect the memory problems.

Both PET and SPECT imaging can help confirm a diagnosis of Alzheimer's. But researchers also are hoping the technologies may help identify individuals at high risk of dementia before the symptoms are evident. PET and SPECT imaging also have been used to help predict which people with MCI will progress to Alzheimer's.

Functional MRI (fMRI) measures brain activity. When asked to perform specific tasks, people with MCI and AD show different patterns of activity, compared with people who are cognitively normal.

Recent research has focused on resting state fMRI, taken when people are not given specific tasks to perform. This technique is useful for understanding how the brain may be altered by disease. More study is needed to see if fMRI can detect memory impairment before any symptoms appear.

Diffusion spectrum magnetic resonance imaging (DSI) tractography is a new technology that reveals the neuron network allowing communication among different parts of the brain. This knowledge may help researchers discern normal cognition and how it may be affected by changes brought on by a neurodegenerative disorder such as Alzheimer's disease.

PET imaging using a radiotracer to show tau accumulation in the brain of a 58-year-old and a 72-year-old individual. Tracking the distinctive buildup of tau in a living brain may prove invaluable to understanding the cause and progress of Alzheimer's disease.

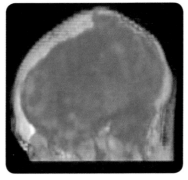
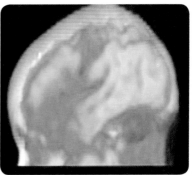

58 years

72 years

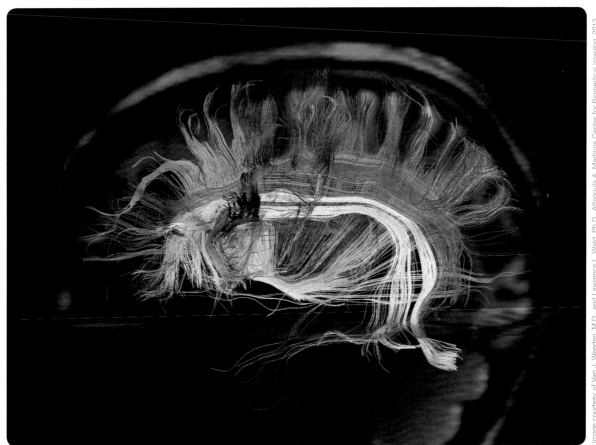

A specialized form of magnetic resonance imaging known as DSI tractography shows the neural pathways connecting different parts of the cerebral cortex. The study of these images may help researchers understand changes taking place in the brain due to Alzheimer's that disrupt neural communication.

Treatment and prevention

The conventional treatment for Alzheimer's disease includes medications that stabilize cognitive functions, such as memory and language use, if only for a short period of time. The drugs help reduce or slow symptoms, but they're unable to treat the underlying disease or stop it from progressing. These medications are described in Chapter 8.

Many new drugs under development are referred to as "disease-modifying" because they're focused more on the underlying disease and not just on the symptoms. Many scientists hope one of these drugs may eventually prove to be a truly effective strategy.

Another therapeutic goal involves early intervention in the disease process. Research indicates that Alzheimer's disease begins decades before a person experiences any signs and symptoms. Increasingly, as investigators work to diagnose the disease at its earliest stage, they're also looking to intervene and stop its progress when effects may still be reversible or even prevented. Drugs based on meeting these goals are currently in clinical testing.

Alzheimer's vaccine

After researchers showed that a vaccine injected into cognitively impaired mice could improve cognition and reduce memory loss, excitement grew about the possibility of developing an anti-Alzheimer's vaccine in humans. Investigators began preliminary studies, but these trials were halted after some participants developed brain inflammation as a side effect.

Even after stoppage, researchers continued to follow the group of participants who hadn't developed inflammation. These individuals did better on neurological testing than did participants who had received placebos during the trials. Immunized participants also showed reduced amounts of plaque in brain tissue and decreased levels of tau protein in cerebrospinal fluid.

Scientists didn't lose all hope for the vaccines. They developed second-generation vaccines with fewer side effects for another round of clinical trials. Unfortunately, in 2012, separate trials of bapineuzumab and solanezumab were stopped after results indicated that neither vaccine improved the cognition or daily functioning of participants with mild to moderate Alzheimer's disease, compared with a group taking a placebo. Later analyses suggest that partici-pants in the solanezumab trial may have shown minor cognitive improvement, which may prompt further studies.

The failure of these vaccines has complicated the ongoing question of whether amyloid-beta is the driving force behind Alzheimer's disease. Some researchers postulate that if these medi-cations could be administered in earlier stages of the disease, before symptoms appear, they may be more effective.

Secretase inhibitors

Secretase inhibitors are a class of drugs intended to reduce levels of amyloid-beta by blocking the action of enzymes that clip amyloid fragments. So far, most studies have shown that, while the drugs don't cause harm, they pro-vide much less benefit than hoped.

Based on these results, some research-ers question the role amyloid plays in causing Alzheimer's. Others argue that clearing amyloid from the brain after the disease has progressed to the mild or moderate stages comes too late. New studies are testing secretase inhibitors in the preclinical phase of the disease — similar to the way a cholesterol-lowering drug can reduce the risk of a

heart attack but won't help the symp-toms of the heart attack.

Cardiovascular therapies

Some studies of cholesterol-lowering drugs called statins have indicated that regular use in midlife decreases the risk of dementia. This suggests the pos-sibility of protecting against dementia by controlling cholesterol levels. Other studies, however, have failed to find a benefit for taking these medications.

Another study found that people taking blood pressure medications had a reduced risk of vascular cognitive impairment. Because of the connection with Alzheimer's, controlling blood pressure may improve Alzheimer's symptoms in the same way that con-trolling cholesterol may help.

Antioxidants

Researchers have studied whether antioxidants such as vitamin E can slow Alzheimer's disease. Unfortunately, no evidence proves that the vitamin helps. Scientists continue to investigate its potential risks and benefits for Alzheim-er's. Some research suggests that food sources, such as vegetable oils and seed oils, may be more protective than are supplements. Other researchers point out that high doses of vitamin E may actually be harmful.

Anti-inflammatory drugs

Studies indicate that nonsteroidal anti-inflammatory drugs (NSAIDs), such as ibuprofen (Advil, Motrin, others), naproxen sodium (Aleve) and indomethacin (Indocin), may reduce the risk of Alzheimer's disease. Inflammation is believed to play a role in the disease process. What isn't known is whether the inflammation is a cause or an effect of the disease.

Several years ago, investigators halted a major trial studying the effects of naproxen and celecoxib (Celebrex), another anti-inflammatory drug, in Alzheimer's. The study was stopped over fears, due to findings from another unrelated study, that celecoxib might increase the risk of heart disease. However, investigators continue to examine existing data from this trial.

Because NSAIDs can cause serious gastrointestinal bleeding, more conclusive trials should be conducted before people attempt taking NSAIDs solely to prevent Alzheimer's.

Estrogen

While some studies suggest that estrogen may protect against Alzheimer's, other studies have failed to confirm this effect. In fact, results of the large-scale Women's Health Initiative Memory Study show an increased risk of dementia for women age 65 and older who had taken hormone replacement therapy — either estrogen alone or a combination of estrogen and progestin.

Other studies have more positive results, suggesting that early hormone therapy — usually given when a woman is in her 50s to treat menopausal symptoms — may benefit cognition. Some researchers speculate that early therapy may have protective effects while later use becomes harmful.

In light of these conflicting conclusions, women should get clear guidance from their doctors about taking hormone replacement after menopause.

In a study of the effects of raloxifene (Evista), a selective estrogen receptor modulator, on postmenopausal women with osteoporosis, participants receiving a higher dosage of the drug had a reduced risk of mild cognitive impairment. Raloxifene isn't a hormone like estrogen, but it mimics some of

Participation in clinical trials

It's difficult, if not impossible, to conduct research without volunteers willing to participate in clinical trials. This is how the public plays a meaningful part in the fight against Alzheimer's disease. Still, enrolling in a clinical trial requires careful consideration. In the case of Alzheimer's disease, the decision often rests with an entire family rather than one person. To help families with this important decision, the Alzheimer's Association has prepared the following list of considerations:

- With your doctor, explore the pros and cons of participating in a particular study.
- Be prepared to answer questions about your loved one's condition.
- Expect further screening to determine eligibility. Only some people may qualify.
- Be aware of the time commitment and other responsibilities, such as making trips to the study site, administering the drug and reporting health-related changes to the study coordinators. Also ask about expenses.
- Understand that clinical studies may involve some risk, as they determine the effectiveness and safety of a drug.
- Be aware that not all participants are given the treatment being tested. In almost every study, one group receives an inactive substance (placebo), while another group receives the experimental medication. This allows researchers to compare the two groups. People receiving the placebo are just as important as those receiving the treatment. If the drug yields positive results, the participants who received a placebo may be given the option of receiving the experimental drug.
- Ask questions. Researchers should answer satisfactorily. If you feel uncomfortable at any point, you always have the option of not continuing with the study.

Find out more about clinical trials for Alzheimer's disease by visiting these websites:

Alzheimer's Association
www.alz.org/research/clinical_trials/find_clinical_trials_trialmatch.asp

National Institute on Aging
www.alzheimers.org/clinicaltrials/search.asp

National Institutes of Health
www.clinicaltrials.gov

estrogen's effects. It may be that the drug provides cognitive benefits while avoiding other harmful effects. For example, unlike estrogen, raloxifene isn't associated with an increased risk of stroke or other cardiovascular events.

Lifestyle factors

Some studies point toward the importance of healthy living, intellectual stimulation and social relationships in preventing cognitive loss. For example, some researchers believe that lifelong mental exercise and learning may promote the growth of neural synapses and delay the onset of dementia.

Other researchers argue that advanced education simply gives a person more experience with the types of memory and thinking involved in the tests used to measure dementia. Some people may simply have a stronger cognitive "reserve" that compensates for any deficit.

Evidence suggests that being physically fit, maintaining good dietary and sleep habits, and staying socially connected may help maintain cognitive performance and reduce the risk of dementia. Read Chapters 14 and 15 to learn more about things you can do that may help keep your brain healthy and active.

Research results in perspective

With all of the ongoing research on Alzheimer's disease taking place worldwide, staying informed of the results can be a challenge. The studies sometimes contradict each other, which may leave you wondering whether any of this effort will ever truly help.

New strategies for diagnosis and treatment take time to develop. After an initial discovery, many studies must be undertaken to support the findings and test the safety and effectiveness of a medication or procedure. This long time frame can be discouraging. But people whose lives are affected by a neurodegenerative disease have the opportunity to advance this research by participating in clinical trials.

With recent passage of the National Plan to Address Alzheimer's Disease and the significant increase in research funding, many scientists expect to see major progress in unraveling the causes of Alzheimer's and in developing the means to treat and prevent this devastating disease.

Part 3

Causes of dementia other than Alzheimer's

Chapter 10

Frontotemporal degeneration

Frontotemporal degeneration (FTD) refers to a diverse group of neuro-degenerative disorders that primarily affects the frontal and temporal lobes of your brain. These regions are associated with reason, analytical thinking, personality and behavior. Frontotemporal degeneration is also known as frontotemporal dementia.

FTD often results in problems with executive skills, such as decision-making, problem-solving, organizing and using good judgment. These skills help you work and communicate more effectively. FTD also interferes with movement, language comprehension and interpersonal skills. Memory loss — one of the earliest symptoms of Alzheimer's disease — also occurs in FTD but it usually develops at a later stage of the disease than in Alzheimer's.

Frontotemporal degeneration also tends to develop at a younger age than does Alzheimer's disease — generally between the ages of 40 and 70. Alzheimer's is typically diagnosed after age 65.

The disease affects men and women equally. Up to half the people who have FTD also have a family history of some type of neurological disease, not just FTD. After a diagnosis of FTD, the disease may run its course for two to 10 years before resulting in death.

People with FTD, Alzheimer's and other causes of dementia face similar challenges in terms of available treatments and practical care. But the specific behavioral and language symptoms associated with FTD, and its earlier age of onset, pose different therapeutic concerns.

Types of FTD

Identifying which diseases fall under the umbrella designation of frontotemporal degeneration is complex, as signs and symptoms may vary greatly. Scientists have classified FTD subtypes based on these differences.

Behavioral changes. One subtype of FTD is known as behavioral variant frontotemporal dementia (abbreviated as bvFTD), or simply as

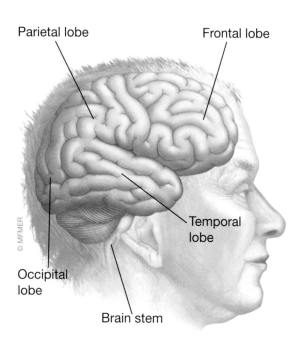

In frontotemporal degeneration, neuron loss occurs predominantly in the frontal and temporal lobes of the brain, unlike Alzheimer's disease where neuron loss starts in the interior and spreads across most of the brain.

frontotemporal dementia. It's marked by extreme changes in behavior and personality. These include:

- Increasingly inappropriate actions
- Lack of judgment and inhibition
- Apathy
- Lack of empathy
- Repetitive compulsive behavior
- Decline in personal hygiene
- Changes in eating habits, especially overeating
- Lack of insight or awareness

Speech and language comprehension. Other subtypes of frontotemporal degeneration involve aphasia — difficulty expressing and understanding verbal and written language. They fall under the general term of primary progressive aphasia (PPA):

- **Nonfluent variant PPA.** People have trouble conveying meaningful sentences and pronouncing words correctly. They may use incorrect grammar, struggle with spelling, or leave out short words, such as "the" or "his," when speaking. Although behavior and personality changes occur, many people continue to function normally and perform daily activities. Eventually the condition may result in the person not being able to speak at all.

Example of behavioral variant FTD

At the age of 63, Linda began experiencing paranoia and delusions that her husband was being unfaithful. Her husband noticed she wasn't paying as much attention to household chores and that she had become socially withdrawn. Linda denied having any problems. She had no memory difficulty and continued to manage the household finances and drive a car with little trouble.

Eventually, Linda's gradually progressive paranoia led her to purchase a gun, which she carried in her purse, despite her husband's protests. One night, while she was sleeping, he slipped the gun out of her purse and hid it, but she soon purchased a replacement.

Testing revealed some impairment in problem-solving and intellectual flexibility, but her general intelligence, memory and visuospatial skills were normal. A magnetic resonance imaging (MRI) scan of Linda's brain showed noticeable shrinkage of the frontal lobes.

Over the next three years, her delusions continued. She became increasingly apathetic and also developed urinary incontinence. Her situation demonstrates many characteristics of the behavioral variant frontotemporal form of dementia.

- **Semantic variant PPA.** This condition is characterized by speech that's grammatically correct but bears little relevance to the conversation that's taking place. People with semantic variant PPA often can't recall the names of familiar people and don't understand the meaning of infrequently used words. Their comprehension of statements spoken to them is often impaired. People with this subtype usually retain the ability to read and write, but they may not recognize familiar objects around them. As the disease progresses, behavioral changes and additional language difficulties may develop.

Movement disorders. These subtypes primarily cause problems with movement rather than memory or language.

- **Corticobasal degeneration (CBD).** CBD affects the brain's frontal and parietal lobes. Signs and symptoms resemble those of Parkinson's disease, including poor coordination, rigidity, impaired balance, tremor and muscle spasms. Some people with CBD also experience alien hand syndrome — they're unable to control movement in one hand. They may lose their ability to carry out purposeful movements, such as getting dressed or combing hair. Simple calculations, such as adding or subtracting, also can become difficult. Cognitive changes happen

Example of semantic variant PPA

For two years, John, age 53, had struggled to find the words for ideas he wanted to express. He decided to seek help from his doctor. John and his wife felt that all of his other intellectual functions were intact, including memory and language comprehension. His personality remained unchanged. His wife even noted John's continued ability to tinker in the workshop and fix small engines — a task requiring considerable skill and patience.

John was fully aware (and frustrated by) his difficulties with language, sometimes making self-deprecating remarks about the problem. A mental status examination showed some difficulty with abstract thinking, general knowledge awareness, construction tasks and verbal recall. Though he couldn't remember the specific words for various items on a naming test, he could describe details about them. He also had trouble understanding spoken words such as "pyramid" and "compass."

An MRI of John's brain showed prominent shrinkage in the left temporal lobe, while the hippocampus appeared relatively normal. These factors are fairly typical of a person with semantic variant PPA.

later in the course of this subtype if at all. CBD is sometimes referred to as corticobasal syndrome (CBS).

- **Progressive supranuclear palsy (PSP).** Similar to CBD, this disorder can resemble Parkinson's disease. Vision problems, frequent falls, slowed movement and thinking, and stiffness in the neck and limbs are the main signs and symptoms of PSP. The frontal lobes are often affected, resulting in many of the behavioral changes described in earlier subtypes.

- **Frontotemporal degeneration with motor neuron disease (FTD/MND).** People with this form of FTD experience signs and symptoms characteristic of amyotrophic lateral sclerosis (ALS, or Lou Gehrig's disease). These include weakness, muscle shrinkage, muscle cramps and swallowing difficulties. Along with these issues, the typical symptoms of FTD occur. The ALS-type symptoms may develop before the FTD symptoms or vice versa.

People with frontotemporal degeneration can also develop movement abnormalities like those seen in Parkinson's disease (parkinsonism). Some people develop FTD and parkinsonism due to a mutation in one of the genes associated with familial FTD.

What goes on in the brain

To help diagnose FTD, doctors must carefully examine the brain's overall shape, structure and function. Neuropsychological, speech and language tests can reveal strengths and weaknesses in thinking, reason and language. Advanced imaging technology, such as MRI and PET, can identify shrinkage (atrophy) of the brain's frontal and temporal lobes and areas of decreased brain activity.

Tests and imaging can often identify FTD subtypes. For example, people with behavioral variant frontotemporal dementia may do poorly on tests for attention and executive functioning, while MRI and PET scans may show shrinkage and decreased activity in both frontal lobes.

People with nonfluent variant PPA typically struggle on language tests and often show mild or no atrophy on an MRI, although a PET scan typically shows abnormalities in the left frontal region. An MRI or PET scan of semantic variant PPA often shows abnormalities in the left temporal lobe. MRI and PET imaging is useful for showing progression of the disease over time.

The genetics of FTD

Some cases of FTD are sporadic, meaning that no history of any form of dementia runs in the family. But in up to half the FTD cases, a family member has (or has had) a neurological disorder at some time. These forms of FTD are known as familial. Some familial forms of FTD have been linked to mutations in specific genes, including the tau gene, progranulin (PRGN) gene and C9orf72 gene. There are other genes associated with FTD, but mutations in those genes are exceedingly rare. Testing is available to screen for genetic mutations in people with strong family histories of FTD to help to determine their risk level.

Because of the difficulty of obtaining adequate biopsy samples, a definitive examination of the brain usually must wait until an autopsy. By comparing the brain tissue of people who had exhibited signs and symptoms of frontotemporal degeneration during life, scientists have concluded that the disease typically involves:

- Loss of neurons in the frontal and temporal regions
- Overgrowth of neuronal support cells, forming scar tissue in the brain
- Formation of tiny holes on the brain's surface, a process known as microvacuolation

Like Alzheimer's, FTD is associated with abnormal protein deposits in the brain. Instead of the amyloid protein,

as in Alzheimer's, about 40 percent of all cases of FTD show changes in the tau protein, causing nerve cells to collapse and die. Other FTD cases show changes in a protein known as TDP-43 rather than in tau.

Signs and symptoms

Many combinations of signs and symptoms fall within the spectrum of frontotemporal degeneration. At the same time, the various subtypes share enough characteristics in common to allow for a general description of FTD. These commonalities are helpful in diagnosis and in planning appropriate treatment.

As with other forms of dementia, not everyone experiences all the signs and symptoms of FTD in the same way, to the same degree or in the same sequence as the disease progresses. Changes usually occur gradually, although some forms of the disease progress more rapidly. Generally, in all the subtypes, behavioral and emotional changes occur before cognitive skills decline. Memory and visuospatial orientation may be preserved for a relatively long time after diagnosis.

Following are some of the general signs and symptoms of FTD. For more information, visit The Association for Frontotemporal Degeneration website, *www. theaftd.org*.

Emotions

Emotional changes occur early in the disease and typically include:

- Apathy toward people, surroundings and events
- Loss of emotional warmth, sympathy and empathy toward others, including loved ones
- Abrupt mood changes
- Exaggerated high spirits and enthusiasm (euphoria)

Behaviors

Changes in behavior are early signs of FTD. These changes gradually and progressively worsen and can be especially difficult for family and friends. Behavioral changes may include:

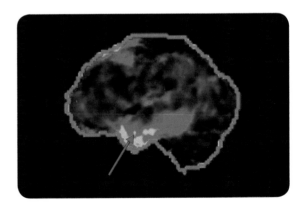

Two PET scans using a radiotracer to detect levels of glucose metabolism in different regions of the brain — lower metabolism means less brain activity — can help with diagnosis. In the color scheme, blue is normal metabolism while green, yellow, orange and red indicate a progressively severe reduction of activity. In behavioral variant FTD (left), severely reduced metabolism occurs in the frontal lobe. In semantic variant PPA (right), severe reduction is focused in one section of the left temporal lobe.

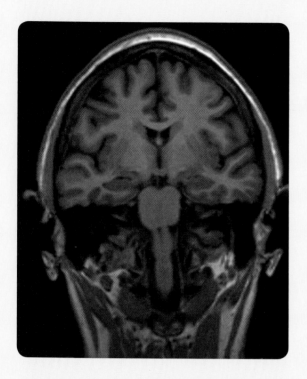
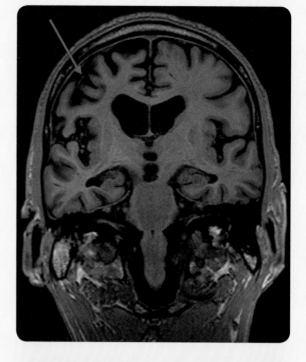

Careful examination of MRI scans may help the doctor identify a subtype of frontotemporal degeneration during the diagnostic process. That's because several of the subtypes follow characteristic patterns as atrophy takes place in the brain due to cell damage. Compare the coronal MRI of a normal brain (upper left) with the image (upper right) showing atrophy in the right frontal lobe (red arrow). This pattern is typical of the behavioral variant of FTD. Another image (lower right) shows atrophy occurring in the left temporal lobe (red arrow). This pattern is more typical of the semantic variant of FTD.

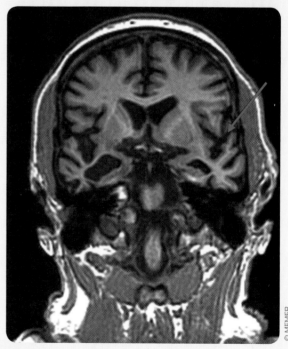

- Loss of social skills — decline in tactfulness, manners and observance of social norms
- Loss of personal awareness — decline in hygiene, such as choosing not to bathe and change clothes
- Oral fixation — obsession with certain foods, overeating, excessive drinking and smoking
- Repetitive behavior — reading the same newspaper over and over, hand rubbing and clapping, humming the same tune repeatedly
- Hypersexual behavior — loss of inhibition, explicit sexual comments, obsession with pornography
- Impulsivity — impulsive buying or shoplifting, grabbing food before it's served or off someone else's plate
- Hyperactivity — agitation, pacing, vocal outbursts, aggression

Language

In primary progressive aphasia, language problems tend to be the main symptoms. But a decline in language can occur with any FTD subtype. Language problems may include:

- Not speaking as much or speaking very softly
- Difficulty speaking because of muscle weakness or incoordination
- Inability to speak grammatically, such as problems with tense and number

- Inability to recall the names of familiar people or objects
- Decreased comprehension with regard to reading and writing
- Repeating words and phrases
- Gradual loss of all speech

Cognition

In frontotemporal degeneration, the cognitive skills that tend to decline first are executive skills — decision-making, problem-solving, organizing, judgment and planning. Cognitive skills such as recent memory and visuospatial orientation may not decline until later. Common cognitive symptoms include:

- Difficulty focusing on a task or becoming easily distracted
- Mental inflexibility — becoming stuck in familiar patterns and having difficulty adapting to new circumstances
- Difficulty in planning daily chores, errands and appointments or coordinating a schedule
- Poor financial judgment
- Taking things literally — difficulty detecting sarcasm or irony

Neurological signs and symptoms

In subtypes such as corticobasal degeneration, FTD/MND and familial FTD, movement disorders may occur earlier than other symptoms. But other FTD subtypes also can cause movement-related symptoms. Some are similar to those of Parkinson's disease:

- Decreased facial expression
- Slowed movements
- Rigidity
- Instability with maintaining posture

People with corticobasal degeneration may also experience:

- Difficulty with coordination of an arm or leg
- Difficulty with eye movements
- Lack of normal muscle tone
- Involuntary hand movement

People with FTD/MND may experience signs and symptoms similar to those seen in amyotrophic lateral sclerosis:

- Muscle weakness
- Muscle atrophy
- Muscle spasms
- Swallowing difficulties and choking

Psychiatric symptoms

People with frontotemporal degeneration may experience depression, delusions, euphoria or hallucinations. These psychiatric symptoms may cause someone with FTD to be diagnosed initially with some form of mental illness, such as a bipolar disorder.

Diagnosis

Diagnosing frontotemporal degeneration is similar to diagnosing Alzheimer's disease. No single test can confirm FTD, so the doctor tries to identify characteristic features while excluding other possible causes for the symptoms. For various reasons, a correct diagnosis of FTD is often delayed, and early misdiagnosis is common. Because FTD affects behavior and personality, it can be mistaken for a mental illness, and the person may be referred to a psychiatrist.

To diagnose frontotemporal degeneration, a doctor will:

- Evaluate signs and symptoms and create a detailed medical history
- Conduct a neurological exam to test awareness and responsiveness, vital signs, reflexes, sensory responses, coordination and gait
- Assess memory, executive skills, problem-solving skills, language skills and visuospatial orientation
- Use imaging to check for shrinkage of the frontal and temporal lobes and to evaluate brain activity

Lack of response to a particular treatment may help distinguish between disorders having similar signs and symptoms. For example, corticobasal degeneration or progressive supra-nuclear palsy are sometimes confused with Parkinson's disease. If someone with Parkinson-like symptoms doesn't respond to Carbidopa/Levodopa — a combination medication used to treat Parkinson's — he or she may have either of the two FTD subtypes.

Going through the diagnostic process can be a frustrating experience and usually requires a great deal of patience for the person with the condition. But working with an experienced health professional can help determine what's causing the signs and symptoms and lead to appropriate treatment.

Challenges for family members

Frontotemporal degeneration affects areas of the brain involved in regulating personal behavior, such as determining what are appropriate responses in social situations. At a restaurant, a person with FTD might be overly honest and say things that should not be said in that context, for example, informing a server, "You're too fat." Or the person may be unable to restrain impulses and kiss the server's hand. Such inappropriate responses can be a source of embarrassment and anger for family members.

Holding people with this disease fully responsible for their behavior isn't fair since they may have lost areas of the brain that allow them to differentiate what's right from what's wrong. And yet, the other extreme — ascribing no responsibility for their actions — also can be harmful. Find a middle ground by encouraging people with FTD to work on strategies for controlling their behavior. At the same time, families need to recognize the difficulty for people with FTD to choose appropriate responses.

Another source of distress for family members can occur when a person with FTD loses the ability to empathize, unable to consider himself or herself in another person's position and see the world from that perspective. People with FTD may also lose their ability to detect sarcasm, taking what others say quite literally.

Treatment

Currently there's no cure for fronto-temporal degeneration and no effective way to slow its progression. Treatment relies on managing the symptoms and maintaining or improving quality of life. Some therapies that may be prescribed include:

Selective serotonin reuptake inhibitors (SSRIs). People with frontotemporal degeneration have a decreased level of serotonin, a neurotransmitter that influences mood and behavior. Some people with FTD may benefit from SSRIs — antidepressant drugs that typically increase serotonin levels. SSRIs may improve signs and symptoms such as apathy, overeating and compulsive behavior.

Antipsychotics. Antipsychotic drugs block the effects of dopamine, a neurotransmitter associated with psychosis. Using them may help with managing delusions and aggressive or hypersexual behavior, but the drugs are linked with an increased risk of death in older people.

Sedatives or hypnotics. A small dose of a sedative or hypnotic medication such as trazodone may be helpful for agitation or other difficult behaviors.

Cholinesterase inhibitors. This class of medications, developed to treat symptoms of Alzheimer's disease, hasn't been found to help people with FTD and sometimes worsens symptoms. Therefore, cholinesterase inhibitors are generally not used to treat FTD.

Comparing FTD and Alzheimer's

Characteristic	FTD	Alzheimer's
Age when condition starts	Between ages 40 and 70	Less common before age 65
Area of the brain initially affected	The frontal and temporal lobes, which control personality, behavior and speech	The hippocampus, an internal structure important to memory
Progression	In early stages, personality and behavior changes; memory may not be affected until later	In early stages, increasing and persistent forgetfulness; later stages produce personality and behavior problems

Memantine. Memantine (Namenda) modestly improves functional abilities in people with moderate to severe Alzheimer's. While this drug has been shown to be ineffective in FTD, doctors may recommend it for some people with the disorder.

Other medications. Behavior problems such as aggression, socially inappropriate behavior and hypersexuality can be very difficult to manage in some people with FTD. When other medications haven't provided a benefit, beta blockers such as propranolol (Inderal) and anti-epileptic drugs, such as carbamazepine (Carbatrol, Tegretol), topiramate (Topamax) or valproic acid (Depakene), are sometimes used.

Speech therapy. Speech therapy can help someone with primary progressive aphasia adjust to language difficulties and learn alternate ways to better communicate.

Nutritional support. A person with FTD/MND who is having difficulty swallowing may benefit from consulting a dietitian. A dietitian can recommend foods that are nutritious but easy to swallow. As the disease progresses and eating difficulties increase, a feeding tube inserted into the stomach may be considered.

Behavioral interventions. Medications can be helpful for easing symptoms of FTD, but a caregiver's practical support often becomes necessary for everyday activities. For example, dietary restrictions — even locks on cupboards and refrigerators — may be needed to prevent excessive weight gain. Predictable routines and supportive guidance can be calming, while distraction and redirection of attention can help avoid potentially difficult situations caused by aggressive behavior. For more on challenging behaviors, including practical tips for dealing with them, see the Action Guide for Caregivers in this book.

Occupational and physical therapy. Occupational and physical therapy can be helpful for managing some of the cognitive aspects, and particularly motor aspects, of FTD. It's important for caregivers to participate in therapy sessions. Recommendations for managing many problems with feeding, dressing, toileting, walking safely and transferring can improve quality of life for loved ones and their families.

Caring for someone with frontotemporal degeneration can be distressing because of the extreme personality changes and behavioral problems that frequently develop. If you're a caregiver, it's vital that you seek assistance from local resources. You may get help from other family members and friends, a support group, or respite care provided by adult care centers or intermittent home health care. You need time for yourself and a break from the stress of caregiving. The Action Guide for Caregivers has more information and tips on becoming a caregiver and finding support.

Moving ahead

As scientists reach a better understanding of and diagnosis for the many subtypes of frontotemporal degeneration, they hope to also discover more-effective treatments. Several drugs are being studied in animal trials, and human clinical trials have recently started. Many people with FTD are participating in research to aid scientists in identifying biomarkers and preparing for future treatment trials. These combined efforts will contribute greatly to our knowledge of this challenging and diverse group of diseases.

Chapter 11

Dementia with Lewy bodies

Earlier chapters of this book identified an abnormal buildup of protein in the brain as a characteristic feature of many neurodegenerative diseases that cause dementia. For example, hardened plaques formed from fragments of the amyloid precursor protein are hallmarks of Alzheimer's disease. The neurodegenerative disorder described in this chapter features distinctive structures called Lewy bodies, which are deposits of alpha-synuclein protein.

Alpha-synuclein protein is normally abundant in the brain, although its exact function is unclear. With abnormal function, deposits of excess alpha-synuclein protein build up within deteriorating nerve cells (neurons) to form the abnormal structures. Lewy bodies become widespread as the disease progresses throughout the brain.

Dementia with Lewy bodies (DLB) can occur alone or concurrently with Alzheimer's disease. With or without the presence of Alzheimer's disease, DLB is one of the most common causes of dementia. According to the Lewy Body Dementia Association, it affects an estimated 1.3 million Americans.

DLB is more common with age, and men are slightly more likely to have it than are women. Although there are several cases of DLB being diagnosed in various members of the same family, so far genes linked directly to the disorder have been difficult to identify.

The existence of alpha-synuclein protein buildup often cannot be confirmed until brain tissue is examined directly during an autopsy. While the person is alive, diagnosis and treatment are based on a careful interpretation of diagnostic tests and the monitoring of signs and symptoms.

In addition to the cognitive decline that characterizes most dementias, people with DLB usually have visual hallucinations and signs and symptoms similar to Parkinson's disease (parkinsonian symptoms), such as rigid muscles and slowed movement. These signs and symptoms fluctuate, especially in early stages of the disease. Often, people with DLB act out their dreams at night — a condition known as rapid eye movement sleep behavior disorder (RBD).

Because the signs and symptoms of DLB are so similar to those of other disorders that cause dementia, particularly Alzheimer's disease, obtaining an accurate diagnosis is important. Some medications commonly used to treat psychiatric symptoms, such as haloperidol (Haldol), may make a person with DLB extremely ill. The person may also be sensitive to certain anti-parkinsonian medications called dopamine agonists, which may increase hallucinations.

On the other hand, a person with DLB may respond better to cholinesterase inhibitors than does a person with Alzheimer's, the condition for which these medications are commonly prescribed.

Signs and symptoms

The changes in the brain caused by dementia with Lewy bodies vary substantially from one person to another, as can the timing of the appearance of signs and symptoms. This makes it difficult for doctors to predict how the disease will progress. Still, scientists have identified characteristic patterns of the disease. Common signs and symptoms can be grouped into the following categories.

Cognitive impairment

The type of cognitive decline characteristic of dementia with Lewy bodies is marked by forgetfulness, attention deficit and difficulty with focusing on a single train of thought. The person appears disoriented and confused and often misidentifies people, including loved ones. He or she may have problems with depth perception and spatial orientation. Apathy and slowness of thought may be present. All of these problems progressively worsen.

Distinctive fluctuations in alertness and in the ability to perform complex cognitive tasks and solve problems are features of DLB, especially early in the disease process. Confusion, disorientation, reduced attention span or even severe sleepiness may last for minutes, hours or days, interspersed with periods of normal or near-normal function.

Psychiatric symptoms

People with DLB often have visual hallucinations involving vivid, colorful images of people and animals — although no sounds usually accompany the images. The hallucinations may range from funny to frightening for the people having them. Some individuals attempt to talk to or shoo away these perceived images and become upset if someone tries to convince them that what they see isn't real.

Other people are aware that their perceptions are false and manage to carry on as normal. Hallucinations may occur during the day and night, but they're more often experienced in the early morning, late afternoon and evening.

Delusions, which are false beliefs, are common with DLB. People may become paranoid and susceptible to conspiracy theories, believing that someone is stealing from them or that an impostor has replaced a spouse or partner.

Visual illusions may occur, in which the person believes a real object is something other than what it is, such as perceiving an ornate lamppost to be an animal or a person.

As with other forms of dementia, depression and anxiety also commonly occur. However, these conditions may improve with treatment.

Why dementia with Lewy bodies causes psychiatric symptoms is unclear, but it may be associated with a lack of certain neurotransmitters in the brain, such as dopamine, acetylcholine and serotonin. Sleep disorders that typically accompany DLB also may play a role.

Motor symptoms

At some point during the course of the illness, many people with DLB develop parkinsonian signs and symptoms. They primarily affect muscle function and may include:

- Slowed movements
- Stooped or leaning posture
- Difficulty manipulating facial muscles, resulting in blank expressions
- Tendency to drool
- Muscle stiffness and rigidity
- Balance problems

- Shuffling walk (gait)
- Difficulty with refined motor skills, for example, buttoning a shirt
- Tremor or shaking (not as common as in Parkinson's disease)

Although all of these cognitive, psychiatric and motor symptoms are common with DLB, some people may never experience all of them during the illness. When they don't occur, it may be easy to mistake DLB for another cause of dementia.

Sleep disorders

Sleep disorders — in particular, a condition known as rapid eye movement sleep behavior disorder (RBD) — are common to illnesses involving a buildup of alpha-synuclein protein in the brain, such as DLB, Parkinson's disease and multiple system atrophy.

RBD is a disorder in which people act out their dreams — the dreams often involve being chased or attacked. Those with RBD may yell, scream, punch, kick or try to defend themselves from the attacker, which may be dangerous to the dreamer as well as to a spouse or partner in the same bed. When awakened, their vivid descriptions usually match the actions of the dreams. RBD tends to precede other signs and symptoms of dementia with Lewy bodies by several years.

Other sleep disorders associated with this dementia include insomnia, excessive daytime sleepiness (drowsiness), sleep apnea and restless legs syndrome.

Sleep disorders can be treated separately from DLB. Treatment may help improve alertness and lessen periods of confusion. In some cases, treating the sleep disorder decreases or eliminates visual hallucinations.

Autonomic nerve dysfunction

In DLB, the autonomic nervous system — which controls involuntary muscle movements such as blood vessel or bladder contractions— is frequently impaired. This may result in:

- Lightheadedness or dizziness when standing up, the result of a dramatic drop in blood pressure
- Fainting
- Frequent falls, resulting from dizziness or fainting
- Impotence
- Urinary incontinence
- Constipation

Diagnosis

Doctors diagnose dementia with Lewy bodies based on the presence of signs and symptoms from among the ones described in the preceding section. The results from additional diagnostic tests (described below) may further support or refute the diagnosis.

No single test can positively identify DLB — a definitive diagnosis is possible only at the time of autopsy. However, the presence of certain signs and symptoms combined with the results from certain tests can be highly accurate for determining the presence of the underlying disease.

A determination of cognitive decline from previous levels of function along with two of the following features must be present for a doctor to be fairly certain of DLB — this is known as a "probable" diagnosis.

- Noticeable fluctuations in cognition with varying levels of alertness
- Recurrent visual hallucinations
- Spontaneous parkinsonian symptoms (there's no evidence these symptoms are caused by medications or any other identifiable factor)
- Rapid eye movement sleep behavior disorder (RBD)

If at least one feature in this bulleted list is present, along with the cognitive decline, the physician may consider the possibility of DLB — this known as a "possible" diagnosis.

Although additional signs and symptoms aren't essential to the diagnosis, their presence may provide a more complete picture. Some of this information may come from family and friends willing to share their observations.

Tests that support a diagnosis of DLB are similar to those in use for other causes of dementia. People with DLB often have greater problems with attention, concentration and visuospatial skills, but less trouble with naming objects and verbal memory.

Computerized tomography (CT) and magnetic resonance imaging (MRI) scans reveal that atrophy of the hippocampus area of the brain is frequently less severe in DLB than in Alzheimer's or in vascular cognitive impairment.

While not used routinely in a diagnosis of suspected DLB, positron emission tomography (PET) may be of assistance. Typical results with DLB are abnormalities in the occipital lobes at the back of the brain. This is not always the case, however, as some scans show abnormalities in the frontal lobes or in a pattern more typical of Alzheimer's disease, while at other times, the images appear normal.

Other imaging involves single-photon emission computerized tomography (SPECT) technology with a radioactive tracer that identifies dopamine — known as a DaTscan. Dopamine is the key neurotransmitter in the brain regulating muscle control and movement.

DLB and Alzheimer's

Dementia with Lewy bodies causes many of the same cognitive signs and symptoms that are commonly associated with Alzheimer's disease. In fact, DLB is often mistaken for Alzheimer's in a diagnosis.

Autopsies reveal that the brain tissue of most people with DLB contains one or both of the abnormal structures characteristic of Alzheimer's — amyloid plaques and neurofibrillary tangles — in addition to Lewy bodies. Doctors may refer to this combination as "DLB coexisting with Alzheimer's disease."

Scientists note that people with DLB who have fewer tangles in their brains tend to show primarily the symptoms of DLB, while people with a greater number of tangles exhibit symptoms closer to those of Alzheimer's.

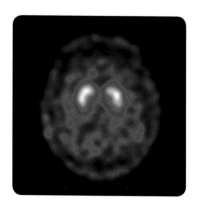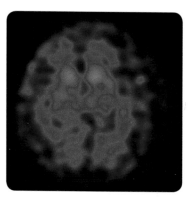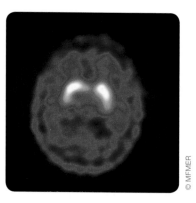

A DaTscan uses SPECT technology to measure dopamine levels in the brain. In the color system for the scans, cool colors (blues and greens) indicate low levels while warm colors (oranges, reds and whites) indicate high levels. For a person with AD (right), the scan typically registers dopamine usage in the brain similar to usage in an normal brain (left). A scan of a person with DLB (center) typically indicates much lower dopamine usage in the brain.

On the other hand, the brain tissue of some people with Alzheimer's will contain Lewy bodies, even though no symptoms of DLB are apparent. This complicates the question, still unanswered, of how closely DLB and Alzheimer's are related.

DLB and Parkinson's

Lewy bodies can appear in the brainstems of people with Parkinson's disease. Dementia also can develop with Parkinson's, usually referred to as Parkinson's disease with dementia (PDD). This form of Parkinson's is similar to DLB, differing only in the timing of when symptoms occur. If parkinsonian symptoms occur more than a year before dementia symptoms begin, doctors generally consider this to be PDD rather than DLB.

Scientists debate whether the mechanisms of disease that underlie DLB and PDD are the same or if they represent two distinct disorders. Most evidence suggests that DLB and PDD are variants of the same disease. With so many uncertainties and possible connections to other conditions, a diagnosis of one condition or the other may change during the course of the illness or even after death.

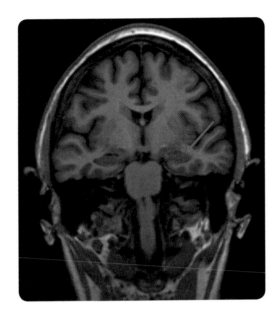

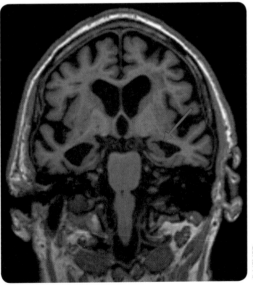

© MFMER

Along with the similarities between DLB and AD, there also are important differences. As these MRIs illustrate, the hippocampus of an AD brain typically appears shrunken (arrow on lower image) while the hippocampus of a DLB brain (arrow on upper image) remains relatively equal in size to the hippocampus of a normal brain.

Treatment

Because the underlying cause of dementia with Lewy bodies is still unknown, treatment is aimed at lessening the impact that symptoms have on quality of life. This typically involves a combination of caregiving, nondrug interventions and possibly medications. People with DLB and their caregivers can play important roles in therapy by identifying the symptoms that they feel need the most attention, even as symptoms and needs change over time.

Caregiving

As with treating all causes of dementia, caregiving is one of the most important and humane components of DLB therapy. Caregiving can provide fundamental physical, emotional and spiritual support. Most of all, caregiving can ensure that the doctor's recommendations for treatment are carried out and can improve quality of life.

Because of the rigorous demands of the task, it's essential for caregivers to obtain education and support — from doctors, community health centers, dementia support groups or other sources of assistance. For more information, see the Action Guide for Caregivers at the back of this book. For information about DLB, visit the Lewy Body Dementia Association's website at *www.lbda.org*.

Nondrug treatment

Much can be done to improve the quality of life of someone with DLB without the use of medication. This is where education and awareness play vital roles. Resources can be selected from the ones that are available and adapted to suit your specific situation.

For example, someone with DLB may complain of lightheadedness as an ongoing concern in treating the condition. Low blood pressure leading to orthostatic hypotension can be managed in several ways — by increasing dietary salt intake, by using thigh-high compression stockings or elastic abdominal support garments, and by elevating the head of the bed about 30 degrees.

To decrease risk of injury from nighttime concerns, such as rapid eye movement sleep behavior disorder, consider moving lamps, nightstands and other furniture away from the bed and placing padding or cushions on the floor beside the bed, in case of a fall. If a bed partner is at risk, sleeping in separate beds should be considered.

The doctor may request a careful sleep history or monitor sleep patterns to determine if sleep apnea is present. This can be done by using a machine that delivers air pressure through a mask placed over the nose (continuous positive airway pressure, or CPAP, therapy). Rearranging the dosing periods of drugs known to cause insomnia, such as cholinesterase inhibitors, also may help improve sleep.

Occupational and physical therapy can be helpful for managing some of the cognitive issues brought on by DLB. It's important for the caregiver to participate with the loved one in therapy sessions. The recommendations for managing the problems of feeding, dressing, toileting, walking safely, transferring and other challenges of living with the disease can greatly improve the quality of life for people with DLB and their families.

Medications

Medications are often necessary to help treat the cognitive, psychiatric and parkinsonian symptoms of DLB. Medications intended for sleep disorders, insomnia and low blood pressure — which often are concurrent, treatable conditions — also may improve the quality of life for a person with DLB.

It's worth repeating the need for an accurate diagnosis, ideally from a doctor experienced in treating dementia, such as a neurologist or neuropsychiatrist. That's because some common medications for treating general psychiatric and parkinsonian symptoms can actually make DLB symptoms worse. The dosages and side effects of various drugs must be continuously adjusted and balanced for optimal benefit.

Here are medications that may prove helpful in treating DLB:

Cholinesterase inhibitors. A sharp drop in the level of acetylcholine, a neurotransmitter in the brain that's important for thinking and memory skills, characterizes both Alzheimer's disease and dementia with Lewy bodies.

Cholinesterase inhibitors were originally designed to treat the cognitive losses of Alzheimer's by obstructing actions of acetylcholinesterase. This enzyme breaks down acetylcholine immediately after the neurotransmitter has done its primary job — triggering a nerve cell to send an impulse.

In effect, the enzyme's action cancels out the acetylcholine's availability to trigger additional messages between nerve cells. By blocking this enzyme, cholinesterase inhibitors allow the acetylcholine to remain available and trigger more nerve impulses, thereby improving cognition.

Interestingly, cholinesterase inhibitors appear to be more effective in treating dementia with Lewy bodies than in treating Alzheimer's. This may be because the damage to neurons may be less severe in DLB than in Alzheimer's.

In DLB, the cholinesterase inhibitors help temper the fluctuating nature of the cognitive deficits and improve problems with hallucinations, apathy, anxiety and sleep. However, these drugs may cause gastrointestinal side effects and excessive salivation. They may also increase the risk of falls.

Antipsychotics. Conventional antipsychotic medications such as haloperidol (Haldol) — often used to treat hallucinations, delusions and agitation — can provoke severe reactions in individuals with DLB, leading to irreversible losses of certain motor skills.

Some newer antipsychotics — quetiapine (Seroquel) and clozapine (Clozaril) — may cause fewer side effects while improving symptoms. But their use requires careful monitoring, as there are reports of negative reactions to these medications as well, and of slightly increased risk of death.

Caregivers and doctors should make sure that all health care providers are aware of the loved one's condition and that prescriptions of antipsychotics are monitored appropriately.

Anti-parkinsonian drugs. Medications commonly used to treat parkinsonian symptoms need close monitoring in people with DLB. Two examples are Carbidopa/Levodopa and dopamine agonists — drugs that convert to or mimic the effects of dopamine.

Unfortunately, these drugs may also worsen psychotic symptoms and orthostatic hypotension. As a result, these medications are given at a dose that provides the most benefit and causes the least side effects.

Antidepressants. Depression is common in people with DLB, likely due to a declining level of the neurotransmitter serotonin. One class of antidepressants will increase the level of active serotonin in the brain — selective serotonin reuptake inhibitors (SSRIs). A related class of drugs known as selective norepinephrine reuptake inhibitors (SNRIs) also is effective at treating depression and anxiety.

Example of dementia with Lewy bodies

At age 72, Robert, a physician, began to experience difficulties in dictating notes, counseling patients and writing prescriptions. This caused him to retire from his profession the following year. Shortly afterward, he started having trouble expressing himself in conversations and frequently lost his train of thought. He would forget recent events and miscalculate numbers in his head. His thinking slowed, as did his normal walking pace. His wife noticed that some days were better for Robert than were other days.

Of some concern was the fact that both his sister and maternal uncle had developed dementia in their late 60s. Robert also had a history of depression, for which medical therapy was only moderately effective. More recently he began to feel light-headed when standing up, nearly fainting on several occasions. Testing revealed that Robert had low blood pressure.

His wife noted that, beginning nine years earlier, Robert would often yell, curse and vigorously shake his legs while sleeping, as if he were "acting out his dreams." If she woke him, he often described being chased in the dreams. Tests revealed rapid eye movement sleep behavior disorder, as well as sleep apnea. His doctor prescribed therapies for both, which improved his alertness, concentration and mood.

His doctor also prescribed a cholinesterase inhibitor traditionally used for Alzheimer's, which improved some cognitive symptoms. Therapy normally intended for Parkinson's was then added, which improved his motor symptoms.

Recently, Robert left on a vacation with his wife. Shortly after checking into the hotel, he began to experience visual hallucinations and delusions. At the emergency room, the medical staff gave Robert haloperidol, a conventional antipsychotic, because his symptoms were worsening. Hours later, he developed extreme sleepiness and muscle stiffness.

Robert was started on a low dosage of a newer antipsychotic that has fewer adverse effects than haloperidol on people with DLB. After making the switch, his mental state improved significantly, although the muscle stiffness persisted.

In the rare instances when an SSRI or SNRI cause worsening of REM sleep behavior disorder, an alternative medication may be prescribed. Tricyclic antidepressants aren't helpful in treating DLB, as they reduce an already depleted reserve of acetylcholine.

Memantine. Memantine (Namenda) has modestly improved the functional abilities of people with moderate to severe dementia from Alzheimer's. Memantine has recently been shown to help some people with DLB, but the effects are generally quite modest.

Wake-promoting drugs. Some people with DLB have symptoms similar to narcolepsy, which is a disorder that causes people to struggle staying awake during the day and maintaining good sleep at night. Visual hallucinations and RBD also are common with narcolepsy.

Medications that promote wakefulness, such as modafinil (Provigil), armodafinil (Nuvigil), methylphenidate (Concerta, Ritalin), methamphetamine (Desoxyn) and dextroamphetamine can help people with narcolepsy.

These same medications may be used to treat people with DLB who are very sleepy despite other sleep disorders being treated. In some people with DLB, alertness improves as well as memory, concentration, and other problems, such as hallucinations.

Use of these medications is controversial due to their potential side effects, such as rash, an increase in blood pressure and pulse, and agitation. There's also the high cost of some of these agents. These medications should be considered only for select individuals and prescribed only by clinicians experienced with their use.

All for one, one for all

Unraveling the enigmatic mysteries that may link dementia with Lewy bodies to Alzheimer's disease and to Parkinson's disease remains a perplexing issue for scientists. As research progresses in the search for more-effective treatments for Alzheimer's and Parkinson's, the advances may ultimately end up being of considerable benefit to people with DLB. Conversely, any advances made in the understanding of DLB may be applicable to the treatment of Alzheimer's and Parkinson's.

Chapter 12

Vascular cognitive impairment

Vascular cognitive impairment stands out from many other conditions associated with dementia, including Alzheimer's disease, because its cause is relatively well understood. The condition stems from chronic damage to the complex network of blood vessels that supply the brain.

When blood flow in the brain is disrupted or blocked, not enough oxygen and nutrients reach brain cells. The result is cell damage or death. Areas of damaged or dead cells (infarcts) form permanent scar tissue and are not replaced by new cell growth. The infarcts can cause problems with reason, judgment, memory, personality, emotions and other cognitive functions, depending on the location of the damage in the brain and on the cognitive functions that are affected.

Vascular cognitive impairment (VCI) used to be called vascular dementia. The name change reflects the fact that vascular disease can cause milder forms of cognitive impairment that don't necessarily meet the strict criteria for dementia.

Your risk of VCI is linked to the health of your blood vessels. Conditions such as high blood pressure and atherosclerosis can damage blood vessels anywhere in your body, increasing the risk.

Factors that increase your risk of heart disease and stroke — including diabetes and smoking — also raise your risk of VCI. The good news is you can take steps to reduce all of these risks and prevent further damage if the symptoms of vascular cognitive impairment begin to appear.

Your brain's vascular system

As the operational control center for your entire body, your brain requires a substantial supply of blood — about 20 percent of your heart's total output. Four main arteries (carotid arteries) converge at the base of your brain. From there a network of progressively smaller blood vessels reaches deep inside brain tissue. Any interruption in the blood supply deprives brain cells of essential nutrients, such as oxygen and glucose. Without these nutrients, the cells are rapidly damaged or die.

Stroke is a common result of vascular disruptions in the brain. Stroke may occur if a blood clot blocks an artery or if an artery leaks or ruptures, bleeding into surrounding tissue. This disruption of blood flow — even for a few seconds — can dramatically affect brain function.

Most people think of stroke as a major event that causes severe and instantaneous impairment of movement and speech. A stroke such as this is an emergency situation that can permanently damage structures important to cognition and lead to vascular cognitive impairment.

Stroke and VCI

Vascular cognitive impairment commonly occurs in people who've had a major stroke. According to some estimates, between 20 and 30 percent of people who've had a stroke go on to develop cognitive impairment, usually within several months of the event. One study found that having a stroke doubles a person's risk of dementia.

At the same time, all strokes clearly don't lead to VCI. Although stroke can cause confusion, memory loss, and difficulties with language and perception, these effects are typically severe immediately after the stroke but then gradually improve with time. This temporary impairment isn't the same thing as having VCI — in which the signs and symptoms of dementia get progressively worse, never better.

But strokes may also occur on a milder, "silent" level with few or no symptoms. A series of these minor strokes may damage enough brain cells over time to cause cognitive impairment.

In addition, if the small blood vessels throughout the brain weaken and narrow due to vascular disease, the reduced blood supply may damage or destroy tissue, even if the blood vessels aren't completely blocked or ruptured.

It's hard to estimate how prevalent VCI is. Years ago, doctors believed most cases of dementia resulted from diseased arteries in the brain. Research now suggests that neurodegenerative conditions such as Alzheimer's, which are the primary causes of dementia, are a result of multiple factors, some of which are not vascular in nature.

It's also difficult to estimate the number of new cases (incidence) of VCI. Definitions of the condition vary, and different sets of criteria are used for diagnosis. Symptoms of VCI often overlap those of other causes of dementia, especially Alzheimer's disease. VCI and Alzheimer's disease frequently occur together, so diagnosing one may not rule out the other. As a result, estimates of the prevalence range widely, from one-tenth to one-third of all dementia cases.

Causes

Vascular processes that lead to VCI may include:

Multiple infarcts. When someone experiences a series of strokes — whether small or large — the damage creates areas of dead brain tissue. Even if they're small, multiple infarcts create enough damage to cause cognitive impairment. In fact, VCI was formerly known as "multi-infarct dementia." But associating VCI with multiple events is

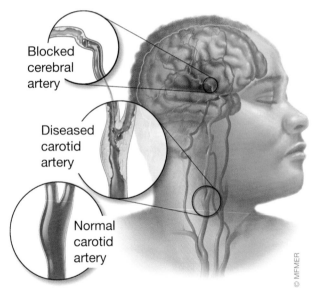

Blocked cerebral artery

Diseased carotid artery

Normal carotid artery

© MFMER

The formation of a blood clot in one of the carotid arteries of the neck may set the stage for a stroke. If the blood clot breaks free, it will travel through the vascular system and may become lodged in an artery of the cerebrum, blocking blood flow and causing the stroke.

not considered accurate since a single, strategically located infarct (see following entry) can also impair cognition.

Single strategic infarct. Sometimes a single infarct affecting a critical area of the brain — such as the thalamus or parietal lobe — can cause the sudden onset of dementia. The thalamus acts as your brain's switchboard for processing information, while the parietal lobe receives sensory information and supports visuospatial skills. Severe damage to either one of these areas can dramatically affect cognition.

Small vessel disease. As its name implies, this disease affects the small blood vessels deep within the brain and is closely linked to high blood pressure. Widespread damage from narrowed vessels and reduced blood flow leads to a slow, subtle onset of cognitive impairment. Some scientists believe that this "microvascular" disease may be more damaging to the brain than larger strokes involving the major arteries.

A rare cause of small vessel disease is called cerebral autosomal dominant arteriopathy with subcortical infarcts and leukoencephalopathy (CADASIL), an inherited condition caused by a genetic defect on chromosome 19.

Combined Alzheimer's disease and VCI. Autopsy reports indicate that many people diagnosed with dementia had both Alzheimer's disease and VCI. It appears that when the two conditions occur together, the effects are compounded, leading to a more severe form of dementia.

Risk factors

As described earlier, many risk factors for VCI are the same as those for heart disease and stroke. They include high blood pressure, high cholesterol, tobacco use, obesity, physical inactivity and high blood glucose (diabetes).

You may change or manage some factors to help reduce your risk of VCI or your risk of further vascular damage. But some risk factors are beyond your control — including advancing age, male sex, family history and African-American ethnicity.

As you age, your blood vessels are more prone to the accumulation of fatty deposits containing cholesterol and other substances. When compounded by diabetes, high blood pressure, smoking or obesity, plaque buildup leads to a narrowing and hardening of your blood vessels (atherosclerosis). It's more difficult for blood to flow through the stiffer, narrower vessels. In addition, chronic high blood pressure makes the walls of your blood vessels weak and more susceptible to rupture.

Signs and symptoms

People with vascular cognitive impairment experience many of the same signs and symptoms of dementia as do people with Alzheimer's disease. For example, memory loss is a common complaint — although people with VCI may respond better to memory cues and reminders than someone with Alzheimer's would. Other signs and symptoms include:

- Apathy
- Confusion
- Wandering or getting lost in familiar places
- Difficulty with problem-solving, organizing and planning
- Difficulty with walking
- Loss of bowel or bladder control
- Sudden, involuntary fits of laughing and crying
- Hallucinations and delusions

A classic pattern of VCI symptoms may reflect the occurrence of a series of strokes. That's because changes to the symptoms occur in noticeable steps. Cognition drops when one stroke occurs, then plateaus or remains steady until the next stroke, causing further damage and increasing severity.

The symptoms that do appear and how severe they are depend on which parts of the brain have been damaged by the infarcts. Some cognitive functions may become impaired while others stay the same. You may, for example, have trouble following instructions or calculating numbers and be fully aware of your impairment. This can be frustrating and lead to depression — a condition that often accompanies VCI.

Compared with the early stages of Alzheimer's disease, people in the early stages of VCI may experience greater physical disability and problems with movement. In general, people with Alzheimer's live longer than do those with VCI, who are more likely to die of heart disease or stroke.

Sometimes, VCI progresses in a fashion similar to Alzheimer's disease, featuring a slow but steady rather than a step-like decline in cognitive and, eventually, physical functions.

Jean, an independent-minded, 80-year-old woman living on her own, experienced a stroke. From the location of an infarct that was evident on a CT scan, the stroke appeared to have affected the occipital lobe of her brain — often known as the visual cortex. Although Jean's symptoms improved immediately after the stroke, her son observed a noticeable decline in her ability to think clearly and to take care of herself. One year after her stroke, Jean could dress and feed herself but needed help with most other activities of daily living, including bathing. She could no longer drive, pay bills or do household chores. She also became increasingly quiet and withdrawn. Although she could write and name a few simple items, she lost the ability to read.

Another imaging test — this time an MRI with more detail — showed that the stroke had damaged not only Jean's occipital lobe but also the hippocampus and thalamus, parts of the brain important in memory and information processing. This helped explain her dementia symptoms. Her doctor could not discern if she had pre-existing cognitive impairment that either contributed to the dementia or was exacerbated by her stroke.

Diagnosis

Diagnosing VCI is similar to diagnosing other forms of dementia. Your doctor will likely:

- Review your medical history
- Assess your signs and symptoms
- Conduct exams to evaluate memory and cognitive function
- Order brain imaging tests to detect areas of vascular blockage or rupture

Although different doctors may use different criteria to diagnose the symptoms of vascular cognitive impairment, three characteristic features are typically included in whichever standards a doctor might use:

- Cognitive problems that begin or worsen within three months of the person having a stroke
- Evidence of one or more strokes on imaging tests, for example, infarcts

- Signs and symptoms similar to what has occurred after previous strokes, such as nerve problems limited to a specific location or a problem with speech or fine motor skills

Distinguishing between vascular cognitive impairment and Alzheimer's disease may be one of the most challenging aspects of diagnosis.

There may not be a clear connection to a stroke. Symptoms of VCI can be very similar to symptoms of Alzheimer's, and without evidence of a stroke, it may be virtually impossible to discern a vascular cause of dementia. Imaging, such as CT or MRI, is key to diagnosing VCI because it often provides evidence of stroke even if you don't show any external signs and symptoms.

Vascular cognitive impairment may develop as a result of infarcts so small that they're undetectable even with brain imaging. Frequently, a diagnosis of Alzheimer's is made, and VCI may not be recognized until brain tissue is examined during autopsy. Since it's possible to have both VCI and Alzheimer's at the same time, one diagnosis doesn't necessarily rule out the other.

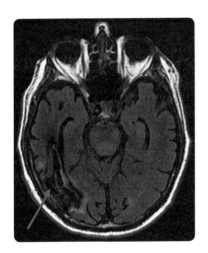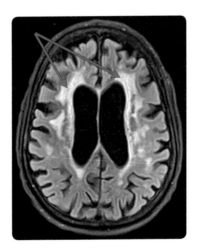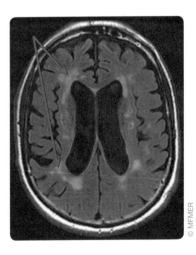

© MFMER

Sections of dead tissue (infarcts) shows up on MRI imaging as white, clouded areas of the brain. The location of an infarct may correlate with the signs and symptoms of dementia that a person exhibits. The axial image on the left shows damage to the parietal lobe due to stroke (red arrow). The center image reveals large infarcts in the interior of the brain, causing VCI. The image on the right shows the effects of Binswanger's disease, with faint indications of cell damage due to atherosclerosis in small blood vessels deep within the brain, producing symptoms of dementia.

Treatment and prevention

Damage to brain tissue can't be reversed — what's done is done. So the treatment of vascular cognitive impairment is focused on preventing any additional damage. This means trying to avoid more strokes by tackling certain risk factors that you can control, such as blood pressure and diabetes. Taking control may help limit the severity of VCI, slow its course or be purely preventive in nature.

Although scientists are uncertain about any relationship between vascular risk factors and the development of Alzheimer's disease, one appears to be related to the other. As previously mentioned, having VCI may increase the severity of Alzheimer's disease. So, it's possible that taking steps to prevent stroke may, in some way, be beneficial to Alzheimer's symptoms, as well.

Preventing stroke

Whether or not you've experienced a stroke in the past, it's important to know where you now stand in terms of your risk of having one (or another one). Ideally, prevention should start early — before any damage to brain tissue can happen and symptoms begin. Work with your doctor to learn how to reduce your risk of stroke and VCI. It may require you to change behaviors and lifestyle.

These steps may help reduce your risk of stroke and VCI:

Control high blood pressure. One of the most important things you can do to reduce your risk of stroke is keeping your blood pressure under control. If you've already had a stroke, lowering blood pressure can help prevent another stroke. Exercising, managing stress, maintaining a healthy weight, and limiting salt (sodium) and alcohol are all ways to keep blood pressure in check. In addition, your doctor may prescribe blood pressure lowering medications.

Don't smoke. Stopping smoking reduces your risk of stroke. Several years after stopping, a former smoker's risk of stroke is about the same as that of a nonsmoker.

Control diabetes. You can manage diabetes with diet, exercise, weight control and medication. Strict control of blood glucose (blood sugar) may reduce the damage to your brain if you do have a stroke.

Maintain a healthy weight. Being overweight contributes to other risk factors for stroke, such as high blood pressure, cardiovascular disease and diabetes. Weight loss of as little as 10 pounds may lower blood pressure.

Exercise regularly. Aerobic exercise improves the health of your blood vessels and heart, and can reduce your risk of stroke. This type of exercise can also lower blood pressure and help you lose weight, control diabetes and reduce stress. Gradually work up to 30 minutes of aerobic activity, such as walking, jogging, swimming or bicycling, on most, if not all, days of the week.

Manage stress. Stress can cause a temporary but sharp spike in your blood pressure — a risk factor for brain hemorrhage — or chronic high blood pressure. Stress also increases your blood's tendency to clot, which may raise your risk of a blocked artery and stroke. Consider a variety of stress-reduction approaches, such as simplifying your life, exercising and learning to relax.

Drink alcohol in moderation. Alcohol can be both a risk factor and a preventive measure for stroke. On one hand, binge drinking and heavy alcohol consumption increase your risk of high blood pressure and stroke. On the other hand, drinking small to moderate amounts of alcohol may decrease your blood's tendency to clot — but you can lower your risk of stroke without drinking at all.

Take B vitamins. B vitamins — B-6, B-12 and folic acid (folate) — can work together to reduce blood levels of homocysteine. Excessive levels of this protein in your blood may increase your risk of blood vessel damage. However, there's no direct evidence that B vitamins can prevent stroke or VCI — so taking this step may have little effect other than improved cardiovascular health. If you take B vitamins, avoid more than 100 milligrams of B-6 a day.

Don't use illicit drugs. Many street drugs, such as cocaine, are associated with a high risk of stroke.

Dementia medications

Studies have found that the Alzheimer's medications galantamine (Razadyne) and donepezil (Aricept) may be effective in treating vascular cognitive impairment — although these drugs do not provide enough benefit to have received approval from the Food and Drug Administration. They are thought to be most helpful for people who have both VCI and Alzheimer's. As with Alzheimer's, the medications may slow the progress of VCI, but they can't cure the condition.

Cholinesterase inhibitors help raise the level of the neurotransmitter associated with memory function (acetylcholine). People with Alzheimer's experience a dramatic drop in acetylcholine as the disease progresses. In VCI, damage from high blood pressure may reduce the production of acetylcholine.

One of the best ways to maintain vital cognitive functions, such as memory and reason, is to prevent VCI from ever developing. That's why it's so important to know your risk factors for stroke. Ask your doctor's advice about how best to control these factors.

As imaging technology improves, doctors will be able to identify the strokes causing VCI, resulting in a more accurate diagnosis and appropriate treatment. They may be able to view microscopic changes in the brain that aren't visible with current technology. In addition, as researchers unravel the complex relationship between vascular cognitive impairment and Alzheimer's disease, doctors may develop joint methods for diagnosis and treatment.

Chapter 13

Other causes of dementia

In addition to the neurodegenerative and vascular disorders described in preceding chapters, there are other conditions that can damage nerve cells in the brain, impair cognition and cause dementia. These diverse conditions have been grouped in a single chapter because, as dementing disorders go, they are less common than conditions such as Alzheimer's disease and vascular cognitive impairment.

However, being less common doesn't make these conditions less worthy of attention or less devastating for the individual who has one of them. Furthermore, it's entirely possible that study results from one of these conditions may provide insight into the onset and development of dementia or provide clues to a new treatment that has applications for other causes of dementia.

There are, nevertheless, some common features among the various and seemingly disparate conditions that are described in this chapter. A few of the conditions are genetic, passed on from parent to child. And with several of these conditions, the onset of dementia symptoms may be secondary in nature — complications of the primary symptoms of the illness.

Most of these causes of dementia are intractable and irreversible, and treatments of the conditions are focused primarily on managing the signs and symptoms. But there are exceptions that may be treatable, such as normal-pressure hydrocephalus. When dementia symptoms are the complications of such an illness, then treating the underlying cause may help stop or delay the progression of cognitive loss.

Normal-pressure hydrocephalus

Hydrocephalus is a condition in which the cerebrospinal fluid that surrounds and cushions the brain doesn't resorb into the bloodstream as it should. Instead, the fluid builds up in brain cavities (ventricles), causing an abnormal enlargement of the ventricles and putting increased pressure on the brain. It's most commonly recognized as a disorder existing at birth.

In adults, a variation of hydrocephalus called normal-pressure hydrocephalus may occur. In this variation, the resorption of cerebrospinal fluid may be defective even though pressure measurements fall within a normal range. This causes the ventricles to enlarge, but not under high pressure. The enlargement compresses brain tissue and can cause cognitive impairment.

This type of hydrocephalus is most often seen in older adults. It may be the result of an injury or illness, but in a majority of cases, the cause is unknown. Sometimes normal pressure hydrocephalus may be treatable.

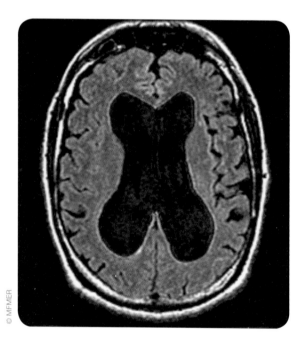

© MFMER

With normal-pressure hydrocephalus, the resorption of cerebrospinal fluid in the brain is defective, causing a buildup of fluid in the ventricles. The greatly enlarged ventricles (at the center of the above image) compress brain tissue, causing cognitive impairment.

Signs and symptoms

The characteristic features of normal-pressure hydrocephalus include:

Difficulty walking. Usually the earliest sign of this condition may be walking slowly with short, shuffling steps. A person with normal-pressure hydrocephalus will tend to walk with feet spread wide. Difficulty turning and starting to move, lack of balance and frequent falls also are common.

Urinary incontinence. Deformation of the nerve fibers that control the bladder can lead to stronger and more-frequent urges to urinate, which may cause incontinence. Some people may instead develop the sudden urge to urinate (urinary urgency) rather than incontinence. These signs and symptoms usually follow the appearance of walking difficulties.

Dementia. Dementia often shows itself in normal-pressure hydrocephalus as an overall slowness in thinking and mental processing, as well as inattention and lack of spontaneity. The signs and symptoms may not appear as severe as those of the dementing disorders described elsewhere in this book. Unlike Alzheimer's disease, for example, people with normal-pressure hydrocephalus usually can answer a question correctly, although it may take a bit longer than normal to reply.

The signs and symptoms of normal-pressure hydrocephalus are common to other causes of dementia, which can sometimes lead to misdiagnosis. However, careful evaluation by a neurologist or neurosurgeon will often reveal a distinctive pattern in the way the signs and symptoms develop — particularly from Alzheimer's. Imaging tests and a spinal tap can help rule out other possible conditions. With early diagnosis, treatment for normal-pressure hydrocephalus can be started immediately for those who might benefit from it.

Treatment

Draining excess cerebrospinal fluid from the brain through a shunt system is typically used to treat normal-pressure hydrocephalus. To do this, a surgeon places the end of a long, flexible tube in one of the brain's ventricles. From the ventricle, the tube is tunneled beneath the scalp and under the skin along the neck and chest down to the abdomen, where the fluid is allowed to drain into a container. Drainage normalizes the fluid level in the brain and may help to relieve symptoms.

Although treatment can help many people with this condition, the shunt procedure carries significant risk with it, even when undertaken at an excellent medical center.

Not many well-designed trials have been conducted on normal-pressure hydrocephalus. It's difficult to estimate the outcomes but improvement of the symptoms may range anywhere between 50 and 90 percent of individuals having the procedure — and not everyone who improves will sustain that improvement over the long term.

In general, people with a known cause for the hydrocephalus — trauma, for example — have a better chance of successful treatment. So do those who have experienced the signs and symptoms for only a short time.

Your doctor may conduct a test before placing a permanent shunt, to see how you respond to fluid drainage. For example, the doctor may check if your walking gait improves within 30 minutes of a simple test.

Huntington's disease

Uncontrolled movements, emotional disturbances and mental deterioration characterize Huntington's disease. Huntington's disease is an inherited disease that usually develops in middle age. Men are as likely as women to develop the condition. Younger adults with Huntington's disease often have more-severe symptoms, and these symptoms may progress more quickly. In rare instances, children develop this condition.

Signs and symptoms

Some of the earliest signs and symptoms of Huntington's disease are associated with emotional changes such as irritability, anger and paranoia. Signs of depression are common. Impaired cognitive skills include difficulties with decision-making, learning new information, responding to questions and remembering facts.

Early movement disorders associated with Huntington's disease may include mild balance problems, clumsiness, and involuntary facial movements such as twitching and grimacing.

As Huntington's disease progresses, other physical signs and symptoms develop, including sudden jerky, involuntary movements throughout the body; a wide, prancing gait; halting or slurred speech; and dementia.

Huntington's disease usually develops slowly, and its severity relates to the amount of cell damage that has occurred in the brain. Death occurs about 10 to 30 years after the symptoms first appear. Typically, the earlier the symptoms appear, the faster the disease will progress. Death is often caused by a pneumonia-related infection or injuries related to a fall and its complications.

Screening and diagnosis

A single abnormal gene on chromosome 4 is the cause of Huntington's disease. Normally, this gene controls the production of a protein called huntingtin (note the difference in spelling between the protein and the disease). It's possible that the mutated gene produces a toxic form of huntingtin, leading to the destruction of neurons.

To determine whether Huntington's disease is causing your symptoms, the doctor performs a physical exam and obtains your medical history and a family medical history. He or she may ask about recent changes that may have occurred with your emotions or intellect. Computerized tomography (CT) or magnetic resonance imaging (MRI) may show changes to brain structure, reflecting the loss of neurons.

A blood test is available to determine whether a person carries the defective Huntington gene. Your doctor may suggest this test to confirm that Huntington's disease caused the signs and symptoms. Some people with a family history of the disease choose to take the test even before symptoms develop.

Deciding whether to be tested early for the gene is a personal decision. If you're uncertain about whether to have the test, consider contacting a genetic counselor. Doctors who specialize in medical genetics can help you weigh the pros and cons of testing and understand the implications of a positive or negative result. If you choose to be tested, consider paying for it with your own money so that the test results remain within your control.

Treatment

No treatment is available currently that can stop or reverse the development of Huntington's disease, but several approaches can be used to manage its signs and symptoms.

Antipsychotic drugs such as haloperidol help you manage uncontrolled movements, violent outbursts and hallucinations. Antipsychotics aren't prescribed in the presence of dystonia — abrupt muscle contractions that may be caused by Huntington's — as these medications may worsen the contractions, causing stiffness and rigidity.

Preliminary studies suggest that newer types of antipsychotics, such as olanzapine (Zyprexa) and quetiapine (Seroquel), may be more effective and cause fewer side effects.

Tranquilizers such as clonazepam (Klonopin) can help lessen anxiety. Various antidepressants, including fluoxetine (Prozac, Sarafem), sertraline (Zoloft) and nortriptyline (Pamelor), can help control depression and the obsessive-compulsive rituals that some people with Huntington's disease develop. Medications such as lithium can help control extreme emotions and mood swings.

Psychotherapy, physical therapy and speech therapy also may be helpful, particularly in the early stages of Huntington's disease. These therapies may reduce the risk of side effects associated with taking any of the medications listed above. At the same time, these forms of therapy can greatly improve your quality of life.

People with Huntington's disease may burn as many as 5,000 calories a day — which is much higher than normal. Therefore, it's important that they get adequate nutrition and maintain a healthy body weight. They may require assistance with meals. Allow plenty of time for eating. Cutting food into small pieces or serving pureed food may make it easier for the person to swallow and avoid choking. Extra vitamins and supplements may be a consideration, but check with your doctor first.

Creutzfeldt-Jakob disease

Creutzfeldt-Jakob disease (CJD) is a degenerative brain disorder that affects about 1 person in 1 million worldwide. It's believed to occur when misshapen proteins (prions) attack brain cells, creating sponge-like holes in brain tissue. The disorder leads to dementia and, ultimately, death.

CJD typically occurs around the age of 60. Once a person becomes sick with CJD, the course of the disease is swift. He or she usually dies from complications within months of developing the first symptoms of CJD. Currently no treatment is able to stop or slow progression of the disease.

CJD captured the public eye in the 1990s when a form of the disease — named variant CJD (vCJD) — developed among a number of people in Great Britain who had eaten contaminated beef from cows that had bovine spongiform encephalopathy, the medical term for mad cow disease.

CJD and its variants belong to a group of diseases known as transmissible spongiform encephalopathies. The name derives, in part, from the appearance of the spongy holes, visible under a micro-scope, in affected brain tissue.

Signs and symptoms

The main characteristic of CJD is the rapidly progressing symptoms of dementia. In the beginning, a person with the disease may experience:

- Problems with muscle coordination
- Personality changes
- Insomnia
- Blurred vision
- Unusual sensations, such as a sense that the skin is sticky

The symptoms become dramatically worse, resulting in severe mental im-pairment. The person may develop involuntary muscle jerks, difficulty moving and speaking, and blindness.

Many people with CJD eventually fall into a coma. Heart failure, respiratory failure, pneumonia or other infections are generally the cause of death. The disease usually runs its course in about five to seven months after signs and symptoms first appear.

The variant of CJD associated with mad cow disease usually begins with psy-chiatric symptoms, such as depression, anxiety, apathy and delusions. Cogni-tive impairment usually occurs in the later stages. The variant form affects people at a younger age than standard CJD does and has a slightly longer du-ration — 12 to 14 months.

Causes

Prion proteins occur naturally in the brain. Normally they're harmless, but when misshapen in form, they can cause disease. They perform their intended function once they're folded into a specific three-dimensional shape. Most proteins fold spontaneously during or just after they're manufac-tured inside body cells.

Protein folding isn't foolproof, how-ever, and many proteins made by the cells aren't usable. The rejects are sent to a kind of recycling center, where they're prepared for reuse. But as people age, the recycling process may stop working efficiently. As a result, misfolded proteins start to accumulate in the brain, causing serious problems.

Misshapen prions may enter brain cells and force normal proteins to misfold as well. The infected cells die. Eventually, large clusters of cells die, leaving the brain riddled with holes.

Transmission

Researchers have identified three basic ways through which people can get Creutzfeldt-Jakob disease:

Spontaneously. Most people with CJD develop the disease for no apparent reason. Sporadic CJD accounts for more than 85 percent of all cases.

By genetic mutation. In the United States, about 5 to 10 percent of people with CJD have a family history of the disease or test positive for a genetic mutation associated with CJD.

By contamination. The risk of being exposed to contamination with CJD-related prions is low. CJD can't be transmitted through air or casual touch. A few people have been exposed to infected human tissue during medical procedures such as skin transplants or injections of contaminated growth hormone. Since 1985, all human growth hormone in the United States has been genetically re-engineered, eliminating the risk of CJD.

Misshapen prions aren't affected by standard sterilization methods including heat, radiation, alcohol, benzene and formaldehyde. As a result, there's a very slight risk that instruments used in some types of brain surgery can harbor small bits of infected tissue.

Animal studies suggest that contaminated blood and related products may transmit the disease, but no case of a blood transfusion leading to CJD has been recorded in humans. The CJD variant has been linked primarily to the consumption of beef infected with mad cow disease.

CJD and vCJD have long incubation periods, which means the disease may not show up until years after the initial protein abnormalities have occurred. For vCJD, the incubation period is approximately 10 years.

Diagnosis

Doctors can make a fairly accurate diagnosis of CJD based on a medical exam, personal history, neurological exam and other diagnostic tests. The diagnosis often requires eliminating other possible causes of the symptoms.

MRI scans can show subtle, yet characteristic, abnormalities. Brain wave tests can also display a characteristic series of irregular brain waves referred to as "periodic complexes," although these are not seen in everyone with CJD.

The presence of certain proteins in cerebrospinal fluid also may help confirm CJD in someone who is already showing signs and symptoms of the disease. Samples of spinal fluid can be obtained through a spinal tap (lumbar puncture).

Only an examination of brain tissue after death can confirm Creutzfeldt-Jakob disease with certainty.

Treatment

No effective treatment exists for either CJD or vCJD. A variety of drugs have been tested, including steroids, antibiotics and antiviral agents, with disappointing results. For that reason, doctors focus on alleviating pain and other symptoms and on making people with the disease as comfortable as possible.

Secondary dementias

Sometimes dementia symptoms can be the complications of a chronic disorder affecting movement or other functions in other parts of the body. You may hear these cases referred to as secondary dementias, because the dementia is the result of a disease that's characterized primarily by other symptoms.

Some conditions in which this may occur are Parkinson's disease, progressive supranuclear palsy, human immunodeficiency virus (HIV), multiple sclerosis and Wilson's disease.

Parkinson's disease dementia

Some people with Parkinson's disease may develop dementia in later stages of their illness. Parkinson's disease is a disorder that affects mainly the neurons producing dopamine, a neurotransmitter controlling muscle movement.

People with Parkinson's often experience trembling, muscle rigidity, difficulty walking, and problems with balance and coordination. These signs and symptoms typically develop after age 50, although the disease may affect some younger adults as well.

Symptoms of cognitive impairment may be present when Parkinson's disease is diagnosed, but these are generally mild. In some people, the symptoms may develop into severe dementia. A study suggests that the overall prevalence of dementia in people with Parkinson's may be between 50 and 80 percent — especially as people with Parkinson's live longer and dementia becomes better understood.

Signs and symptoms. The following cognitive signs and symptoms, some of which may fluctuate in intensity, characterize Parkinson's disease dementia.

Impaired executive skills. These functions include the ability to plan, organize, problem-solve and make decisions, as well as to understand complex concepts and follow internal cues for behavior.

Attention difficulties. A person with Parkinson's disease dementia may have difficulty paying attention during a conversation or staying focused on a simple task.

Memory problems. A person with Parkinson's disease dementia may retain the ability to store new information, but accessing that information can be a challenge. Thus, the person may have difficulty remembering things unless given a visual or verbal cue. General forgetfulness is not as severe as it is with Alzheimer's disease.

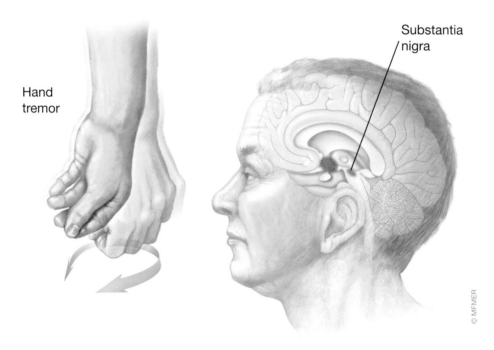

Hand tremor

Substantia nigra

© MFMER

Problems associated with Parkinson's disease, such as physical instability and tremor, are caused primarily by inadequate levels of dopamine, a neurotransmitter that relays messages from the substantia nigra to other parts of the brain.

Psychotic symptoms. Hallucinations similar to those experienced in dementia with Lewy bodies are a common symptom of Parkinson's disease dementia. The hallucinations usually involve vivid, colorful images of people or animals, although sounds are not included. Delusions and paranoia are less common symptoms.

Causes. Because Parkinson's disease dementia is so similar to dementia with Lewy bodies, some experts believe both disorders may be rooted in the same disease mechanism.

Currently the only difference between a diagnosis of Parkinson's disease dementia and dementia with Lewy bodies is the timing of the onset of symptoms. If problems with balance and coordination occur more than a year before cognitive difficulties begin, the disorder is considered to be Parkinson's disease dementia. If cognitive impairment occurs within a year of the balance and coordination deficits, the diagnosis becomes dementia with Lewy bodies.

Lewy bodies — the name for abnormal deposits of the alpha-synuclein protein — are present in the brains of most people with Parkinson's disease. When there's no dementia involved, the Lewy bodies are restricted to an area of the brain called the substantia nigra. When there is dementia, Lewy bodies are found in other parts of the brain.

A prominent theory is that the presence of Lewy bodies in areas associated with intellect and emotions is what causes the dementia in Parkinson's disease. New information continues to emerge, however, suggesting that Lewy bodies may not be the only factor involved.

In addition, at autopsy, people with Parkinson's disease dementia frequently show amyloid plaques and neurofibrillary tangles in brain tissue. This suggests that Alzheimer's disease may be a cause of the dementia and raises the possibility that Alzheimer's and Parkinson's are in some way connected.

It's also possible that the loss of dopamine-producing neurons, the main mechanism underlying Parkinson's disease, may itself cause or at least contribute to cognitive impairment and dementia, in spite of abnormal structures such as Lewy bodies, plaques and tangles.

Treatment. People with Parkinson's disease dementia experience a heavy loss of neurons producing the neurotransmitter acetylcholine, in addition to the loss of dopamine-producing neurons. In fact, the decrease in acetylcholine levels, a characteristic of Alzheimer's disease, is far greater in people with Parkinson's disease dementia than in people with Alzheimer's. Studies indicate that cholinesterase inhibitors, medications that increase the level of acetylcholine in the brain, may be of some benefit for improving cognitive symptoms, although more research is needed to confirm these results.

Newer types of antipsychotic medications — quetiapine is commonly used — may help reduce hallucinations and other psychotic symptoms.

Progressive supranuclear palsy

Progressive supranuclear palsy is a disorder that's often misdiagnosed as Parkinson's disease. It has many characteristics that are similar to those of Parkinson's disease, such as an unsteady gait, stooped posture, muscle rigidity, and difficulty with spoken language and articulation.

People with progressive supranuclear palsy have a tendency to fall backward. They also have a greatly reduced rate of blinking, which often leads to dry eyes and an increased susceptibility to eye infections. Eye movements in general

become slowed. A characteristic symptom is the person's inability to focus his or her gaze downward.

Some people with progressive supranuclear palsy may experience cognitive impairment, ranging from memory loss and personality changes to apathy, depression and anxiety. They often have difficulty with executive skills. Other signs and symptoms may include sleep disturbances, increased irritability, occasional angry outbursts, and unexplained episodes of laughing or crying.

The destruction of neurons in the brain is far more widespread in progressive supranuclear palsy than it is in Parkinson's disease. The cause of the disease is uncertain, but like a number of other disorders — including Alzheimer's disease and frontotemporal degeneration — neurofibrillary tangles characterize it. The relationship among various tau-related diseases, or tauopathies as they're sometimes called, is not understood, but learning how to prevent tau accumulations may lead to better treatments of these diseases.

At present, treatment of progressive supranuclear palsy is geared toward improving comfort and quality of life. Medications used to treat other movement disorders may be of help temporarily. Glasses with prisms can improve a person's ability to see downward, and artificial tears may soothe dry eyes. After the onset of symptoms, the course of the disease runs an average of seven years. Death is usually caused by a pneumonia-related infection or the complications of a fall or reduced mobility.

HIV-associated dementia

Some people infected with the human immunodeficiency virus (HIV) may eventually develop dementia. This occurrence is referred to as HIV-associated dementia (HAD).

Before the widespread use of highly active antiretroviral therapy (HAART), about 20 to 30 percent of people with HIV went on to develop some degree of dementia. More recently, given the success of HAART, the incidence of dementia in HIV-infected adults has decreased to about 10 percent.

HIV-associated dementia is characterized by memory loss; impaired concentration; judgment and motor skills; personality changes; mood swings; anxiety; and, occasionally, hallucinations, paranoia and delusions. At onset, the symptoms are subtle and easy to pass off as fatigue.

People experience the signs and symptoms of dementia at different rates and with different degrees of severity. Some individuals may develop a very mild level of cognitive impairment, known as minor cognitive motor disorder (MCMD). This form does not seriously interfere with their abilities to function in daily life. Other individuals may become severely demented.

What causes the deterioration of brain cells in a person with an HIV infection isn't well understood, but the onset of dementia is correlated with the number of cells infected by the virus. One theory, sometimes called the Trojan horse hypothesis, is that the virus enters the central nervous system as a hidden passenger in immune cells. These cells have access to the brain. Once there, the virus-infected cells infect neurons, replicating the virus many times over.

Neuropsychological testing and brain imaging help determine the extent of cognitive impairment. During diagnosis, doctors try to distinguish HIV-associated dementia from other treatable causes of dementia. These causes may include brain infections such as meningitis, nutritional deficiencies, medication side effects, and psychiatric illnesses such as depression and anxiety.

Standard therapy for HIV-associated dementia is the HAART regimen combined with the treatment of any associated mood and anxiety disorders. At the same time that it greatly reduces the number of infected cells in the body, HAART decreases the risk of HIV-associated dementia.

MCMD, the milder form of cognitive impairment, may develop into dementia later, particularly as new treatments extend the life span of a person infected with HIV. Thus, researchers continue to search for ways to protect the brain from the effects of this viral infection.

Multiple sclerosis

About half of all people with multiple sclerosis (MS) experience some degree of cognitive impairment. The impairment usually isn't as severe as it is in Alzheimer's disease and other forms of dementia, but it can affect a person's work life and social life and impair his or her daily living skills.

In multiple sclerosis, the body incorrectly directs antibodies and white blood cells to attack proteins in the myelin sheath, a protective coating that surrounds nerve fibers in your brain and spinal cord. This causes inflammation and injury to the sheath and ultimately to the nerves that it protects. The result may be areas of scarring (sclerosis). Eventually this damage slows or blocks the nerve signals that control muscle coordination, strength, sensation and vision.

In multiple sclerosis, different types of cognitive impairment are believed to result from damage to nerves deep in the brain's white matter. Signs and symptoms may include:

- Difficulty remembering things
- General forgetfulness
- Slowed reaction time
- Difficulty with executive skills
- Personality changes that include carelessness, irritability, lack of judgment and lack of responsiveness
- Difficulty with words
- Depression

These signs and symptoms generally occur in episodes (attacks) that last for weeks or months and are separated by periods in which the problems improve or disappear (remission). The types of symptoms and their severity roughly correlate to the areas of the brain that are affected and to the degree of nerve damage. Cognitive symptoms are more likely to occur in people with a chronic, progressive form of multiple sclerosis.

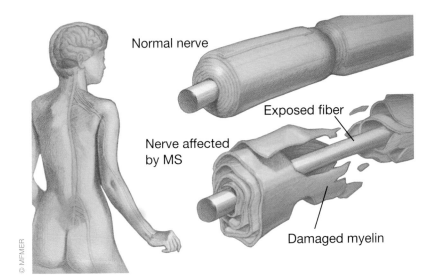

Normal nerve

Exposed fiber

Nerve affected by MS

Damaged myelin

In multiple sclerosis, the protective coating on nerve fibers (myelin) becomes detached and eventually destroyed. Depending on where the nerve damage occurs, MS can affect vision, sensation, coordination, movement, and bladder and bowel control.

Treatment of the underlying cause can reduce new nerve damage and prevent or minimize associated cognitive decline. Studies suggest that some medications used to treat Alzheimer's may be beneficial in treating the cognitive symptoms, but more studies are needed to confirm the drug's efficacy.

Wilson's disease

Wilson's disease is a hereditary disorder that causes too much of the mineral copper to accumulate in your liver, brain and other vital organs. Bile, a fluid that assists in digestion, normally carries excess copper away from your liver. In someone with Wilson's disease, the liver doesn't release the mineral into bile as it should.

The resulting buildup of copper in the liver injures the liver tissue. Eventually, some of the excess copper travels throughout the body, where it may damage your brain, eyes, kidneys and red blood cells. If left untreated, Wilson's disease is fatal.

In some people, Wilson's disease can cause abrupt personality changes and inappropriate social behavior. Tremors, muscle spasms and speech problems also may occur. Later complications of the disease include mood swings, depression, agitation, memory loss and periods of confusion.

With early diagnosis and prompt treatment, the progression of Wilson's disease can be stopped, and existing symptoms may be improved. Treatment involves taking medications that either remove the deposited copper from tissues or render it harmless.

The two medications approved for this purpose are penicillamine (Cuprimine, Depen) and trientine (Syprine). Taking zinc acetate (Galzin) helps block copper absorption from the stomach and intestine and may be an alternative treatment for pregnant women and people without symptoms or organ damage. Although treatment is lifelong, the long-term outlook and life expectancy are generally good for people with Wilson's disease.

Many causes

Like a finely tuned machine, your brain depends on the harmonious, balanced function of all of its parts in order to maintain maximal efficiency. Even a slight disruption in this balance may have serious consequences.

As described in previous chapters, your brain and nervous system are vulnerable to a wide variety of injuries. Degeneration of nerve cells causes illnesses such as Alzheimer's disease. Interruption of the blood supply to the brain causes strokes.

The conditions described in this chapter broaden the picture considerably with regard to disorders that may affect or destroy cognition, memory, mental processing and learning. The causes include genetic mutation, protein buildup, chemical imbalance, viral invasion and an excessive amount of cerebrospinal fluid that cushions the brain.

Neurologists and other medical specialists must try to determine a cause for your signs and symptoms and prescribe appropriate treatment. Diagnosis may be difficult because the symptoms can be so diverse. Many of the symptoms are associated with cognitive loss in general and not exclusive to a specific condition. A careful assessment of the character and pattern of these symptoms is sometimes necessary to reach an accurate diagnosis.

Part 4

Promising strategies to improve cognition

Chapter 14

Staying mentally sharp

You may be thinking, "Is there something I can do to prevent Alzheimer's disease?"

Whether you're caring for a loved one with dementia or you've recently celebrated a birthday with a lot of candles or you're simply thinking about the future, this may be a question on your mind. You may be wondering what you can do to improve or retain memory and minimize cognitive loss as you age.

Unfortunately, the answer isn't so simple. Although the popular press has extolled the brain-boosting powers of a variety of products — from wild salmon to coconut milk — there's no proven way to reduce your risk of developing abnormal structures in your brain, such as the plaques and tangles of Alzheimer's, which impair cognitive function.

But another part of the answer is this: There are a variety of steps you can take to cultivate good memory habits and sharpen recent memory (the part of memory that's quickly impaired with the onset of dementia). The earlier you take these steps the better, before you're diagnosed with a memory problem. Healthy lifestyle habits also can enhance brain function and prevent memory problems.

It's believed that some of these steps may increase your *resilience* to Alzheimer's disease. Research shows that two people with comparable amounts of plaques and tangles, measured by brain imaging, may experience very different symptoms. For one person, the plaques and tangles are debilitating; for the other person, they cause little change in cognition. How is this possible?

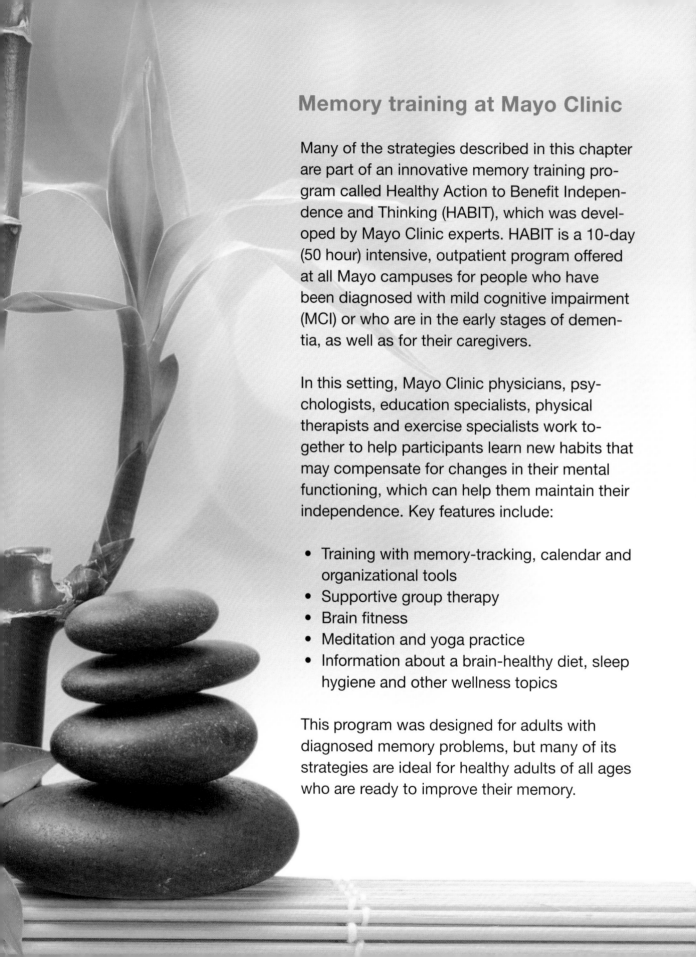

Memory training at Mayo Clinic

Many of the strategies described in this chapter are part of an innovative memory training program called Healthy Action to Benefit Independence and Thinking (HABIT), which was developed by Mayo Clinic experts. HABIT is a 10-day (50 hour) intensive, outpatient program offered at all Mayo campuses for people who have been diagnosed with mild cognitive impairment (MCI) or who are in the early stages of dementia, as well as for their caregivers.

In this setting, Mayo Clinic physicians, psychologists, education specialists, physical therapists and exercise specialists work together to help participants learn new habits that may compensate for changes in their mental functioning, which can help them maintain their independence. Key features include:

- Training with memory-tracking, calendar and organizational tools
- Supportive group therapy
- Brain fitness
- Meditation and yoga practice
- Information about a brain-healthy diet, sleep hygiene and other wellness topics

This program was designed for adults with diagnosed memory problems, but many of its strategies are ideal for healthy adults of all ages who are ready to improve their memory.

One explanation is that some people are simply more resilient to the physical damages taking place in the brain, perhaps because their neural connections are just a little bit stronger. This resilience — also known as cognitive reserve — may be something you're born with, or it may be something you develop through lifelong mental stimulation and other lifestyle choices. More research is underway to better understand these factors.

In the meantime, make the most of your intellect and memory. In this chapter, you'll find practical strategies that may improve your retention and processing of information, as well as mental activities to stimulate your mind. In the next chapter, you'll learn about lifestyle habits that can benefit your brain.

Effects of aging on brain function

Do your mental abilities change as you age? Research indicates the answer is probably yes. Just as you notice changes in vision, hearing or balance as you get older, you may also experience the following changes in brain function:

- It may take you a little longer to learn new things. Compared with when you were younger, you either learn less in the same amount of time or you need more time to learn the same amount.
- It may be harder for you to recall some names, faces, dates, places and other facts.
- It may be more difficult for you to handle more than one task at the same time. You may need to focus on a single task and accomplish it well before turning your attention to the next task.
- You may experience memory lapses, such as forgetting where you parked the car or where you put your keys. This is a common complaint of people age 50 and older.

All of these changes can be unsettling or scary, so it's worth noting that there are many parts of the brain that generally remain untouched by age. This includes the areas that store language and word meanings, and the areas associated with creativity and wisdom. There's also procedural memory, which stores the skills you develop because you've done them over and over again. These are skills such as riding a bicycle or playing the piano. Once you master them, they tend to stay with you. And procedural memory deteriorates little with age.

It's also important to remember that no two people age in the same way. There are older adults who live into their ninth decade with their golf swing and memory intact. But that's probably not a realistic or likely goal. Most people experience at least some subtle changes in memory as they age.

Whatever your mental strengths and weaknesses are as a young adult, they will likely continue as you get older. For example, if you've always been good at remembering people's names, you're likely to maintain this skill. If you've always had trouble remembering names, you'll likely not get much better at it with age. In fact, this type of problem may even get worse.

Fortunately, most experts believe that you can improve memory if you're motivated to change some everyday habits. This is great news, but it isn't always easy to accomplish.

Despite good intentions, many people don't find the time or motivation to work on memory until an early-stage dementia diagnosis spurs them into action. By reading this book, you're already taking a proactive step toward protecting memory. Now, it's time to roll up your sleeves and get started on actively making changes.

Stimulating strategies

It's never too early to develop good habits that may help offset age-related cognitive loss. Here are practical strategies that may improve your everyday memory and information-processing abilities. These strategies may also help you keep your brain in shape.

Keep a calendar

You may find yourself bombarded with lots of facts coming from all directions — names, numbers, passwords, to-do lists. If you feel like your brain isn't particularly well designed to lug this type of information around, you're right. When you're trying to track too many tedious details, you're actually more prone to memory lapses.

An effective calendar and organization system can help you avoid information overload. Developing this habit at a young age may help you cope better as you get older — but you can never be too old to start.

In fact, this type of system is the foundation of the Mayo Clinic memory training program. Participants in the program

More than memory lapses?

In the typical aging process, memory lapses and forgetfulness are an annoyance and may be a source of frustration or embarrassment. You forget a name at a dinner party, but you remember it later. You misplace things from time to time. You miss a bill payment but are able to fix your mistake.

If memory lapses begin to disrupt daily life or interfere with personal safety, then that's not a typical part of the aging process. Cognitive changes that get in the way of a normal routine may be a warning sign of dementia. Other warning signs of dementia may include:

- Poor judgment and decision-making
- Difficulty performing familiar tasks or solving problems
- Difficulty holding a conversation
- Trouble understanding visual images or spatial relationships

If you notice any of these signs or symptoms in yourself or a loved one, see your health care provider for an evaluation.

learn to use a highly structured calendar and note-taking system. The goal is to establish this system as a habit that's stored in procedural memory, because this type of long-term memory is preserved in the aging process.

As an established habit, the system can become a substitute (prosthesis) for memory. It works the same way as a physical prosthesis, such as a walker. Rather than fixing or changing brain function, the system provides a way to compensate for loss of memory, just as a walker compensates for loss of balance.

The success of this system hinges on its training program. But you can apply key concepts to a calendar system of your own. There's a variety of tools that can help you organize and remember appointments and tasks — from paper calendars to smartphones to applications (apps) for tablets and computers. Whatever tools you choose, follow these key ideas:

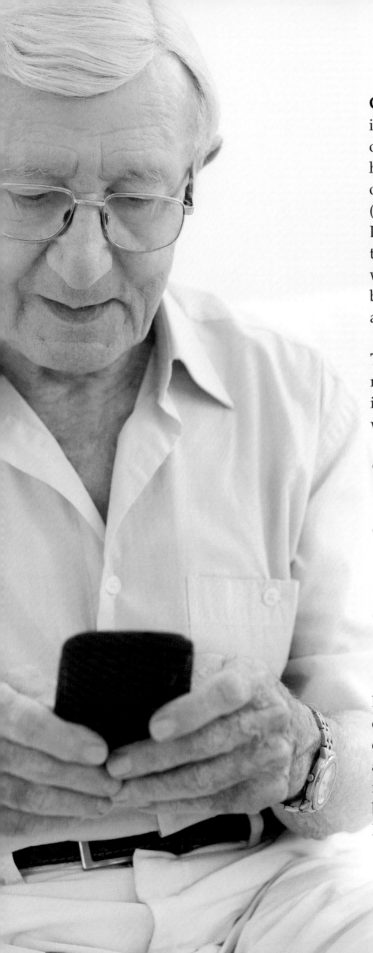

Choose one tool. Rather than relying on piles of sticky notes and slips of paper scattered throughout your house, purse and pants pockets, pick one comprehensive tool that you can (and will) take with you at all times. Look for something that's small enough to fit into a man's breast pocket or a woman's purse. It can be a paper datebook or a smartphone with multiple apps — whatever suits your style.

Track the information. Develop a method to track the different kinds of information on a daily to-do list. Most will fall into one of three categories:

- Events that must happen at a particular time, such as appointments and meetings
- Tasks that need to get done, though not at a scheduled time, including routine work tasks, home chores and medications to be taken
- Addresses, phone numbers and other contact information for people in your life

Designate a separate section in your datebook or phone to track each kind of information. It's easier to remember and process information when it's separated according to category, rather than being jumbled together into one big list. You may also benefit from a short journal or note-taking area, where you record events happening throughout the day, such as the details of an important phone call.

Regularly use the system. Frequent use is the best way to turn your calendar system into an established habit. Set a regular schedule for reviewing your calendar system, at least three times a day. You can associate the reviews with other routine tasks, for example, right after breakfast. The reviews are in addition to each time you schedule or complete a new meeting, appointment or task.

Mark completed tasks. Put an X or some other notation right by the entry. This makes it easier to track unfinished items and leaves no question about whether routine tasks, such as taking medications, were done on a particular day. If you think your memory is still sharp enough to skip this step, think again. It's wise to establish this habit early. And you'll likely feel a motivating sense of accomplishment as you mark off each task.

Over time, you'll surely develop personal strategies, shortcuts and abbreviations that make your calendar system work best for you. That's great! Experts agree that there isn't one right way to keep a calendar. The best calendar system is the one that suits your personal needs and takes the least amount of time and energy to maintain.

Organize the clutter

Nowadays, there are whole stores devoted to selling bins, baskets, cases, containers, hooks and hangers. So there's no shortage of organizational options and inspiration for your home. You don't have to alphabetize every drawer and shelf. But keeping your environment clutter-free can help minimize distractions and improve memory.

Create a system for belongings. Just as you did with information, you can develop a system for organizing your belongings, whether at home or at work. Store frequently used items in the same place. Carry car keys or house keys in the same pocket or handbag every time you use them, and always return them to a designated spot when you're finished with them.

Here are more ideas: Keep kitchen utensils that you use for certain tasks together in convenient locations, for example, mixing bowls with measuring cups or knives with cutting boards. Use a toolbox to store tools that you need once in a while, such as a hammer, pliers and wrench. Always return the tools to the box when you're done with them so that you know where they are for the next time you need them.

Put correspondence in order. It's not easy to stay ahead of the endless stream of letters, bills, bank statements, meeting notices and special announcements that you receive each week. Instead of letting correspondence and junk mail accumulate in miscellaneous paper piles or long email lists, sort mail and other documents as soon as you get them. As you sort, ask yourself: "Will I ever need this document again?" If the answer is yes, keep it. If the answer is no, get rid of it.

Next, separate the correspondence in the "yes" pile or list into designated folders, files or baskets for the following categories:

- *Information that requires a response or action.* This category includes bills that need to be paid and invitations that need an RSVP. Put these to-do items into a special folder or basket as they arrive. Then set aside time to address these tasks at least once a week.
- *Information that you'll need to consult occasionally.* Examples are tax records; statements for your checking, savings and investment accounts; insurance policies and other key contracts; and owner's manuals for appliances, cars and other possessions. Create files to keep these items safe. At least once a year, review the files and purge anything that's irrelevant.
- *Information to read at your leisure.* Collect magazines, newsletters and brochures into a "to-read" pile or folder that can be read at any time. Save these items for bedtime reading or weekend relaxation or even your next plane trip.

Focus your attention

Attention happens when you focus on an object, task, interaction or event. This skill is an important part of memory processing — it takes concentration to input information into your brain so that it can be stored properly as memory and be retrieved when you need it. However, as you age, it can become more difficult to sustain attention.

Slowing down and focusing on the present can help. Before you start a conversation or activity, take a deep breath. Then look closely at the person or task in front of you. You can also use your senses (sight, hearing, taste, touch and smell) to help you focus on the present. Thinking about smells or sounds around you can create awareness of your surroundings and help you concentrate. Here are some other tips for improving attention.

Minimize distractions. Turn off the radio or TV or pull the "buds" out of your ears when you're reading instructions or trying to concentrate. Control your work environment to reduce interruptions, such as shutting the office door when you need to focus. And what about the chimes, rings and alerts from your phone or other technology devices? Consider silencing your phone and computer for a couple hours each day — or at least while you're working on a project.

Do one task at a time. Whenever possible, do one thing at a time. Focus on that task for a set period of time and then take a break.

Use selective attention. You often rely on this type of attention anytime you're having a conversation in a noisy, crowded restaurant. You tune out background noise and conversation to focus on a select task — in this case, whatever your dinner companion is saying. You can use this same technique to be selective about what you're trying to remember.

Remind yourself of what's truly important and what's a lesser priority. When meeting a number of new people at the same time, for example, focus on retaining just a handful of key names — better to remember a few people than to be confused about everyone. When reading a news article, give it a skim to consider what facts or ideas may be the most important to remember, then read it again for the full details.

Use memory tricks

Memory techniques may be useful aids. Most prompt you to encode information more efficiently — that is, to focus on information when you first encounter it and manipulate it in a way that helps you recall it later. Approach these memory techniques as if playing a game — have fun with them. Being creative (or even outlandish) may make them more effective. Note that you must practice these techniques until they become automatic. Until then, they can actually be a distraction that worsens memory.

Make associations. One way to remember something new is to associate it with something that you already know. Making intentional connections gives information meaning and makes it more likely that you'll remember it. You did this as a child when you learned to recognize Italy on a world map by remembering that the country is shaped like a boot or that the state of Michigan resembles a mitten.

Association can also work for learning definitions and people's names. For example, to remember that the port side of a boat is the left side (and not the right), connect the fact that the words *port* and *left* both have four letters — whereas as right has five letters. This links *port* and *left* in your memory.

Make associations to learn new names:

- Think of other people you know well with the same name, such as an uncle or close neighbor.
- Associate the new name with an image, if one comes to mind. For example, link the name Robin with a bird. Or picture Robert Green covered in green paint.
- Associate the new name with a noticeable feature of that person or some information about how you know each other, for example, Tall Timothy or Concert Catherine.

You can use association to retrieve memories. Say that you're trying to remember the name of a person you worked with 10 years ago and haven't

seen since. If that name doesn't pop immediately into your mind, try to think of something associated with that person that you do remember. Visualize the building you both worked in, the location of your offices or the name of your supervisor.

Prompting your memory with related details helps you retrace your mental path to look for information, just as you might retrace your physical path to look for your keys. And it often yields the information you want.

Repeat, rehash and revisit. Repeating new information helps you pay attention to it and encode it properly. It helps to repeat factual information, such as names and numbers, several times when you first learn it. For example, when you meet new people, use their names in conversation right away. The same technique works for directions. Repeat directions out loud to properly process the information and the order of steps.

Similarly, when you want to remember key concepts or ideas, talk about them with other people. If you want to remember the main ideas of a book you've just finished, summarize them in a conversation with family and friends. Turning your thoughts into words will help you pinpoint the most important information and formulate your opinions.

You may want to review relevant information in advance of a special event — such as paging through your yearbook before attending a class reunion to help remember names and faces.

Other memory techniques.
These tricks of the trade may help you remember new information:

- *Break it down.* Divide large amounts of information into meaningful, manageable chunks. You do this already when you break down a 10-digit phone number into the area code, three-digit exchange and four-digit personal number, for example, 800-555-1212. Apply the same technique to remember your driver's license ID, computer password or other long numbers. You can also chunk a long list of items or directions into smaller groups. For example, rather than trying to remember a grocery list of seven random items, think of the list as four vegetables and three fruits.
- *Picture it.* Create a vivid mental image of the information you want to remember. Creativity works particularly well with this technique.

For example, if you store your roasting pan on a shelf in the basement closet between holidays, you might remember its location by mentally imagining a turkey running around inside that closet.

- *Write it down.* Making notes or lists can help you remember information. In addition, just the act of writing involves mental actions that often stay with you. So writing down the name of a restaurant you want to try may help you remember the restaurant even if you misplace the note. Recording a sequence of events and your feelings about them in a journal may help you remember the experience, even if you never reread the passage.
- *Use a cue.* A cue is anything that signals you to do something, be it an object, a sound or even a smell. Many people like to place objects in uncommon locations in order to help them remember. For example, place letters to mail in your pathway to the front door so that you don't forget them as you leave the house. Or stick reminder notes on the bathroom mirror or the refrigerator at night to make sure you do something the next morning. You can also use auditory cues, for example, setting your watch alarm a few minutes before appointments.

Cross-train your brain

One way to keep your mind sharp may simply be by exercising it. Just as regular physical activity improves your heart and lung capacity, regular brain training may improve your brain function.

Early research on science-based brain-training programs — which include a structured set of exercises designed to train specific areas of the brain — is overall very positive. These brain training programs may increase your ability to focus and your mental processing speed — and may even help build the cognitive reserve described at the beginning of this chapter.

The Mayo Clinic memory training (HABIT) program includes a scientific, computerized brain fitness technique, which consists of listening exercises that get progressively trickier. Participants wearing headphones are asked to distinguish between high- and low-pitched sounds, for example. To start, the sounds are slow and distinct. Then, the sounds go faster and faster, until they end up sounding almost like a single click. Another exercise asks participants to distinguish between similar syllables such as "doe" and "toe." The goal of both exercises is to improve speed and accuracy of sound (auditory) processing in the brain. Revving up this type of processing may improve overall brain function in older adults.

You'll find a wide range of available online brain training programs, computer software programs and smartphone apps with scientific merits at varying price points. Do your homework before you purchase any program. Or start with brain exercise books and free online games that are designed to stretch and strengthen your brain. Crossword puzzles, number and word games, and a host of everyday activities also provide opportunities for mental aerobics.

Keep these general guidelines for brain training in mind — they're similar to those you might employ for physical fitness training:

- *Be consistent.* It takes regular physical activity to get your body in shape and reduce your risk of heart disease. The same is likely true of brain training. To make a noticeable change in brain function, you need regular mental workouts, not just occasional card games. In fact, in one successful study of cognitive training, participants trained for one hour each day, five days a week, for a total of eight weeks.

- *Vary your routine.* A good fitness program mixes different exercises designed to work the whole body. The same concept applies to brain training. So, if you're about to start your 100th crossword puzzle, it's time to try something else. Aim for a combination of exercises and activities to stimulate the whole brain, including the areas that control visual processing, sound processing, sequencing, spatial relationships, language and more.

- *Target a range of skills.* Or seek out everyday activities that work different parts of the brain. For example, try jigsaw puzzles to sharpen spatial relationship skills. And attend classical music concerts or lectures to test your sound processing.

- *Challenge yourself.* The brain fitness software used at Mayo Clinic automatically adjusts the difficulty of the program, based on users' responses, so that everyone always gets about 85 percent of answers correct. As a

Resources for brain training

If you're interested in brain training, you'll find hundreds of options, including books, websites, smartphone applications and computer software programs. Here's a small sample of the available options:

Paid online programs and computer software
- Brain Fitness: *www.positscience.com/products*
- MindFit: *www.mindfit.com*
- Happy Neuron: *happy-neuron.com*
- Lumosity: *www.lumosity.com*

Free online games and puzzles
- AARP games: *games.aarp.org/*
- Enchanted Mind: *www.enchantedmind.com*
- MazeWorks: *www.mazeworks.com*
- Ravensburger Web Puzzles: *www.ravensburger-webpuzzles.com/*
- Your Amazing Brain: *www.youramazingbrain.org/testyourself/default.htm*

result, the program is always challenging but does not disillusion participants. Follow the same principle in your own brain-training efforts. Choose a level where you can't get everything right, and move to more advanced exercises, as needed.

- **Focus on speed.** Dedicate time to improving the speed at which you process information, since speed is a part of memory that typically slows with age. Think Slapjack instead of Solitaire. The former is an easy childhood card game, but you can't win without quickly slapping the Jacks as they're placed on the pile. Test yourself against one of your favorite five-year-olds, or seek out other fast-paced brain games, such as Concentration or Minesweeper. Or try your usual crossword puzzles against a timer.

Try new things

Lifelong learning and mental stimulation are sure to make life more interesting and enriching. And it's possible that these activities may reduce your risk of memory loss. Although you may not be able to do some things as well as you did them before, age shouldn't stop you from pursuing new frontiers. Studies show that older adults learn new skills as well as younger adults do. While younger adults may mentally process faster, older adults can apply more wisdom and experience.

Don't be afraid to test your limits. Excitement is an important part of learning. Former president George H. W. Bush celebrated his 75th birthday by sky diving. The first time he made a parachute jump was when his plane was shot down over the Pacific Ocean during World War II. After that experience, he promised himself he would one day jump out of a plane for fun.

If you're not one for sky diving, creative work may be more your style. Artist Georgia O'Keefe, after discontinuing her work for years, returned to painting at the age of 86 and went on to receive the Medal of the Arts. Director Clint Eastwood was nominated for three Academy Awards in his seventies. One of the films earned Eastwood a directing Oscar, along with an Oscar for 68-year-old Morgan Freeman as best supporting actor.

More recently, at the age of 88, actress Betty White became the oldest person to guest host "Saturday Night Live," and she won a Primetime Emmy Award for her efforts. Architect Philip Johnson worked into his 90s and continued to exert influence on architectural design and aesthetics. Quite simply, it's never too late to turn out some of your best work.

On the other hand, it doesn't take celebrity status to expand your horizons. Here are ways to get you started:

- Stay curious. Take continuing education classes. Learn yoga or Pilates, or try your hand at painting or creative writing.
- Volunteer at a local school or to a civic or charitable organization.
- Stay up to date on new technology, such as computers, cameras and telecommunications. You can do this cheaply by reading trade journals and visiting specialty stores.
- Use the Internet to access information on a topic that's interesting to you. Research new recipes, gardening or golf trends, or genealogy.
- Travel to new places, be it a far-flung destination or a new ethnic restaurant in your hometown.
- Stay in touch with family and friends and look to expand your circle of acquaintances with new stimulating friendships.
- Join a book club or discussion group.

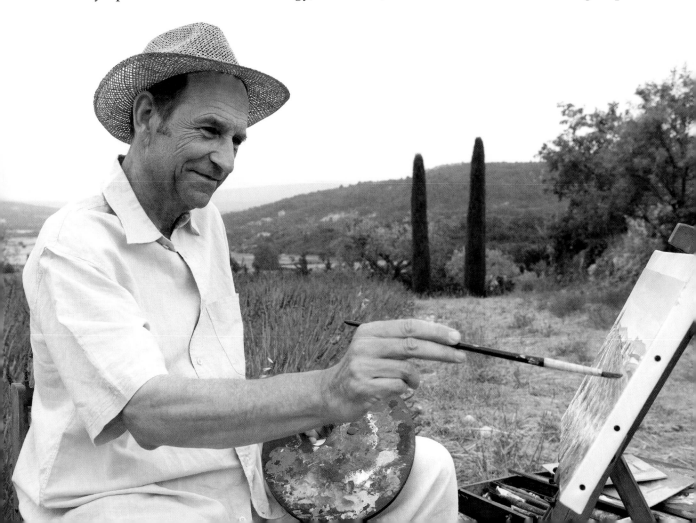

- Attend local concerts, lectures and plays to explore the cultural life of your community.
- Research family history and publish your account.

The experience of age provides a rich backdrop for developing skills, embracing change and integrating new knowledge into your life.

Putting it all together

You're not expected to incorporate all of these strategies into your daily or weekly routine overnight. You might find that some of the strategies are easy, or even fun, to carry out. (You've always wanted to take a painting class and now you have a good reason!) However, changing some daily habits — such as the way you organize your home or track your schedule — may be a bit more challenging.

It takes time and practice to develop new behaviors that can improve and protect your memory. Start by reviewing the strategies described above in relation to your current habits and lifestyle. Are you already using some of

the strategies described here — at least to a degree? Are there some techniques that you've tried in the past and liked or discarded? Are there certain strategies that seem like they'll easily fit into your routine?

Identify all of the things that you're already doing right. Give yourself credit for small successes — for example, note that you keep meticulous financial records, even if you can't claim that your whole house is tidy.

At the same time, list behaviors that could use improvement, based on your newfound knowledge from this chapter. Identify new habits you want to try and incorporate on a regular basis.

Select one strategy that you'd like to work on first. Trying to tackle all six strategies at one time is likely to feel overwhelming and increase the chances that you won't be successful. Focus instead on just one.

Which strategy? That's up to you. You can select the one you're most excited about or the one that you feel the most confident you can achieve. Or you can choose a strategy that you feel you need the most help with right away, such as remembering people's names or remembering important tasks.

Medications and memory

If you've become concerned about memory lapses, ask your doctor about any side effects from the medications you may be taking. Some medications, including the examples below, can interfere with your ability to remember. When you talk to your doctor, mention everything you're taking, including vitamins, minerals, over-the-counter drugs and herbal supplements.

A couple of points to remember: Just because you're using one of the medications listed below doesn't mean that you're going to develop memory problems. In addition, some people may experience forgetfulness related to medications that aren't on this list.

Medications with possible memory side effects

Category	Generic name (brand name)	
Anti-anxiety medications	• Alprazolam (Niravam, Xanax) • Clonazepam (Klonopin)	• Diazepam (Valium) • Lorazepam (Ativan)
Antidepressant medications	• Nortriptyline (Pamelor) • Amitriptyline	• Imipramine (Tofranil) • Paroxetine (Paxil)
Antihistamines	• Diphenhydramine (Benadryl) • Chlorpheniramine (Chlor-Trimeton) • Hydroxyzine (Vistaril)	• Loratadine (Claritin, Alavert) • Meclizine (Antivert)
Heartburn medications	• Cimetidine (Tagamet) • Ranitidine (Zantac) • Famotidine (Pepcid)	
Pain medications	• Fentanyl (Duragesic) • Oxycodone (Oxycontin, Roxicodone, others) • Tramadol (Ultram)	
Sleep medications	• Flurazepam (Dalmane) • Temazepam (Restoril) • Triazolam (Halcion)	• Zaleplon (Sonata) • Zolpidem (Ambien)
Urinary incontinence medications	• Darifenacin (Enablex) • Fesoterodine (Toviaz) • Oxybutynin (Ditropan)	• Solifenacin (Vesicare) • Tolterodine (Detrol) • Trospium (Sanctura)

Once you set your overall goal, identify small, practical steps that can help you achieve it. For example, if your goal is to get your house organized, the first step might be creating a mail-filing center in the back hallway. If your goal is to use associations to remember names, identify an upcoming event where you can try out this strategy.

As you experiment with new techniques, take a moment to consider the impact your attitude may have on memory. The fact is, many people who claim to have trouble with memory actually don't. But they've developed such a poor attitude about their memory that they continually doubt themselves. They may know someone's name but are afraid to speak out for fear they might be wrong.

The alternative is to trust yourself. Instead of telling yourself, "I never remember names," say "That name will come back to me in a minute." Instead of thinking "I'm such a scatterbrain," substitute "I sometimes forget, but I remember the things that are really important." Move from self-blame statements to positive messages. Be patient with yourself, and take it one step at a time.

Chapter 15

Keeping a healthy lifestyle

If you want to do everything you can to maintain your memory as you age, you have to think beyond brainy games and mentally stimulating activities. Your lifestyle matters, too. That includes, overall, what you eat and drink, how much you sleep, how much you move your body, and how well you manage the stress in your life. If these habits are out of kilter, they can affect brain function and make your memory seem worse than it really is.

Are there superfoods or physical exercises that could actually reduce your risk of Alzheimer's disease? That's not so clear. Healthy lifestyle habits are known to play an important role in preventing different disorders, including heart disease and cancer. So there's a lot of interest in determining whether you can control a component

of Alz-heimer's disease by regularly practicing good lifestyle habits.

So far, the accumulating scientific evidence adds up to a big, encouraging *maybe* — and not an indisputable *yes*.

The good news is that the habits that have the greatest potential for reducing your risk of Alzheimer's disease are also the ones that may have the greatest impact on improving your overall health and wellness.

These healthy habits also help prevent other conditions that may play a role in Alzheimer's disease, such as high cholesterol, high blood pressure, diabetes and obesity. Plus, these healthy lifestyle habits may reduce your need for medications, some of which can have a negative effect your memory.

All things considered, improving your lifestyle is good for your brain — even if it isn't a surefire strategy to beat Alzheimer's disease. This chapter gives you a plan for making healthy changes to your daily routine. You'll learn about six lifestyle habits that may be your best bets for maintaining memory.

At the end of the chapter, you'll find a quick-start plan that can help you begin incorporating these healthy changes into your life.

The mind-heart connection

The latest research on reducing your risk of Alzheimer's disease through lifestyle changes seems to boil down to one basic theme: What's good for your heart is good for your brain.

For years, doctors have known that there are many things you can do to keep your heart and blood vessels healthy. This includes increasing physical activity, stopping smoking, eating a healthy diet and getting enough sleep. Now, it turns out that these lifestyle factors may do double-duty and help keep your brain healthy as well.

In addition, there seems to be an important link between your heart health and your brain health. Research shows that people who have some form of heart disease, such as high blood pressure or high cholesterol, are at higher risk of stroke and cognitive decline. On the flip side, preventing or controlling high blood pressure and high cholesterol appear to be factors in maintaining brain health.

That's good news! If you've already been taking steps toward a heart-healthy lifestyle, consider these measures as healthy benefits to your brain as well. On the other hand, if you've been putting off changes to improve your heart health, consider the impact of this delay on your brain health as extra motivation. Now you know that daily lifestyle choices can affect two of the most important organs in your body — your heart and your brain. Every positive change you make can be a double bonus for your health.

Be active

You're probably aware of at least some of the benefits of regular physical activity. It can improve your cardiovascular fitness, muscle strength and flexibility. It can build up your coordination, agility and speed. It can brighten your mood and disposition. It can help control your weight and lower your risk of many conditions, including heart disease and cancer.

Now, mounting evidence puts physical activity at the top of the list of lifestyle factors that are most likely to reduce your risk of Alzheimer's disease.

A growing body of research links regular physical activity to better brain function and lower risk of cognitive decline and dementia. In the Nurses' Health Study, which includes data from women between the ages of 70 and 81, regular physical activity was associated with improved mental functioning equal to being three years younger than the participant's actual age. In another study of adults age 65 and older, the risk of developing dementia was 35 to 40 percent lower for those who exercised three or more times each week.

There are probably several mechanisms at work here. Physical exertion increases blood flow to your brain, which increases the supply of oxygen and nutrients to brain cells. Exercise also tends to boost mood and energy level, which can sharpen mental processing and memory. Physical activity may also promote the regeneration of brain cells or the development of new ones.

In clinical studies involving rats, exercise appears to inhibit some Alzheimer's-like changes in the brain. These studies show that rats with higher levels of physical activity developed fewer amyloid plaques in their brains than rats with lower levels. Plaques are abnormal structures that are a characteristic feature of Alzheimer's disease.

Daily exercise may offer fringe benefits, as well. Physical activity is often an opportunity to learn new things and to socialize with others, both of which can stretch your imagination and exercise your mind. So you may reap additional perks from walking with a friend, joining a group exercise class, or trying new things, such as water aerobics or ballroom dancing.

How much is enough?

You don't need to be a triathlon champion in order to sharpen your memory and enhance other cognitive skills. Activity doesn't have to be strenuous or time-consuming to have a positive effect on your health. In the Nurses' Health Study, women who walked at least an hour and a half each week at a leisurely pace — which would be about 15 minutes daily — saw discernible mental benefits.

That said, it's also fair to say that more activity generally equals greater benefits. To affect your risk of Alzheimer's disease, you'll probably need to engage in exercise that raises your heart rate for at least 30 minutes a day several times a week.

For the greatest health benefits, the Department of Health and Human Services recommends at least 150 minutes a week of moderate-intensity activity for most adults.

In reality, many people — especially older adults — are a long way from meeting this recommendation. If you're one of these individuals, remember that every little bit of activity is better than doing nothing at all.

One study suggests that when it comes to reducing risk of Alzheimer's disease, participating in a number of different activities is more important than the intensity or duration of one activity. Household chores, such as raking and gardening, and leisure activities, such as hiking, yoga and bowling, all count.

Strategies for success

Here are easy ideas for adding more minutes of physical activity to whatever exercise you're already doing:

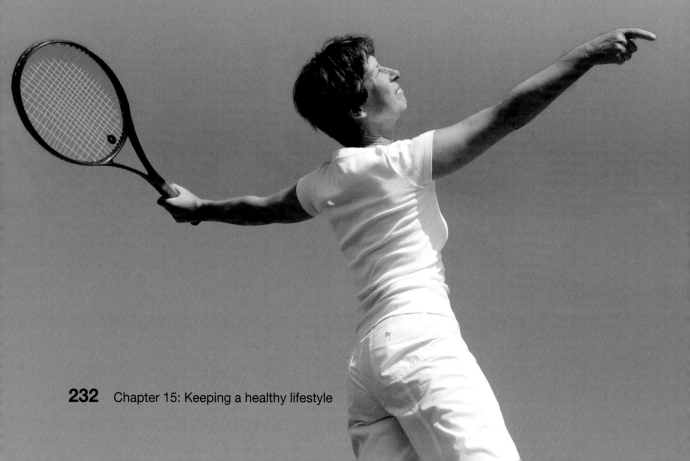

Try a walking program

A regular walking program can help you stay active. But before starting, talk to your doctor if you've been sedentary for a long time or you have serious health issues.

Try to walk at least five times a week. Always start with a five-minute, slower paced walk to warm up and end with a five-minute, slower paced walk to cool down. Start at a pace that's comfortable for you. Then gradually pick up speed until you're walking briskly — the equivalent of about 3½ miles an hour.

While walking, you should be breathing hard, but still able to carry on a conversation with a companion. Each week, try to add a few more minutes to your walking time until you reach at least 150 minutes of moderate aerobic activity for the week.

Walk as much as possible. Walking is a gentle, low-impact exercise that can ease you into a higher level of fitness and health. It's also an excellent way to add short bursts of activity to your regular routine.

Try walking, rather than driving, to locations in your neighborhood, such as the school, a retail store or a friend's house. Intentionally park your car farther from a destination and walk the extra distance. Take the stairs instead of the elevator, or organize a family walk — anything that helps you move and put one foot in front of the other.

Schedule regular exercise time. Identify at least three 30-minute time slots throughout your week that you can set aside for physical activity. Mark these times on your calendar, and treat them as you would any other important appointment. Try picking times of the day or week when you naturally feel most energetic.

Choose activities you enjoy. Sign up for a yoga class. Join a bowling league. Walk the dog along new routes. Take a bike or canoe ride. Dance to music with your grandchildren. As a rule of thumb, you're doing moderate-intensity activity when you can easily carry on a conversation with a companion but not sing during the activity.

Eat healthy

The dietary choices that you make at the grocery store and the dinner table can help prevent heart disease and high blood pressure. Now, studies suggest that food choices may also help your brain function at its prime — and potentially reduce your risk of cognitive decline and Alzheimer's disease.

In addition, a healthy diet combined with regular exercise can help you lose weight if you're overweight. An increasing number of studies are finding links between obesity in midlife and increased risk of dementia and Alzheimer's disease in later years.

To be sure, the link between excess body fat and dementia isn't clear, and there's no guarantee that losing weight protects you from Alzheimer's. But a slimmer you certainly can't hurt your odds — it may even improve them — and provide other health benefits.

Try adding the following brain-friendly fats, vitamins and nutrients to your daily diet. You won't get the same benefit if you try to get these substances in the form of a supplement or vitamin.

Omega 3 fatty acids. This type of unsaturated fat is essential for your brain and nervous system to function at their best. Your body produces this substance naturally, but people who are able to consume more in their diet may experience less cognitive decline and dementia. You'll find omega 3 fatty acids in flaxseeds, walnuts, and fatty fish, such as salmon, mackerel, herring and tuna.

Folate. This type of B vitamin also plays an essential role in brain development and function. Folate occurs naturally in leafy green vegetables, citrus fruits and dried beans. The synthetic form, found in supplements and fortified cereals, is known as folic acid.

Antioxidants. These dietary substances may slow down oxidation, a natural process that leads to cell damage in the brain and elsewhere. There are many delicious options for getting your share of these beneficial food substances, which include vitamins C and E, carotene, lycopene, and flavonoids.

In general, dark-skinned fruits and vegetables have the highest antioxidant levels. This includes kale, spinach, Brussels sprouts, broccoli, beets, blueberries, raspberries and cranberries. Other foods and drinks that are rich in antioxidants include beans, nuts, green tea, red wine, dark chocolate, cinnamon, ginger and turmeric powder.

At the same time that you're loading your plate with the brain foods described above, you also want to limit your intake of the unhealthy fats and cholesterol found in butter, red meat, high-fat dairy products and processed foods. Too much of these foods may cause inflammation and narrowing of the arteries to the brain, which can affect brain function and memory.

Try a plant-based diet

If you like the idea of a brain-healthy diet but you're not up for keeping track of specific nutrients, the Mediterranean diet might be a good fit for you. This diet is bursting with fish, vegetables, fruits, basil and olive oil, following the traditional cooking styles of countries bordering the Mediterranean Sea.

In recent years, the Mediterranean diet has gained popularity in the U.S. because of its ability to reduce the risk of heart disease. Now, research indicates

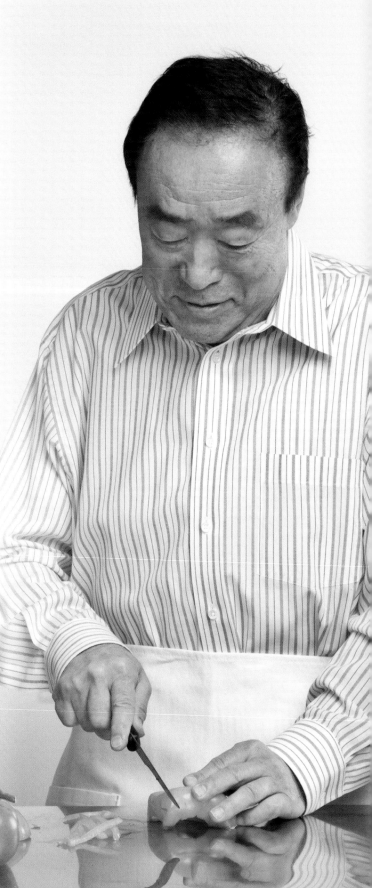

that adherence to the Mediterranean diet may also be associated with decreased risk of dementia and Alzheimer's disease.

This decline in risk may be attributed to the wide variety of individual brain-boosting foods that are at the heart of the Mediterranean diet. As well, there may be something about the specific combination of these foods that makes a difference.

If you want to give the Mediterranean diet a try, follow this basic model for success:

- Eat primarily plant-based foods, such as fruits and vegetables, whole grains, legumes, and nuts
- Replace butter with healthy fats, such as olive oil
- Add flavor with Mediterranean seasonings, such as thyme, oregano, basil, garlic or lemon juice, instead of salt
- Eat fish at least twice a week
- Limit red meat to no more than a few times a month

In true Mediterranean tradition, you may frequently enjoy meals with a large group of family and friends — and perhaps a glass of red wine, if you choose to have one. Participating in a rich, satisfying social life may also protect against memory loss and dementia.

Strategies for success

Although trying out the Mediterranean diet may sound like fun, changing your well-established eating habits isn't always so easy. (There are other plant-based diets you can try, such as The Mayo Clinic Diet.) The following strategies may help you make the gradual switch to more brain-healthy foods.

Make it three. Rather than trying to incorporate a whole list of new foods into your diet, start out with just three — berries, oily fish and dark leafy greens. This trio is packed with fatty acids, folate and antioxidants, and you can easily add these ingredients to meals you may already eat.

For example, sprinkle a handful of blueberries or strawberries on your morning cereal or yogurt. Toss spinach into a stir-fry or pasta. Or top your favorite salad with grilled salmon for a hearty, healthy dinner.

Pile on the vegetables and fruits. According to some research, eating lots of vegetables and fruits may be key to reducing your risk of cognitive decline.

Try filling the biggest part of your plate with vegetables at dinnertime, while moving meat to the side.

Snack on vegetables and fruits that require little preparation, such as baby carrots, cherry tomatoes and grapes. And be sure to start your day with a fruit or vegetable. Blend a smoothie with plain low-fat yogurt and any combination of fresh or frozen fruits. Or sauté red peppers, tomatoes or spinach into your scrambled eggs.

Make some days meatless. Making some of your meals vegetarian is a great way to reduce the amount of unhealthy fats and cholesterol you're eating — and naturally up your vegetable consumption. Start by challenging yourself to skip meat on Mondays, and then move to a couple of meatless dinners each week. Many soups, pastas and casseroles can probably be made without meat. Swap in beans, extra vegetables or legumes, if needed.

Sleep well

Sleep is one of life's basic necessities, right there at the top of the list with oxygen, food and drink. A good night's sleep allows your body to rest and leaves you feeling refreshed, alert and ready to tackle the day ahead of you.

Sufficient sleep is also important for keeping your brain and nervous system working properly. Some experts believe that sleep provides an important opportunity for some neurons in your brain to shut down and repair, even while other vital neuron connections are exercised during sleeping hours. Sleep also appears to have an impact on learning and memory processing.

When you're not getting enough sleep, you may feel less alert and more confused, irritable and fatigued. Sleep deprivation can also lead to forgetfulness and problems with attention and concentration — which can make the normal changes in memory and brain function that occur with age even worse.

Most adults need seven to nine hours of sleep each night to stay healthy and function at their best.

Unfortunately, a good night's sleep may be harder to get with each passing decade of life. Many people get fewer hours of sleep — or fewer hours of quality sleep — as they age. Older adults often wake up easily, which makes it difficult to spend time in the deepest, most restful stages of sleep.

Establishing good sleep patterns can help prevent problems. Healthy habits may also reduce the need for sleep medications, which are commonly associated with memory side effects.

Strategies for success

You'll never sleep like a baby again — and you don't need to. But it's a mistake to think that you can get away with less sleep as you age. The following tips can improve the quantity and quality of your sleep:

Stick to a sleep schedule. Try to go to bed at about the same time every night, and try to get up at about the same time every morning. Your sleep schedule should include the weekends.

Establish a bedtime routine. Make a habit of spending the time before bed in a quiet, soothing environment. Take a hot bath, or unwind with a magazine. Get rid of anything in your bedroom that might distract you from sleep, such as an old, worn-out mattress or anything that causes loud noise or bright light. Keep the television and computer out of your bedroom.

Avoid sleep stealers. Caffeine, nicotine, alcohol and large, late-night meals can all interfere with sleep. So can naps after 3 p.m., as well as certain medications. If you're having trouble sleeping, see if you can identify any obvious reasons and eliminate them.

Manage stress

Stress is your body's natural alarm system. When your brain perceives a threat or challenge, it signals your body to release a burst of hormones that allow you to respond — a reaction known as the fight-or-flight response.

Some stress can be useful, mentally stimulating or even fun — for example, when you're about to participate in a competitive game, undergo a job interview or go on stage for a big speech.

However, stress is not useful or fun if your natural alarm system is a constant siren. A steady stream of hassles, demands and responsibilities can leave you on edge. Long-term stress has harmful implications for your health.

A persistent feeling of being overwhelmed by life's challenges can interfere with your cognitive processes, such as reasoning, analyzing and decision-making. Stress may cause actual shrinkage of the hippocampus, an area of the brain that's important to memory. Damage to the hippocampus can exaggerate memory lapses that you may already be experiencing. Ongoing stress can also harm the immune system, leading to fatigue, depression, anxiety, anger and irritability.

You can't eliminate every source of stress in your life, but you can control the perception and management of the stressors you face. This perspective may help reduce the negative effects on your brain structures and memory.

Strategies for success

Some of the habits discussed in this chapter can help you manage the impact of stress in your life. For example, exercise can release muscle tension, improve sleep and boost levels of endorphins, your body's natural painkillers. Here are other positive ways to manage your stress:

Identify your stressors. Make a list of the top 10 things causing stress right now, which can range from major life changes to work deadlines and morning traffic. Recognize the stressors you may have some control over and others that you don't. Come up with simple ways to resolve the problems you can fix. For some stressors that you can't change, you may need to be more accepting. For others, it may be a matter of letting go — maybe you don't need to waste time and effort dealing with them.

Pursue positive and meaningful activities. Devoting more of your time to the things that mean something to you may reduce the amount of time and energy you spend worrying about the things you can't control. Meaningful activities can also bring inner peace and a sense of purpose.

Try meditation or yoga. These relaxation techniques can work wonders for improving your stress level, your ability to breathe deeply, and your power to cope with new challenges or unexpected surprises.

Stop smoking

Tobacco harms just about every organ and tissue of the body — and the brain is no exception. Several studies have found that current smokers have an increased risk of cognitive decline, dementia and Alzheimer's disease, when compared with those individuals who have never smoked.

Unfortunately, this message isn't being heard loud and clear. Some scholarly journals and popular magazines have propagated the incorrect notion that nicotine is somehow a beneficial brain stimulant that might protect people from Alzheimer's disease.

If you've heard — and believe — this claim, you should know that the idea has been debunked by new research.

Smoking appears to be an independent risk factor for Alzheimer's disease — which means it raises your risk of the disease by itself without having to interact with something else.

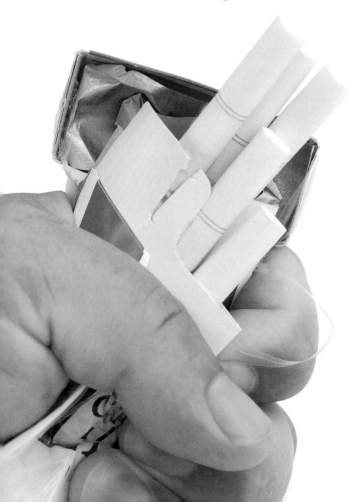

But, in reality, the impact of smoking may be a double blow on your risk of Alzheimer's. Smoking is a known contributor to many cardiovascular diseases by raising blood pressure, narrowing blood vessels and increasing the risk of blood clots. Research is beginning to reveal the connection between these vascular problems and an increased risk of Alzheimer's disease.

However, this risk seems to apply only to current smokers, not to former smokers. This may mean that the effects of smoking on the brain fade away once you stop smoking, just as the risk of stroke and heart attack lowers within years of quitting smoking.

The bottom line is this: If you smoke, a higher risk of Alzheimer's disease should provide you with yet another powerful reason to stop smoking.

There are many resources, products and medications that can help you break the habit. Unfortunately, there isn't sufficient room to cover all the information you need in detail in this book. But you can find the knowledge, tools and support you need from trusted online organizations and local groups within your own community. Some of these resources are listed in the sidebar on the accompanying page.

Resources to quit smoking

Toll-free tobacco quit lines are available in every state in the United States and many countries throughout the world. Call the national quit line at 800-784-8669 to find the best fit for you. These online resources also can help you:

American Cancer Society
www.cancer.org

American Heart Association
www.heart.org

American Lung Association
www.lungusa.org

Ex
www.becomeanex.org

Mayo Clinic Nicotine Dependence Center
www.mayoclinic.org/ndc-rst

National Cancer Institute
www.cancer.gov

Nicotine Anonymous
www.nicotine-anonymous.org

QuitNet
www.quitnet.com

Smokefree.gov
www.smokefree.gov

Drink alcohol in moderation

Drinking a light to moderate amount of alcohol — such as an occasional glass of red wine at dinner — may lower your risk of Alzheimer's disease and dementia. Something in red wine appears to provide some benefit to your heart and your brain. It may be the presence in red wine of anti-oxidants called polyphenols. Even so, the evidence isn't certain, and alcohol consumption may not benefit everyone who drinks.

In sum, if you don't consume alcohol already, doctors agree that you shouldn't start drinking alcohol just for the health benefits. And if you do drink, do so in moderation.

Drinking too much alcohol negates any health benefits you might receive. Excessive alcohol consumption can have immediate effects on your brain, causing poor concentration and judgment and impaired motor skills.

Heavy drinking has additional long-term consequences. People who regularly drink alcohol in excess can experience permanent brain damage due to poor nutrition. They're also at higher risk of developing memory problems and dementia.

How much is too much?

The guidelines for moderate drinking are based on age and gender. So it's important to adjust your level of alcohol consumption as you age.

The National Institute of Alcohol Abuse and Alcoholism recommends that men who are age 65 and younger should have no more than two drinks a day. Women and people older than age 65 should have no more than one drink a day. The stricter amounts for people older than 65 reflect that, with age, your body processes alcohol more slowly.

One standard drink equals 12 ounces of regular beer, 4 to 5 ounces of wine or 1 to 1.5 ounces of 80-proof spirits. If your glasses are oversized, you may be pouring two "drinks" at a time.

Pay attention to how much alcohol you're really drinking, and look for opportunities to cut back. If you have a hard time sticking to this guideline, talk to your health care provider about programs that may help.

Eat 5, Move 10, Sleep 8

You can get started on a path to better brain health with this easy, two-week, quick-start program. A quick start is just what it sounds like — it means you can begin immediately. Eat 5, Move 10, Sleep 8 are daily goals upon which you take action for the next two weeks:

- **Eat 5** servings of vegetables and fruits every day.
- **Move 10** minutes more than you typically do every day.
- **Sleep 8** hours every night.

Sure, there's much more you can do to protect your brain. As you learned in this chapter, eating omega-3 fatty acids, reducing your stress and stopping smoking are important, too. But you don't have to tackle everything at once. These quick-start goals are important steps you can take right now.

During these two weeks, you'll learn that the process of improving your memory and protecting your brain doesn't have to be complicated. Simple, everyday actions can make a difference. The key is turning these actions into long-term habits.

Congratulate yourself that you're taking these initial steps. This effort can lead to a healthier, more confident you — and it can prepare you to make other lifestyle changes.

Step 1: Take a baseline quiz

Answer these three questions to give yourself a starting point for Eat 5, Move 10, Sleep 8. Your responses don't have to be exact — an estimate will do:

- **How many servings of vegetables and fruits do you eat every day?** Give your answer within a range of one to 10 servings.

  If your answer was five servings or more, you're in great shape for the quick start — and the higher the number of servings, the better. If your answer was four servings or fewer, you'll need to increase the number of servings.

- **How many minutes each week do you take part in moderately intense physical activity?** Give your answer as follows: 0 = none, 1 = less than 30 minutes, 2 = 30-69 minutes, 3 = 70-109 minutes, 4 = 110-149 minutes, and 5 = 150 minutes or more.

  The more active you are, the better for your brain and overall health. If your answer was 4 or 5, it means you're already pretty active. An answer of 2 or 3 means you could benefit from being more active. An answer of 0 or 1 means you're not very active at all.

- **How many nights of the week do you get adequate sleep?** Give your answer from zero to seven days.

  In truth, this is a subjective question — what feels like adequate sleep to one person may not be adequate sleep to the next person. For the purposes of this quiz, "adequate" means you awaken easily in the morning feeling refreshed, alert and able to carry out daily activities without being tired or dozing off.

Tips for success

There's a whole science dedicated to figuring out why some people are able to make long-term behavior changes, while others fail. Here are some additional tips for staying motivated and meeting your goals:

- **Be confident and positive.** Believe in yourself. You believe what you hear yourself say, so you have more control over your habits than you think. Remind yourself of this frequently with positive statements.
- **Create a supportive environment.** Surround yourself with things you need to succeed. Keep a bowl of berries in your refrigerator so it's easy to add them to your breakfast or lunch. Pair up with an "exercise buddy" who keeps you motivated for neighborhood walks.
- **Create a support team.** Ask your family and friends to cheer you on. Tell them about your goals and give them specific ways to assist you.
- **Celebrate small successes.** Reward yourself when you meet your goals. Choose a reward that means something to you — whether it's a new, best-selling book or a tee time on your favorite golf course.

Ideally, you want adequate sleep on most days of the week. If your response is four days or fewer, getting more sleep should be a priority.

Step 2: Work on your goals

It's true that everyone eats, moves and sleeps on most days. The quick start attaches specific numbers to these activities — and the numbers stand for daily goals you want to reach.

Follow these goals for two weeks, using the strategies for success you learned throughout this chapter. Use results from your baseline quiz to point out your strengths and weaknesses at the beginning of your program.

Use a simple log or scorecard to track your progress during the quick start. This can be a simple notebook page marked off in columns and rows. For each day, put a check mark under each goal, if you've achieved it, or leave it blank if you didn't achieve it. Writing down and tracking your progress can help you succeed.

Step 3: Check your scorecard

After two weeks of the program, it's time to analyze your scorecard. The results may give you a better idea of what's most effective for establishing new habits or breaking old ones.

Add up the total number of days you achieved each goal.

- Which goals were strengths for you?
- List reasons why you did well on those goals.
- Which goals were difficult for you?
- List reasons why these goals were more challenging.
- Think of strategies for doing better with the challenging goals. Come up with at least one strategy you can use right away. Use ideas in this chapter to help you.

Add up the total number of goals you achieved each day.

- On which days of the week did you do better?
- List reasons why you did better on those days.

- On which days did you struggle to achieve your goals?
- List reasons why those days were more challenging. Try to identify patterns. Are there days of the week that pose special challenges?
- Think of strategies for doing better. Come up with at least one strategy you can use right away. Use ideas in this chapter to help you.

Being perfect in this quick-start program is unlikely and perhaps unnecessary. At this point, you're aiming for consistency rather than perfection — achieving most of your goals on most days. Don't become discouraged if you didn't hit every goal on every day.

And remember: The quick start is only the beginning of a lifetime effort. Use this time to make a firm break from old habits while establishing new ones. Enjoy your successes and learn from your experience. Figure out ways to improve and do even better.

At the end of two weeks, you may be ready for a new goal. Or you may want to try out a new strategy for doing better on a goal that was challenging for you. There's no going back! Stay on the long and rewarding road to better brain health!

Take the long view

When you take steps to lose weight, you can often see some results within a few weeks. And you can gauge success with a scale or a tape measure.

When you take steps to help improve memory and reduce your risk of Alzheimer's disease, it's more difficult to measure your progress. It may take years — or even decades — to know just how well you've succeeded.

This lack of certainty can get discouraging, especially if you're anxious about the future. Stay positive by taking note of small victories. If you eat more fruits and vegetables than you did a few weeks ago, that's progress. If you exercise more and your blood pressure or cholesterol numbers drop, you're definitely making headway.

Count success any way you can — whether it's more hours of sleep at night or more names remembered at a neighborhood potluck last week. Also pay attention to your overall health and wellness. As you change habits, take time to assess your mood, energy level and sense of satisfaction. These are measures of success, too.

In the end, nature and nurture probably both play determining roles in how well your mind functions as you age. Focus on those factors you can control, just as you would with risk factors for heart disease or any other illness.

Excess stress occurs when you spend time ruminating about the past, worrying about the future and resisting what you cannot control. This internal battle uses precious energy. Living with a mind focused on acceptance and gratitude for what you have offers greater joy in the inevitable aging journey.

And try living in the moment, rather than worrying about the future. If you're doing everything you can to protect your memory and other cognitive skills, your life is bound to be a rich, stimulating and fulfilling journey.

Action Guide

For Caregivers

The structure of this action guide represents, in very general terms, the pathway that caregivers might follow with a loved one on their journey through the disease process of dementia. You can read the tips and strategies from the various sections all at once or selectively at different times. The better your understanding of the caregiving journey, the better you'll be able to cope today and the years ahead. As the dementia progresses, you'll likely interpret and adapt this content in new and different ways.

In this section, as in the rest of the book, we use the term doctor in reference to the person who provides medical care. However, we recognize that there are many health care professionals, including nurses, therapists and nurse practitioners, who care for individuals with Alzheimer's disease.

Sections

Receiving a diagnosis

You've just learned from the doctor that a loved one — parent, sibling or friend — has been diagnosed with mild cognitive impairment or Alzheimer's disease. You may have been hoping to hear something else, perhaps that the forgetfulness and confusion were due to aging or that the symptoms would disappear with a change in medication. You're flooded with disbelief. It's hard to imagine something like this happening to someone so close to you.

Leading up to this moment, it may have been difficult to acknowledge your concerns, and then to bring those concerns to a doctor's attention. Because the onset of dementia is often gradual, the symptoms can be passed off as part of growing old. Plus the word *dementia* is associated with some of your worst fears: untreatable and unrelenting, loss of awareness and self-identity, total dependence on others.

These are strong emotions to work through. Your loved one may not have agreed that something was wrong or may have resisted the doctor visit. Now you and your loved one must face the diagnosis together.

Coming to terms

Family members generally play key roles in a diagnosis of Alzheimer's. They're generally the ones who first notice the memory disruption, disorientation and mood swings in a loved one. They may also be the ones receiving the brunt of those changes. Family members often initiate a doctor visit out of concern that something's wrong.

Range of emotions

A diagnosis of Alzheimer's disease or another cause of dementia may trigger any of the following moods and emotions:

- Disbelief
- Shock
- Fear
- Relief
- Embarrassment

- Anger
- Sadness
- Devastation
- Loss
- Numbness

There's generally a lag between the time family members first begin to notice worrisome symptoms and when an appointment with the doctor is scheduled. The delay may be due to confusion about what are normal age-related changes and what are more-serious developments. Often times, the delay is simply a part of the process — the gradual realization that the symptoms aren't getting any better and they may be getting worse.

Denial is often the earliest and strongest emotion that family members feel. It's a normal response to a difficult situation — as family members become aware of a progressive, incurable disorder in a loved one, they worry about what the future holds and their ability to cope. Denial provides a protective buffer from the uncertainty.

Sometimes, instead of denial, family members experience anger. Emotions such as fear and anxiety are often mixed in. They may think, "If only she (or he) would try harder!" — essentially placing blame on the person with the disease. Anger expresses the perceived unfairness of getting the illness: "Why us? Why now?"

The journey from denial to acceptance isn't a straight path. The person receiving the diagnosis, family members and friends will find themselves at different places along the path at different times. People will work through their feelings and adjust emotionally to the changes at their own pace.

In the past, it may have seemed pointless to see a doctor if Alzheimer's was suspected. What was the use? There was little that could be done to treat the disorder. But that's no longer the case. Medications to help manage dementia symptoms are most effective when they're started early, and they can greatly improve quality of life.

Sometimes, a diagnosis of Alzheimer's actually brings a sense of relief. Family members can understand why their loved one's memory has been so unreliable. They can make sense of other changes that have occurred.

If you ever feel like you're the only one in this situation, remember that you're never alone. Millions of people around the world are dealing with the impact of Alzheimer's disease and other neurodegenerative disorders.

Early symptoms of dementia

People generally schedule the initial appoinment with a doctor because the changes in behavior or mental function have started to noticeably disrupt life. Listed below are some of the most common symptoms of the early stages of dementia. Because everyone is different and the causes of dementia are so

varied, most people will not experience all of these symptoms. In addition, the symptoms may show themselves in different ways and to different degrees.

Memory loss. A person with dementia will frequently forget things, often recent events.

Difficulty performing familiar tasks. A person with dementia will have problems completing tasks he or she may have done before with ease, such as following a recipe, using an appliance or keeping files organized.

Problems with language. A person with dementia often forgets simple words or substitutes the wrong word. He or she may respond by talking less.

Disorientation to time and place. A person with dementia may become lost or confused in familiar places and unable to return home.

Poor or decreased judgment. A person with dementia may buy items that he or she doesn't need or spend large sums of money irresponsibly.

Problems with abstract thought. A person with dementia may forget what the numbers in a bank account represent or how to use the account.

Is knowing necessary?

A doctor has just diagnosed my elderly mother with Alzheimer's disease. Her short-term memory is already impaired. Should I tell her about the diagnosis? If so, how much should I tell her?

In deciding whether to tell your mother that she has Alzheimer's disease, consider the effect that this information may have on her general disposition. Does your mother recognize that she has memory problems? If she's frustrated by her inability to remember things and calls herself dumb or stupid, the diagnosis may remind her that the problems are due to the disease. Telling her, "Mom, you're not stupid, you have Alzheimer's disease" may reduce self-blame and negative moods.

On the other hand, if your mother doesn't think she has memory problems, trying to convince her that she has Alzheimer's may only frustrate the both of you. You may choose not to say anything. Some caregivers feel distress about keeping secrets and withholding information. Other caregivers don't want to upset their loved ones. It's OK to do what feels right to you.

If you decide to tell your mother, she may not respond in the way you expect. Alzheimer's makes people forget they have the condition — so you may have to tell your mother more than once. The disease may impair your mother's ability to fully grasp the diagnosis, and she might have no response at all. Don't be surprised if this is the case.

If you decide not to tell your mother, it still may help to talk about her memory problems instead of ignoring them. You can say, "Mom, we bought a weekly pill organizer to help you keep track of your medicines. This will make life easier and help with your memory problems."

Misplacing things. A person with dementia may put things in unusual places, such as storing an iron in the refrigerator or a watch in the sugar bowl.

Changes in mood or behavior. A person with dementia may experience extreme mood swings for no apparent reason or behave inappropriately.

Changes in personality. A person with dementia may seem different from his or her usual self in ways that are difficult to pinpoint: suspicious, irritable, anxious or short-tempered.

Loss of initiative. A person with dementia may become passive and withdrawn, sleeping more than usual and watching television for hours.

Informing your loved one

There are no formal guidelines on how to break the news to a person who has been diagnosed with Alzheimer's. Factors to consider are how advanced the dementia symptoms are and how well the person comprehends what's being said. In most cases, telling the whole truth should be the usual practice.

The Alzheimer's Association believes that people have a moral and legal right to know their diagnosis if they have the capacity to understand it. Ironically, even in the disease's early stages, some people fail to remember what they've been told. In more-advanced stages, an explanation may have little value if people have lost their ability to comprehend.

Generally in the early stages, knowing the diagnosis allows individuals to take more-active roles in planning their future. With this knowledge, they can:

- Plan life experiences that give them comfort and pleasure
- Prepare legal documents that specify care in advanced stages
- Consider enrolling in research programs and clinical trials
- Participate in support groups
- Participate in drug therapy that's generally effective in early stages

Health care professionals and family members have struggled over how to break the news about a diagnosis, only to have the individual respond, "That's what I've felt it was all along." People diagnosed with Alzheimer's disease may actually feel a sense of relief because the diagnosis provides a cause for their concerns.

Some individuals will express disbelief and question what their doctors are telling them. It may be more acceptable to describe the diagnosis as "a problem with memory" rather than using words such as *dementia* or *Alzheimer's disease*.

Your goal as a caregiver is to provide information about the diagnosis in a way that's considerate to your loved one and avoids unnecessary despair. If family members feel that their words and actions are in the best interest of the person, then they've likely chosen the best approach.

Informing others

Caregivers wonder whom to tell about the diagnosis and when to tell them. This can be frightening for your loved one — he or she may not want to feel "under the microscope," as people closely watch for signs of illness. You may be torn between protecting your loved one's privacy and sharing parts of the emotional roller coaster you're on. Consider the following suggestions:

- Create a list of people who you feel are likely to support you. Start the process with them. A strong support network is a valuable resource.

- Consider notifying your neighbors. They're likely to contact you or offer assistance if they notice unusual behavior from your loved one or if your loved one appears to be wandering and confused.

- Prepare a letter with details of the diagnosis, signs and symptoms that your loved one is experiencing, and how the disease will progress. The same letter can be sent to many different people.

- The more specific you are about caregiving needs, the better. Rather than hinting that you're uncomfortable driving across town, you might say, "We're looking for help getting to doctor appointments (and here are the scheduled times)." Rather than complaining about lifting and bending or that you don't trust leaving your loved one alone, you might say, "Can you help out once a week with chores and caregiving?"

- Be sure to look out for your own needs as well as your loved one's. You may appreciate visitors who can provide conversation and emotional support as well as assistance.

- Consider posting an update every few months to keep people aware of your loved one's condition. Your local Alzheimer's Association chapter can provide information about the disease that you may include.

Explaining the disease to children

Adults may choose to shield young children from the knowledge that a relative has Alzheimer's. But children generally recognize when something is wrong. Your loved one's behavior may seem frightening or disturbing, especially if the children don't understand why such behavior is occurring. Here are ways to support young children during this time of uncertainty:

- Share information in terms that children can understand. Focus more on behavior and less on the science of the disease. This may help children cope with the personality changes they observe.
- Children may feel scared, confused, embarrassed, angry, sad or guilty about what's happening. Reassure them that it's no one's fault, and that your loved one can't help the way he or she is acting.
- Children often ask blunt questions: "Is Grandma crazy?" "What will she do next?" Answer the questions as honestly as possible.
- Draw out worries and concerns by asking children about the changes they've observed in your loved one.
- Prepare children for changes that may occur later, such as language

problems, challenging behaviors and the inability to perform simple tasks.
- Watch for signs of withdrawal, poor school performance, headaches or stomachaches, indicating that a child may have difficulty coping.
- Suggest ways to help children interact with your loved one: "Grandma has a hard time understanding us, so we need to be gentle and speak slowly to her."
- Provide activities that children can enjoy doing with your loved one, such as looking at pictures, listening to music or doing easy crafts.
- The local Alzheimer's Association chapter may have materials to interest children.

Leaving employment

Some people diagnosed in the early stages of Alzheimer's are able to continue working for a while. But soon, they'll need to leave their jobs. Ending a career can be a painful process. The following tips may help your loved one through this transition with dignity.

- Inform an employer soon after your loved one receives the diagnosis. Ask whether work tasks may be simplified or work hours decreased. It may be easier to phase out employment rather than quit abruptly.

- Dementia affects judgment, reaction time and problem-solving skills. Consider whether the job requires decisions that could jeopardize safety. See if it's possible to reassign your loved one to easier tasks.

- Your loved one may have mixed feelings about telling co-workers. Offer to be with your loved one at the time and, if appropriate, continue keeping co-workers informed of developments.

- A consistent routine may help your loved one to function on the job without relying heavily on his or her memory skills.

- Being unable to work may hasten the loss of self-identity. Reassure your loved one and bolster his or her sense of accomplishment. Compile the highlights of his or her work life, for example, in a collection of pictures, mementos and notes from colleagues.

- Replace some job-related tasks with activities that he or she can still participate in. Ask your loved one for help around the house.

- After leaving a job, it may be helpful to maintain the regular hours of a work routine. For example, if your loved one previously went to the office at 8 a.m., you might leave the house together around that time and go for a cup of coffee.

- Your loved one may be able to attend elder care programs during regular work hours. Many caregivers find it helpful to describe this time as "going to work."

- Watch for signs of depression as work skills deteriorate. These signs include changes in appetite and sleep patterns. Other characteristic signs are excessive crying and anger.

Becoming a caregiver

Your spouse or parent has just been diagnosed with Alzheimer's disease. You have many questions. The doctor may have counseled you and referred you to local resources that provide caregiver support, but it will take time to assimilate the news.

Often, it's not clear exactly when caregivers become caregivers. Maybe you feel like you've been in a caregiving role for some time already. Or maybe you never thought of yourself as a caregiver before — and, even now, you're not sure if you can become one.

It may be that you assumed the caregiver role as soon as you noticed the first symptoms. It may have occurred even if you weren't prepared to believe the memory loss was anything more than normal aging. Perhaps your father could no longer pay his bills or keep track of medications. Maybe he needed help getting dressed or working a coffee maker. It may have seemed like very little help at the time — but that first gesture quickly turned into more and more responsibilities.

Alternatively, you may have become the caregiver when you heard the diagnosis. Wanting to understand better what is happening may have triggered your desire to assume a caregiving role.

In fact, the point at which people feel they're caregivers varies. It may have been a conscious decision or it may be something that just seemed to happen. But however your decision came about, what's important is that you're working to meet your loved one's needs and best interests.

What is a caregiver?

A caregiver is anyone who takes responsibility for the basic needs of another person, either temporarily or permanently. This may include physical care and guidance as well as companionship and emotional support.

The caregiver may be required to make important decisions regarding treatment, enlist medical services, and represent a loved one's interests legally and financially. Many mundane chores are involved, such as housecleaning, laundry, yardwork, errand running and chauffeuring.

At the same time, a caregiver must tend to his or her own mental and physical health. There may also be career and family responsibilities to maintain.

Caregivers can't control the memory loss and other symptoms, but they can determine how they support their loved ones. Caregivers can also strengthen their coping abilities to deal with the unrelenting, all-consuming responsibilities they're going to assume. You can expect to play a very active role in your loved one's life in the months and years ahead.

Learn everything you can about Alzheimer's disease. The more you understand about the disease, the better you'll be able to guide him or her through the disease process and make a positive impact. Disease-related changes will seem less mysterious, and you may find it easier to adapt caregiving responsibilities to meet them.

Have realistic expectations of the care you can or cannot provide. You'll be at the center of your loved one's life. Strive to provide the highest quality care, but you also need to be ready to adjust, be willing to acknowledge limitations and expect a few missteps.

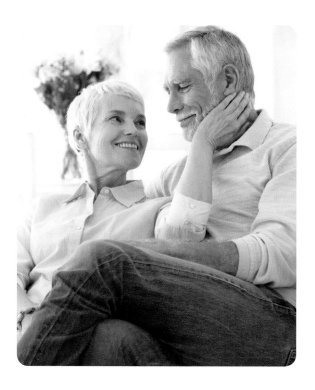

Your loved one may still perform simple tasks with little supervision. But there are some functions — such as managing money and driving a car — that, even at early stages of the disease, are no longer possible without serious risk. Sooner rather than later, you may be involved in stopping or easing your loved one out of these responsibilities.

What if the past relationship between a caregiver and the person with dementia has been rocky? Certainly, previous differences will impact how you think about caregiving now. The truth is, it's important to let go of the past and to forgive yourself and your loved one for whatever may have happened between you. Yes, that may be difficult, but carrying the emotions of the past into the present does no good. It only saps your energy and weighs you down.

There's a story about a son who had a troublesome relationship with his father since childhood. Yet today, the son cares for his father full time and says they've never been closer. The father has forgotten many of the problems. The son realized that he, too, can choose to let go of the past. Of course, he never imagined he would be taking care of his father, a man whom he disliked for much of his life, but, "What's past is past," says the son.

When you reframe a long-standing relationship, even one with a troubled past, you're given an opportunity to let go of that which no longer serves you — most often, your negative thoughts. And you now have an opportunity to create a new and better relationship.

Stages of dementia

Your loved one's physical and emotional health can be gauged by the changing demands placed on you as a caregiver. Many systems have been proposed to describe the natural history of Alzheimer's disease, but each person will progress through dementia in his or her own unique manner. No staging system adequately reflects everyone's experience.

Nevertheless, the following breakdown may help you plan and organize your caregiving duties through the course of the disease:

Mild stage. Individuals in a mild stage of dementia function best in familiar locations, such as at home, and by following well-organized schedules. They can manage many personal-care and domestic responsibilities with minimal supervision, aided possibly by written reminders and memory aids.

These individuals are aware of simple errors or digressions and able to correct them. They can learn new tasks when some instruction is provided. They benefit from home health services and daily checks. They're able to do limited travel outside the home.

Moderate stage. Individuals in a moderate stage of dementia function best with consistent, predictable routines and when minimal expectations are placed on them. They're able to feed themselves and perform simple tasks of personal care.

Attention span is short — generally no more than one to three minutes. Visual cues are often needed for them to begin tasks and continue performing them. Abrupt mood changes and extreme emotional swings are common occurrences. Background noise and visual stimulation should be kept to a minimum because they're unable to mask out these distractions.

Safety becomes a primary concern at this stage. They're able to walk but will tend to wander away and are unable to avoid objects in their paths.

Severe stage. Individuals in a severe stage of dementia will need assistance with the activities of daily living, including feeding, bathing and toileting. They may be able to sit in a supported chair for brief periods and use eating utensils with hand-over-hand assistance. They can hold objects placed in the hand and move body parts in response to gentle touch. Their gaze follows visual contrast and bright colors, and they'll respond to familiar music and sounds. Put yourself in their field of vision before touching them to avoid surprise. Gentle massage may calm them if they become agitated.

Changing roles

When a loved one experiences cognitive loss, a caregiver will often become responsible for making decisions, organizing affairs and managing schedules for that person. When this transition occurs, you may recognize a profound change in the roles that had existed between yourself and a loved one.

Roles are distinct from the responsibilities, or duties, that you and a loved one typically performed. Roles are positions that someone assumes within the family, be it as parent, spouse, homemaker or decision-maker. Roles are established over many years and difficult to transfer from one person to another.

Different roles and responsibilities don't mean the end to a relationship, only that it will change. You may be put in a role that, previously, your loved one had taken particular pride in. Spouses often feel uncomfortable about assuming roles once held by their partners, such as the homemaker. You may struggle to do the laundry or cook a meal if that hadn't been your responsibility before.

You may become responsible for matters that your loved one considers personal and private. You may have to limit or remove something that your loved one holds dear. Children often hesitate to make decisions for a parent, for example, moving from a private home to assisted living quarters.

These changes require emotional adjustments. As awkward and uncomfortable as they may feel, you must come to terms with the fact that people with dementia, even at an early stage of the disease, need someone to step in and help them. Even if your loved one seems resentful or angry for your help, you're responding to demands that the disease has placed on both of you.

The process of adapting to new roles and responsibilities takes on many new dimensions, depending on the manner in which the relationship may have functioned in the past. Over time, this process can be a profoundly positive experience. For some caregivers, it opens unknown reserves of resilience, patience and compassion.

Adjusting your expectations

As your loved one experiences the disease, he or she will require increasing amounts of assistance from you. You may ultimately be "on call" for your loved one 24 hours a day, seven days a week. Activities such as housecleaning, shopping and paying bills may become your responsibility.

You also may become the primary emotional support for your loved one, who will be watching you for cues that indicate how to react or what to do next. Along with keeping your own life on course, that's a lot of pressure for one person to manage!

Realistic expectations of your loved one can make the experience easier. Be aware of what tasks he or she can still perform and what may be too difficult or complex. Expect that confusion and

Avoiding extreme reactions

On a visit, Sarah noticed that her mother was wearing dirty clothes. She also found weeks of unopened mail. Sarah suspected something was wrong because her mother was always meticulous and organized. After a medical evaluation, her mother was diagnosed with Alzheimer's disease. As Sarah became more involved with her mother's care, her mother became agitated and sometimes angry with her.

When people with dementia become frustrated or scared, they often become angry. Other factors may combine to make the reaction more extreme — a reaction termed *catastrophic*. This may be due to feeling insecure or ignored, being made to feel like a child, feeling embarrassed, or being reprimanded. There are things you can do to limit agitation:

- Make sure your loved one gets enough sleep to reduce fatigue.
- Don't expect too much. Tasks that a loved one could do months ago may be too difficult now. Adapt the tasks as necessary.
- Establish routines to provide a sense of purpose and accomplishment.
- Don't argue with or quiz your loved one. Don't say, "Remember what I told you?" Make questions clear and easy to understand.
- Keep the home environment simple and consistent. Even small changes can cause agitation.
- Try not to show irritation or impatience. Respond in a calm manner.
- Provide understanding. Say, "I'm sorry this is so difficult right now" or reassure with a hug or back rub.
- Take the blame. If your loved one blames you for something, recognize this as part of the disease. Don't argue.
- Don't respond with physical force. Consider the five R's: remain calm, respond to feelings, reassure the person, remove yourself, return later.
- Consult a doctor. Agitation can be aggravated by physical symptoms of pain, discomfort, physical illness or depression.

lack of attention can disrupt simple routines on one day but not the next.

Imagine that your loved one is confused and puts shoes on the wrong feet. Instead of asking, "What are you doing?," frame your response in a way that your loved one understands and doesn't feel threatened by.

For example, gently explain that you'd like to see the shoes for just a bit so you can polish them, then help put them on the correct feet. This makes the experience positive.

You can't hope to protect your loved one from hurt feelings in every situation. And each day may have slightly different twists and turns. There will be moments of misunderstanding and tension. Try to view these moments in the context of the disease process and within your expectations.

Of course, realistic expectations apply to you, the caregiver, as well. A daily schedule and to-do list are good to follow, but with all the uncertainties and vagaries of the disease, you cannot expect to accomplish everything you planned or to rush the process and make up time.

Learning from past experience can help you prepare for future changes, which in turn may make it a bit easier to guide your loved one through this journey

Long-distance support

Even if you live far away, your support can be critical to a primary caregiver's ability to function and cope. Stay in frequent contact with the caregiver by telephone, email, Skype or instant messaging. Send cards and letters of support. Try to visit and offer some respite, if that would be helpful. Ask the caregiver for specific situations where he or she could use assistance.

Perhaps the most important way you can support the caregiver is to avoid passing judgment on his or her decisions. Listen closely and ask questions about the situation, but don't assume you know everything that's happening. Your emotional support and encouragement alone are valuable.

Impact on career

Siblings caring for a parent or spouses caring for a partner with an early-onset form of dementia may need to negotiate around demands of a career. You may feel torn between caring for your loved one and attending to work responsibilities. Even if you have satisfactory arrangements during work hours, if your loved one is restless at night, you may suffer sleep deprivation.

- Some caregivers are able to set up an alternate work schedule with their employer by cutting back on hours, job sharing or taking a leave of absence.

- If you worry about your loved one while you're working, check into available community resources that may provide care.
- If you're thinking of leaving your job, consider the outcomes of this action. No longer working may include the loss of income, benefits and security, as well as losing your sense of identity. However, staying with your job may be difficult if you can't arrange alternate care.

Before making a final decision, take your needs into account. Many full-time caregivers have found themselves more stressed and at odds with their loved ones than before they left their

Overcoming denial

Most family members want to be supportive, but some may experience denial about the diagnosis or minimize the impact of the disease on you and your loved one. Denial is a natural reaction that people may use to buffer themselves from painful news. Family members in denial may question your judgment and discourage you from using essential resources. Try to share information with them, but recognize that you may never be able to convince them of the realities of the disease.

Sharing a doctor's written report that details your loved one's diagnosis may help. But the best way to convince people in denial is to have them spend more time with your loved one.

Intimacy

When you care for a spouse with dementia, your sexual relationship will change. Your loved one may experience an increase or decrease in sex drive due to effects of the disease or of its treatment. At the same time, you may experience changes in sexual desire as you take on more roles and responsibilities — your part of the relationship may feel more parental. You may also be uncertain if your loved one is capable of consenting to sex. Build a new relationship slowly, and use your instincts to determine whether the experience is pleasurable for both of you. If either partner becomes uncomfortable with the experience, it should not happen.

Regardless of your loved one's impairment, touch is a powerful tool that you can use to communicate affection and reassurance. Touch can be experienced in many ways, including holding hands and hugging. When used during conversation, touch can indicate that you see and hear your loved one and you care about what's being said.

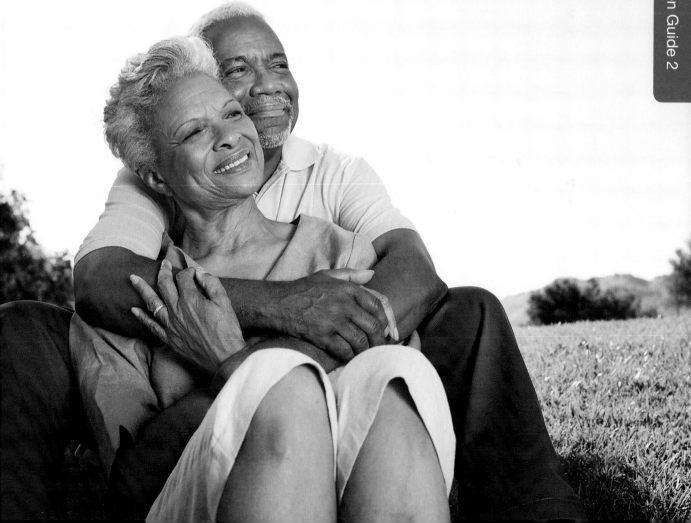

jobs. Placing your loved one in a care facility may be a better solution.

Impact on family

When you transition into a caregiving role, you may find some of the other aspects of your life receiving much less attention. There may be little time and energy to share with your children or spouse. Rather than feeling guilty or trapped by these circumstances, look for ways to integrate the various aspects of your life.

- Consider holding regular meetings to update family members about your loved one's condition and the challenges that both of you face.
- Listen closely and respond to family questions, but at the same time, make sure your voice is heard.
- Provide family members with opportunities to help out if they're willing to do so. Create a list of your needs and your loved one's needs. Work with family members to delegate tasks, but only to an extent that they are comfortable with.
- Be open about the disease with young children and teenagers. They deserve some explanation for the physical and behavioral changes they may be observing.

Some families find it helpful to meet with a social worker, psychologist, nurse or other professional with specific knowledge about the disease. These specialists can assist you in planning for the future, identifying needs and making decisions.

Making a care plan

It's important to put your loved one's personal, legal and financial affairs in order soon after a diagnosis of Alzheimer's is made. A care plan firmly declares your loved one's wishes regarding future treatment and care, makes you aware of the social and financial resources available to you, and clarifies your legal rights and authority as a caregiver.

Prompt focus on the care plan increases the likelihood that your loved one can contribute in a meaningful way. People in the early stages of dementia are often cognizant enough to participate in difficult decisions. Sit down with your loved one — if he or she is able to participate — and over the course of several sessions, learn what you can by way of simple, direct questions. The process is something that shouldn't be rushed. You may also consult other family members as well as a physician, attorney or financial planner.

The following information about your loved one may be necessary to start building a care plan:

- Social Security, Medicare and Veterans Affairs numbers
- Bank and credit card account records, including account numbers
- Will, advance directive and burial arrangements
- Health care provider information
- Insurance records for life, health, homeowner and auto policies, including policy numbers
- Retirement benefits including pensions, annuities, Social Security, IRAs or Keogh plans
- Stock and bond certificates

- Real estate deeds and mortgages
- Leases
- Vehicle titles
- Consumer loans and outstanding debts, especially with credit cards
- State and federal income tax records
- Safety deposit boxes and keys
- Contact information for lawyers, financial advisers and insurance agents

Preparing for the future

These formal documents are a means to communicate how your loved one would like to spend his or her final days and whether measures should be taken to extend his or her life.

Advance directive. This legal document, also known as a health care directive, allows your loved one to express his or her wishes regarding the use of certain medical care and life-sustaining procedures. The document takes effect at a time when your loved one is unconscious or too sick to communicate and participate in medical decisions. There are two primary types of advance directives: health care power of attorney and living will.

Health care power of attorney. A health care power of attorney is a legal document that grants a specific individual — known as a proxy — the authority to make decisions for someone else. For example, you may be given the authority to act for a loved one who is incapacitated by dementia. Often, power of attorney is granted for managing money and property, but there's also power of attorney for medical care.

The person granting power of attorney must be aware and cognizant at the time this action is put in writing — in other words, your loved one can't already be in advanced stages of dementia. The proxy's authority continues after the time when your loved one is no longer competent.

Living will. This legal document specifies the medical treatments that your loved one wants or doesn't want at the end of his or her life. A living will may address issues such as resuscitation, mechanical ventilation and insertion of a feeding tube, which helps sustain life with nutrition and hydration assistance. In order for a living will to be legally binding, it must conform to the appropriate statute — sometimes called natural death act — in the state in which your loved one resides.

Conservatorship. Also known as a guardianship, this legal proceeding grants a conservator, or guardian, the right to make decisions and care for an individual who has been determined legally incompetent and unable to make decisions regarding his or her well being. A judge generally will make such an appointment. This recourse should be considered if your loved one is no longer cognizant and able to grant power of attorney.

Taking the right steps

Consider enlisting an attorney to help you and your loved one prepare an advance directive, although this isn't a requirement. An elder law attorney or special needs law attorney are specialists to consider. Your doctor or hospital staff may provide the necessary forms and resources explaining relevant state law. You also can obtain state-appropriate forms on the Internet.

In case of emergency

What will happen to a loved one if the caregiver is unable to provide care due to illness, injury or death? Be proactive and create a plan that outlines what to do in case of such an emergency.

- Consult family members to create a backup plan, taking into account schedules, capabilities and desire to help.
- Contact local care facilities to find out if you can submit paperwork to have on file for quick admission if you're incapacitated for a long time.
- Inquire if local care facilities will provide short-term respite care if you become ill or need surgery.
- Enlist in a program in which someone calls your house once a day to make sure you're well, or touch base with a friend at the same time every day.
- Consider using a medical alert system that provides you with a bracelet with a call button in case you experience a medical emergency.
- Keep a house key with someone you trust who doesn't live in your home.
- Make a list of important information that an emergency caregiver would need to know.

Advance directive forms should come with directions. If you have questions, ask your doctor or an attorney for help. Whoever is the proxy may be required to sign an acceptance form. Generally, one or more witnesses or a notary should be present.

Once all the necessary forms are filled out, make sure that everyone — the proxy, spouse, adult children, doctors and lawyers — has copies or knows how to get them. At home, keep a copy accessible.

Money management

Because Alzheimer's causes severe impairment to memory and reason, the disease makes people vulnerable to financial abuse. Your loved one may give away or spend large sums of money. You may discover bills that are long overdue or that have been paid several times. Your loved one may not recognize if someone is taking advantage of his or her accounts. To protect your loved one's assets:

- Keep a close eye on bank account balances. Is your loved one withdrawing large amounts of cash, writing many checks or making a lot of debit card transactions? Inquire whether someone at the bank can help watch for unscrupulous behavior and contact you if he or she notices suspicious activity.
- Keep watch for signs that your loved one may be purchasing large quantities of the same item or stowing cash in hiding places around the house.
- Make sure someone reliable has been appointed with durable power of attorney for financial matters. If the disease prevents your loved one from making the appointment, consider becoming a financial conservator or guardian.
- At some point in the disease process, you'll need to take away your loved one's access to cash, bank accounts and financial decision-making. This should be done when you notice your loved one is confused about balancing bank accounts and paying bills or is exercising poor judgment in spending.
- Some caregivers feel reluctant to assume financial responsibility for a parent or another family member. Remember that you still have your cognitive functions, while your loved one may not. It's essential that you step in to help even if the

disease prevents your loved one from recognizing this need.

- Most people with dementia feel more secure if they continue to have a little cash in their wallets or purses. Provide your loved one with a few dollars, but don't give the person more than you feel comfortable losing.
- In case of severe family conflict, consider hiring or having appointed an independent party to manage your loved one's assets.
- Contact the local Area Agency on Aging, Alzheimer's Association or caregiver support group for assistance in taking over financial matters from a loved one.

Financial assessment

The costs associated with caregiving can run high. The Alzheimer's Association reports families often spend several thousands of dollars on caregiving throughout the course of the disease. Personal savings, investments and property generally are sources of income to help meet these costs. You or your loved one also may be eligible for certain financial services that will help defray medical expenses. It's vital that you be aware of all available financial resources.

As you assume control of the financial aspects of your loved one's care, consult with a financial planner, an attorney who specializes in estates or a knowledgeable accountant regarding the payment plans for various care alternatives. Collect all essential information about your loved one's assets. Consider potential expenses associated with caregiving, including medical visits, prescription medications, care services and supplies.

Work with a financial consultant to create strategies for handling investments and assets and to utilize the financial resources available to you. Find out if you or others can gift money or assets because there are specific laws regarding this. You may also learn how much money your loved one may keep.

If you plan to use home health services or another alternative living arrangement, discuss the types and amounts of payment with the agencies before enrollment. Each care option may have specific requirements regarding the type of payment they'll accept.

Financial services

Financial services that may be available to assist you include health insurance, retirement benefits, veterans benefits, tax credits and special programs through Social Security.

Health insurance options. Government-funded insurance such as Medicare and Medicaid — known in some states as medical assistance — and private insurance are among the financial options you may use to pay for medical care and services.

Medicare. Medicare is a federal health insurance program for people age 65 and older who are receiving Social Security benefits. The program covers some costs associated with Alzheimer's, including portions of diagnostic procedures as well as follow-up visits. Under specific circumstances — when your loved one requires skilled care for a condition that is capable of improving — Medicare may cover some costs. Medicare doesn't pay for elder care or respite care, prescription drugs, incontinence supplies, vitamins, or nutritional supplements.

Medicare will pay for up to 100 days of nursing home care but, again, only under special circumstances. Your loved one would have to have been an inpatient in a hospital for at least three days in the last 30 and now must require skilled care daily for the same condition for which he or she had been hospitalized. Meeting these specifications can be difficult, and most people who apply don't receive the full 100 days of coverage. Medicare will also pay for hospice services, which are available during the last months of life.

Medicaid. Medicaid helps pay medical costs for low-income Americans and for people who may have used up their own funds on care. Since Medicaid is administered by states, the benefits and eligibility requirements vary from state to state. If your loved one is eligible, most nursing home costs will be covered, along with many other medical care fees. It's important to plan ahead, even if you still care for your loved one at home. Check with your social services agency for more information.

Private insurance. Private insurance plans vary dramatically in scope and benefit. Some long-term care insurance policies will pay part of the cost of a nursing home but may stipulate the reason for admission and the goal of care. For example, some policies only pay for assistance in a nursing home that's expected to improve your loved one's condition, such as treatment for a broken hip.

Talk to your insurance agent about the policies that your loved one owns. Be aware that good health may be a prerequisite for obtaining a policy. Once a loved one receives a diagnosis of dementia, you may not be able to add any health insurance, long-term care insurance or life insurance policies. And the earlier you enroll, generally the lower the insurance premiums.

Family Medical Leave Act. Remember that you are entitled to job protection if you need to care for a family member with a serious medical condition.

Veterans Affairs. If your loved one is a veteran, check with the Department of Veterans Affairs (VA) and your local VA hospital. He or she may be eligible to stay at a VA hospital rather than a nursing home. The VA may also help pay for up to six months of care in a nursing home or provide respite or family support services. Your local member of Congress can help you secure benefits from the Department of Veterans Affairs, if necessary.

Tax credits. Certain expenses for care or medical treatment may be tax-deductible for your loved one, or for you if you claim your loved one as a dependent. For example, if you work and need to use respite care, you may be able to receive a deduction for part of that cost. Certain nursing home costs that aren't covered by Medicare or Medicaid also may be deductible.

To ensure you are receiving appropriate information about tax deductions, work with a knowledgeable accountant. Contact your local Alzheimer's Association for the latest news on tax-break legislation for caregivers. Contact the Internal Revenue Service for a copy of the booklet *Tax Guide for Seniors* (Publication 554). For more information, go to *www.irs.ustreas.gov*.

Social Security programs. Two special programs administered by the Social Security Administration may be of assistance to you. Social Security disability benefits are available to former wage earners under the age of 65 who are no longer able to work due to disability. Your loved one must have worked five out of the last 10 years and needs specific documentation from a physician that confirms his or her inability to work.

Supplemental security income (SSI) provides minimum monthly income to people who are age 65 or older, blind or disabled, and who have limited assets and income. Much as with Social Security disability benefits, a physician must document your loved one's inability to work.

Funeral planning

Although you may not wish to dwell on the subject of death, you may find it easier to make burial and funeral arrangements while your loved one is still alive. Such planning will allow you, at the time that death occurs, to be with family and focus on coping rather than making difficult, expensive decisions in your grief.

Determine now if you would like an autopsy performed. An autopsy can provide useful medical information for surviving family members and also help advance medical science. There are many misconceptions about autopsy. It won't disfigure the body, and it won't result in additional suffering for your loved one.

A conventional funeral and burial can cost thousands of dollars. For this reason, many people set aside money to cover the expense. Or they enter into contracts with funeral homes and prepay for funeral packages. Either approach will work. It's up to you and your loved one to decide on which approach is preferable.

If you decide to purchase a funeral package — whether it's only a cemetery plot or it also includes a casket, vault and ceremony — it's generally a good idea to shop around. Call or visit at least two funeral homes and cemeteries to compare.

The general services provided by a funeral home may include:

- Preparation of the body for burial
- Copies of death certificates — you may need more than a dozen to settle insurance claims, social security issues and pension benefits
- Transportation of the body to the funeral home and to the burial site
- Use of the facilities for visitation or a memorial ceremony

Some people prefer cremation instead of burial. Although cremation can be less expensive, there are still many costs and options associated with it, such as a memorial spot for the urn. Ask the facility providing the cremation services about various options and costs.

For assistance, contact a funeral director or, if you choose, a member of the clergy. Some financial programs also will allow you to spend a certain amount of money on prepaid funeral arrangements.

Action Guide 4

Being good to yourself

Being a caregiver, you know that your support is an expression of love and respect for someone close to you. You're providing comfort and reassurance to a spouse, parent, sibling or friend who has become dependent on you. Hopefully, you also feel some gratification for the time and effort you put into caregiving.

Nevertheless, Alzheimer's can be as challenging for the caregiver as it is for the person with the disease. One individual thinking and acting for two will demand most of your time and attention. You may find your life revolving completely around the needs of your loved one.

You may wonder if you can still have a personal life, with at least a minimum of privacy. While your loved one may lose the perception that there's a problem, you continually witness the heartbreaking decline.

The demands of caregiving are both physically and emotionally exhausting. At times, you may feel frazzled and overwhelmed. You may develop symptoms that signal you're under stress, such as fatigue, headaches, muscle aches and depression. It's also not uncommon for caregivers to feel guilty, socially isolated and frustrated with the person they're caring for.

Understanding the personal challenges you may face is as important in your caregiving role as knowing how to provide quality care for your loved one. This section is intended to help you recognize these challenges and provides strategies to overcome them.

Focus on yourself

Many caregivers become so focused on the needs of their loved ones that they often forget or ignore their own basic needs. For example, some caregivers don't take time to eat well, get enough exercise, get adequate sleep and take occasional breaks from the daily grind of caregiving.

What's the frequent result? Caregivers often become frustrated, run-down and potentially burned out. Burnout is a state of emotional and physical exhaustion and low morale that often ends with the caregiver giving up his or her duties all together.

Thinking about yourself may seem at odds with your decision to be a caregiver — all your attention is supposed to be directed at someone else, right? But it's not selfish or self-centered to focus on your own needs and desires — in fact, it's a fundamental tenet of a caregiver's job.

Staying healthy is the best way to maintain the levels of physical and emotional energy that you'll need to remain a caregiver for the long term. Staying motivated increases feelings of well-being and reassurance, both for you and for your loved one.

Consider the alternative — what can you contribute to caregiving if you're sick or fatigued? What kind of care will your loved one receive if you're depressed, emotionally drained and no longer willing to participate in decisions related to care? That's why it's critical for caregivers to make self-care a priority and be committed to their own physical and mental health.

Finding a balance

To avoid being overwhelmed by the responsibilities of caregiving, it's important to find balance in your life. One of the biggest challenges you may face is balancing your caregiving duties with other pressing, important responsibilities — those of your family, work and social life.

To avoid potential burnout, here are strategies you may follow to improve your caregiving skills while also attending to your personal needs.

Acknowledge your emotions. Start by accepting the fact that, on many occasions, caregiving will seem difficult and lonely. Rather than being overcome by guilt, try to recognize feelings of anger and frustration as normal. Find healthy outlets for releasing these emotions.

5 tips to help you cope

As you spend time caring for your loved one, you may lose sight of your own health. The Alzheimer's Association recommends these five tips to help you cope with the demands of caregiving:

1. **Manage your level of stress.** Consider how stress affects your body (stomach aches, high blood pressure) and your emotions (overeating, irritability). Find ways to relax.
2. **Be realistic.** Many behaviors can't be controlled. Grieve the losses, focus on positive times as they arise, and enjoy good memories.
3. **Give yourself credit.** You're doing the best you can. For support and encouragement, join a support group or online caregiver community.
4. **Take a break.** No one can do it all by themselves.
5. **Accept change.** Eventually your loved one will need more-intensive kinds of care. Learn about different care options now so you're ready for the changes as they occur.

Share your feelings in a safe setting, for example, with an understanding friend or in a support group. Go for a power walk, punch a pillow, or have a good cry to relieve stress.

Try not to direct your reactions at the person with dementia. Disease has caused the changes in your loved one's behavior — and your loved one has no control over that behavior.

Set your limits. It's probably not hard to come up with a long list of things you intend to do for your loved one —

but good intentions go only so far. You'll be lucky to achieve even a third of what you've put down on that list. In fact, caregiving has no limits, which may only deepen your frustration of never seeming to do enough.

Try coming to terms with the fact that you simply can't do everything yourself. Keep your expectations to what you feel you can achieve safely and comfortably in a day or a week. Be willing to accept that whatever your accomplishments are for that period of time, they're going to be sufficient.

Take regular breaks. A valuable guideline to follow is allowing for respite time — taking regular breaks from the daily grind of caregiving. If you want to take care of others, you need to find ways to keep yourself recharged. It's hard to maintain that energy if you're not getting enough sleep, ignoring your own physical needs and spending every waking hour focused on caring for your loved one.

Consider setting aside personal time for a two-hour break at least twice a week. Spend part of that time in an activity unconnected to caregiving. Even short walks, solitary time at home or a visit to a friend's home can help to revive your spirit.

Without regular breaks, you'll likely burn out, become ill, or lose the ability to support and positively affect your loved one's care.

Get help when you need it. There will be times when you need assistance, even if it's only to run an errand or catch an hour-long break. The obstacle you may need to overcome is your own reluctance to ask for help. You may be worried that your loved one won't feel comfortable with other caregivers. Maybe you think that no one else can provide care as well as you can.

In fact, getting help can make caregiving less burdensome, both physically and emotionally. The assistance can provide resources and skills that you may not possess and allow you to rejuvenate your energy. Your loved one's experience may seem to improve, either because of the opportunity to socialize with more people, or in response to your lowered stress level.

Managing stress

Many different kinds of stress can hit a caregiver from many different directions. The sources of stress may change from day to day, increasing your level of uncertainty. Common sources of stress include:

- Having too much to do
- Added, unforeseen responsibilities
- Routine frustrations of care, which often are beyond your control
- Changes that inhibit your lifestyle, social life and future plans
- Feeling inadequate to the task of caregiving
- Repeated questions
- Mundane tasks
- Sense of personal loss or grief associated with having to assume caregiving responsibilities

Warning signs of stress

Recognizing the early warning signs is the foundation of good stress management. Often, caregivers don't recognize stress overload until they experience one or more signs and symptoms. The Alzheimer's Association lists the following signs and symptoms as common warning signs of caregiver stress:

- Denial about the disease and its progression
- Anger toward the person with Alzheimer's disease
- Social withdrawal from friends and activities
- Anxiety about the future
- Depression
- Exhaustion
- Sleeplessness
- Irritability
- Lack of concentration
- Health problems that begin to take a mental or physical toll, or both

- Disagreements with others regarding care of your loved one
- Uncertainty about what the future holds for you

Take time to reflect on what are the main stressors in your daily life. Then develop a stress management plan to deal with these issues.

Identify your stressors. When you're feeling overwhelmed by stress, jot down the particular circumstances that may have triggered your emotions in a notebook. Over time, look for patterns in your behavior. Realize that stress can be caused by external factors, such as environment, family relations or unpredictable events, as well as by internal factors, such as negative attitudes, unrealistic expectations or perfectionism.

Examine your stressors. Try to identify the causes of stress at their roots. Ask yourself, "How can I change this situation?" or "How can I improve the manner in which I cope with this situation?" Remember that there are some aspects of your life that you can't change — for example, your job responsibilities or dealing with the morning traffic — and other aspects that you can change — for example, simplifying your work schedule.

Select one stressor. It's best to focus your efforts on relieving one stressor at a time. Choose one that you feel most ready to address. When you have some success, systematically move on to the next stressor.

Set achievable goals. Consider several changes you can make in your lifestyle that may help stop or relieve the stressor you've selected. Make the change that you're most willing to make or that seems the most practical and doable. If that doesn't work, try another of your options.

Learn to relax. Develop a strategy that helps you relax whenever you find yourself becoming stressed. Some strategies are described in the section on the next page.

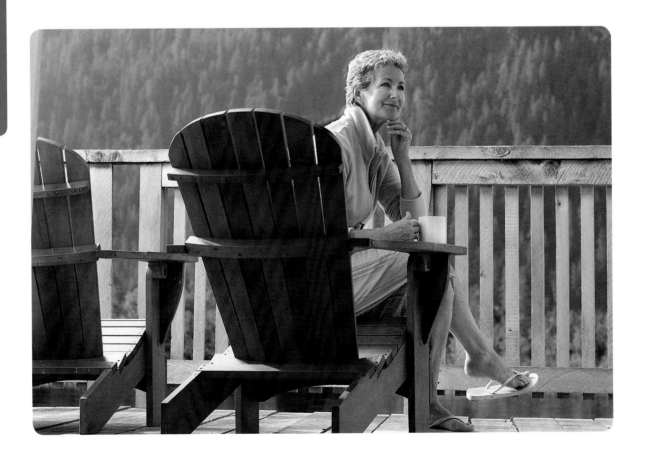

For example, as a caregiver you may feel as if you spend all of your physical energy caring for your spouse or parent. You always used to be able to walk with your neighbor in the mornings, but now it seems like you never have the time. This makes you upset and a little depressed.

Set a goal to make time for regular exercise. Here are practical changes that might help you achieve this:

- Make arrangements for someone to stay with your spouse for 30 minutes to an hour a few times a week.
- If your spouse it OK alone for short periods, walk for 15 minutes a couple of times a day.
- Exercise in the house. You might purchase a treadmill or stationary bicycle or do stretching or aerobic exercises.

Learning to relax

When you feel anxious or stressed, the normal response is arousal — your body prepares to stand and fight the threat or to run from it. Many situations in the caregiving experience can force this response and, if they happen repeatedly, may harm your health. For example, your health may suffer if you

deal with a loved one who frequently becomes stubborn and aggressive.

To prevent these situations, experiment with strategies to help you relax. Relaxation eliminates tension from your body and mind. By using relaxation techniques to reduce the effects of stress, many people gain health benefits, such as the following:

- Fewer symptoms, such as headaches, nausea, diarrhea and pain
- Fewer emotional outbursts
- More energy
- Improved concentration
- Better ability to cope
- More efficient performance

More than skill, relaxation takes patience and practice. Don't be discouraged if you don't feel the benefits right away. They'll come. Following are some techniques that you might use to calm your mind and body:

Relaxed breathing. Also called diaphragmatic breathing, this technique helps you breathe more efficiently, even in stressful situations.

Progressive muscle relaxation. This technique helps reduce muscle tension by having you systematically tense and then relax certain muscles.

Autogenic relaxation. It's a process in which you repeat calming words or suggestions that relax you, reducing tension.

Imagery. Imagery, or visualization, is a technique in which you form mental images of places, environments or situations that you find relaxing.

Tai chi, yoga, meditation and self-hypnosis. These are popular strategies that may help you relax. Talk to your doctor or a nurse about specific techniques and how you can learn them.

Breathing exercise. This exercise helps you do deep, relaxed breathing. Practice it until it becomes natural.

- Lie down on your back on a bed or couch or sit comfortably in a chair with your feet flat on the floor.
- Rest one hand on your abdomen and one hand on your chest. This will allow you to feel the natural movements of your breathing and help you to control the exercise better.
- With your mouth closed and your shoulders relaxed, inhale slowly and deeply through your nose to the count of six. Allow the air to fill your lungs, pushing the muscles in your abdomen out.

- Pause for a second and then slowly release the air through your mouth as you count to six. Make each breath a smooth, wave-like motion.
- Pause for a moment. Then repeat this exercise several times, until you feel better. If you experience light-headedness, shorten the length or depth of your breathing.

Thinking positive

The endless stream of thoughts running through your head every day is called self-talk. When self-talk is critical and negative, it can discourage you to the point of despair.

On the other end of the spectrum is positive self-talk, which can be a powerful tool for building self-confidence and motivation. You use positive self-talk as you bike up a steep hill, repeating all the while, "I can do it! I can do it!"

Some caregivers don't recognize the emotional strain they're under, but the demands of caregiving can seem thankless. Feeling unappreciated and isolated causes negative thinking. You also may be setting yourself up for feelings of anxiety or depression, which sap your emotional strength and diminish your ability to care for your loved one.

Depression: When to seek help

It's not unusual for caregivers occasionally to feel sad, lonely and irritable. After a short time, many people can shake these emotions and begin to feel more positive. But if the feelings persist, you may be experiencing depression. The Alzheimer's Association lists the following as common signs and symptoms of depression:

- Becoming easily agitated and frustrated
- Feelings of worthlessness or guilt
- Feelings of hopelessness
- Disturbed sleep
- Fatigue or loss of energy
- Loss of interest or pleasure in usual activities
- Difficulty thinking or concentrating
- Changes in appetite or weight
- Physical symptoms, such as headaches or pain, that don't get better
- Thoughts of death, dying or suicide

Talk to your doctor if you've experienced any of the above symptoms for a prolonged period of time. If you find yourself thinking about suicide or making a suicide plan, seek immediate medical help.

If you find yourself regularly being critical of yourself or your situation as a caregiver, work at being a little more affirmative. Try one or more of these strategies to change your attitude.

Replace negative thoughts with positive self-talk. During the day, stop for a few moments and evaluate the stream of thoughts going through your head. Question any upsetting thoughts. When you find yourself being critical, replace those thoughts with positive ones. Convince yourself that you're an essential, positive part of your loved one's experience.

Build self-confidence and self-esteem. Focus on the things that you do well. Avoid self-criticism by giving yourself credit for the important work that you do. Make a list of your strengths as a caregiver. Make a list of things that you like about yourself and another list of reasons why others like you.

Share your concerns with a family member, friend, counselor or clergy member. His or her support can be emotional — a shoulder to lean on — or it can be practical. Positive feedback can help you avoid negative thinking.

Self-care strategies

Self-care includes all of the things that you do to keep yourself healthy, happy and functioning well. These actions can be extremely simple or complex. They range from bandaging a cut to taking blood pressure medications and knowing how to respond to a poison emergency; from routinely preparing healthy meals to regularly exercising to avoiding secondhand cigarette smoke.

Self-care is especially important for sustaining your role as a caregiver because your energy and stamina are being shared with another person. Try to incorporate healthy self-care strategies into your daily routine. Keep regularly scheduled medical checkups and dental appointments. Monitor your use of alcohol and medications.

Also, watch for signs of depression and manage your stress. See your doctor if you become concerned or are experiencing any signs of poor health.

From the list below, identify at least four things that you can do to be good to yourself. Remember, if you want to be able to care for your loved one, you need to keep yourself healthy and remain energized.

- Eat at least one healthy, balanced meal every day.
- Get enough sleep.
- Exercise regularly.
- Take your medications as prescribed.
- Engage in daily relaxation activity.
- Schedule regular breaks from caregiving duties.
- Ask for help and accept it when it's offered.
- Participate in a support group and share some of your experiences.
- Seek supportive counseling or talk to a trusted friend when you're feeling overwhelmed.
- Maintain a sense of humor and continue to do things that you enjoy, with or without your loved one.

Online support groups

You may find a variety of chat rooms, blogs and support groups on the Internet. Be cautious of information you receive from these sources. What you find may not be reliable. Use your own good judgment about the Internet and check advice with a trusted medical professional.

Taking care of yourself will enhance your ability to care for your loved one. Even a 10-minute walk can lift your mood, get you into a more positive environment and refocus your thoughts. Your own needs and desires are included in your job as a caregiver. Don't forget about them.

Finding support

There will be times throughout the caregiving experience when you'll need assistance beyond what you alone will be able to provide. Sources of support fall under two broad categories: informal and formal.

Informal support refers to family, friends, neighbors and faith communities. These groups often consist of people who knew your loved one before onset of the disease. They may be very reliable when you need to

arrange respite care. And their visits to your home can be as much for your benefit as for your loved one's by helping to keep you socially connected.

However, some caregivers report that although informal groups are well-meaning, over time they can sometimes drift away, leaving the caregiver without the promised help.

How do you maintain a connection with informal support systems? Be specific as you inform them of your situation and your priorities. Through a phone call, letter, email or personal visit, tell people about the diagnosis, the symptoms and the behaviors of your loved one. Describe your current needs for assistance and offer suggestions for the kinds of activities that may be helpful during visits.

Prepare a list of things that routinely need doing and let your "helpers" choose tasks that are right for them.

Another approach is to list the routine tasks you do in a normal day and assign tasks to indivdual helpers based on the qualities and the resources that they can provide.

You may try assigning tasks based on the qualities you feel individual helpers can provide. Some jobs may involve physical labor, while others may be directed toward paying bills or contacting local resources. Family and friends often find it rewarding to help — it's a way to show they care.

Formal support systems include any nonprofit or for-profit agency that provides assistance to individuals in caregiving settings. Formal support includes home health agencies and elder care centers. Various residential care settings may provide a place where you and your loved one can live so that you can continue to be together, or where your loved one can live in a community setting with others who have dementia.

A support group typically consists of caregivers in similar situations as your own. They regularly meet to share experiences and emotions. Meetings are generally facilitated by a professional or by a trained volunteer.

Using your informal support system

When someone says "Let me know if you need something," you can give the person a list of ways he or she can help:

- Provide transportation to doctor appointments.
- Call or visit once a week.
- Send cards, letters or emails that can be read aloud.
- Help organize and process medical bills.
- Provide a hot meal.
- Shopping or errand running.
- Do housecleaning, laundry or yardwork.
- Inquire occasionally about how you're doing.
- Be a listener or provide a shoulder to cry on.

The support group experience

Members of the Caregiver Support Group for Men, ranging in age from 55 to 90, are businessmen, doctors, farmers, clergy, firemen, carpenters, teachers and veterans. They all have two things in common: Each of them has a loved one with dementia — most often, a wife — and they have decided to share their caregiving journey.

The support group meets regularly twice a month. The men find support and companionship when it feels like no one else understands. It fosters friendships at a time when friends can be scarce. They listen and learn from one another and become more confident caregivers. At different times, they assume the roles of student, mentor and teacher.

Joe has been a student at times, looking to group members for answers. He's been a caregiver for his wife since her diagnosis of Alzheimer's disease several years ago. Joe has also been a mentor and teacher. Joe showed others that caregiving means helping a loved one maintain his or her identity and sense of dignity — even if it involves something unfamiliar. When Joe helps his wife with her hair and makeup, it's important to do it "just right" because his wife was always particular about that sort of thing. When Joe looked at day programs for her, he found a place that was "pretty" because his wife always liked things around her to be pretty. For Joe, caring for his wife meant respecting her for the person she had been — and the person she still is. The group has learned from Joe's example.

Attending a support group didn't come easy for someone like Joe. He's a rather quiet, reserved gentleman who feels most comfortable handling his affairs in a private way. But somehow Joe has found his way and continues to attend group sessions. One of the greatest lessons to learn from Joe may be that asking for help and support isn't the same thing as being needy or dependent.

Attending a support group can be an opportunity for you to hear from others who have dealt with issues similar to the ones that you've experienced. There may also be times when you aren't looking for new ideas or advice — you just want to be among people who understand what you're going through and can relate.

With more emphasis being placed on the early diagnosis of dementia in recent years, support groups for those with early-stage Alzheimer's are becoming more common. To join, generally your loved one must have some recognition of the diagnosis and must want to talk to others who are dealing with similar experiences.

To find support groups in your community, contact the Alzheimer's Association or your local Area Agency on Aging. Some groups may be specifically for Alzheimer's caregivers, while others may encompass broader caregiving issues.

Activities of daily living

The activities of daily living are routine tasks that people do to care for themselves and stay healthy. These activities include such things as bathing, grooming, dressing, toileting and eating. Most people plan to do them every day. When someone with Alzheimer's begins to have problems performing these tasks — activities that were once so routine — frustration and agitation can quickly follow.

The cognitive losses associated with dementia are often accompanied by a loss of fine motor skills — abilities involving small muscles such as the ones in your fingers. This makes buttoning buttons, combing hair, using a toothbrush or eating with utensils difficult.

Loss of reason and judgment make it difficult to choose appropriate clothing for the weather, to select clothing that matches, or even to put the correct shoe on the correct foot. Loss of attention and analytical thinking affects your ability to learn and correct mistakes. Memory loss makes it likely that the day-to-day performance of these tasks will be forgotten.

Early in the disease process, a person with Alzheimer's may still be able to accomplish most activities of daily living with gentle reminders and occasional instruction. In time, a caregiver's help becomes absolutely essential, not just to remind the person that the tasks need to be done and how to do them but also to manually perform them.

Still, your presence for tasks that can be quite intimate may feel to a loved one like an intrusion, increasing the stress

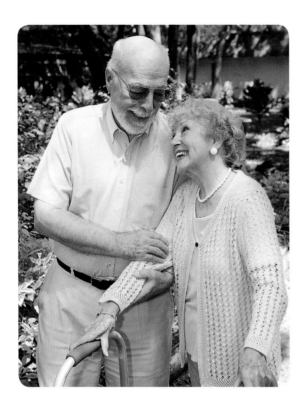

of the moment. Even when it's handled in a gentle, supportive manner, the response to your assistance may be anger, stubbornness and unwillingness to participate, and perhaps even aggressive behavior and striking out.

As you assist your loved one with daily activities, the following guidelines may help make the experience less frightening and burdensome for the both of you.

Take your time. Your loved one may have trouble remembering all of the steps involved in getting dressed or brushing teeth. Trying to rush things will only add to the confusion and slow the process down. Go about the task slowly. If you need to give instructions, break the task down into a series of simple steps.

Keep it familiar. Try to stay with the same routine your loved one has followed in the past and is used to. Did your mom always bathe in the evening? Keep it that way. A familiar schedule makes the effort easier for the both of you. Of course, everyone has good and not-so-good days. Try to be flexible if he or she isn't comfortable with the task at the usual time.

Participate together. Involve your loved one in daily living tasks as much as possible. He or she still can choose an outfit if given two choices — rather than a closetful of clothes. Your loved one may be able to use a toothbrush if you carefully demonstrate how he or she should use it to brush teeth. If nothing else, have your loved one hold an object while you provide the care.

Be respectful. Whether it's helping your loved one with feeding or toileting, make sure his or her dignity is being preserved as much as possible. Even if you're providing full assistance, your loved one may still feel the actions are very personal and private. Keep doors shut during dressing and bathing. Use a napkin to keep your loved one clean while feeding.

Be reassuring. If a particular task is frightening or upsetting to your loved one, respond to the emotion with a calm voice and steady manner. Reassure him or her with empathy and support, not reason. Try to distract your loved one by singing a favorite song, telling a story or providing a snack. Be careful with how intense your distractions are. Sometimes, they may be overstimulating. Use your discretion.

As Alzheimer's disease progresses, the symptoms of dementia will likely worsen over months and years. Situations also change from day to day, and the strategies that worked for you today may not work so well tomorrow. Be willing to take each day as it comes and try different strategies if you need to. You might even retry ones that had failed in the past — their success now may surprise you.

An underlying goal in all you do: patience. Have patience with your loved one and with yourself. You're exploring new territory as a caregiver and you don't also know the direct path.

Bathing and grooming

As dementia progresses, your loved one likely will go from needing reminders to bathe, to requiring hands-on assistance, to being totally dependent on you for help. He or she may find the experience frightening or confusing. Here are tips to help you:

- Maintain a routine. For example, make sure your loved one has a bath at the same time of day. Consider times when your loved one has the most energy — usually in the morning.
- Prepare everything in advance. Have the bathing supplies at hand and the bath water ready.
- Make sure the room temperature is warm enough to be comfortable without clothing. Keep extra towels and a robe handy.
- Provide adequate time to complete each task. Avoid rushing.
- Give simple instructions or commands. Gently tell the person what you're going to do, step by step.
- Allow him or her to participate as much as possible, even if it's simply holding an extra washcloth.
- Provide for privacy. If mirrors are distracting, cover them. Wrapping a towel around the shoulders or placing it on the lap also may help.

- Encourage your loved one to smell the shampoo and soap to trigger a sense of enjoyment.
- Place nonslip strips on the tub or shower floor. Consider installing grab bars for safety.
- Hair care and shaving may be done during the bath. However, an electric razor may be easier to use.
- Trim fingernails and toenails as necessary.
- Apply lotion to any areas of dry skin. Avoid using powder except lightly under the arms. Powder tends to cake in body creases.
- Apply the toothpaste to a toothbrush and have your loved one brush his or her teeth. Demonstrate the motion if you need to.
- Comb or brush your hair and have your loved one do the same. You can perform the final touches, if needed.
- Have your loved one apply a favorite cologne or perfume.

Dressing

Your loved one will have increasing difficulty with choosing what clothing to wear. There will be problems putting on and taking off clothing — especially when there are buttons, zippers, snaps and buckles. To make everyone's life a little easier:

- Emphasize comfort over appearance. Look for items that are durable, can be easily cleaned, and have easy fasteners or elastic waists.
- Replace challenging fasteners with fabric fasteners. Attach key chain rings to zippers for easier opening.
- Dress at the same time each day so it becomes part of the daily routine.
- Buy clothing a size larger than needed if dressing is difficult.
- Avoid overwhelming your loved one with clothing selection. Provide just two choices rather than several.
- Hang coordinated outfits together, or buy clothing that always matches.
- If your loved one wants to wear the same outfit every day, launder it in the evening or buy multiples of the same item.
- Lay out clothing in the order that it's put on, for example, first the undergarments, then blouse or shirt, pants, socks and shoes.
- Avoid nylon stockings, which are a challenge to put on and easily torn.
- If your loved one needs prompting, provide clear instructions, one step at a time. Demonstrate if necessary.
- If he or she insists on it, allow your loved one to layer clothing. You can always remove extra pieces if they become uncomfortable.
- Be tolerant of clothing that is mismatched, stained or worn inside out.

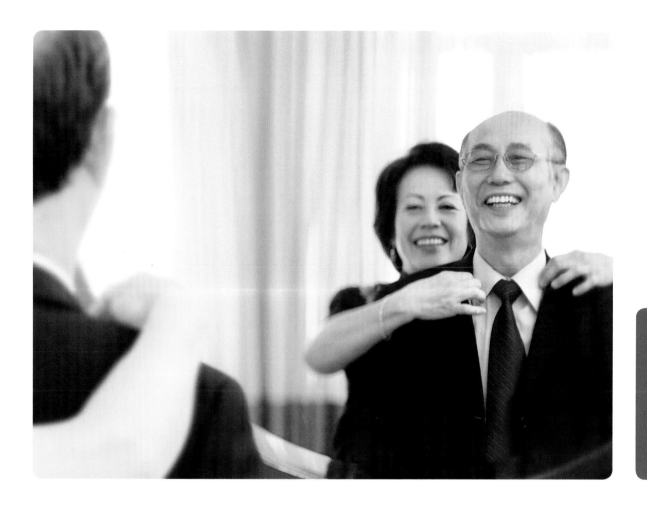

- Undershirts are suitable in place of bras if extra support is not required for your loved one's breasts.
- If your loved one resists moving arms or legs to put on clothing, consider the possibility that he or she may be in pain.
- If your loved one refuses to change his or her clothes, provide comfortable outfits such as sweatsuits, which can be worn during the day and while sleeping.

Eating and nutrition

It's essential that your loved one has a balanced, healthy diet through the course of the disease. Malnutrition and dehydration may increase confusion and stress, trigger physical problems, and reduce your loved one's ability to cope with disease symptoms.

In early stages of Alzheimer's, a person — especially someone living alone —

may forget to eat or how to prepare meals. As the disease progresses, the person may forget table manners and eat directly from others' plates or from serving bowls. Sometimes, the person loses impulse control and tries to eat anything in sight, including items not intended as food.

In late stages of the disease, loss of appetite is common. At this time you should allow your loved one to eat for comfort and pleasure. Provide foods and liquids that are appealing and easy to ingest — there should be few dietary restrictions. During end stages of the disease, he or she may be unable to chew and swallow properly and may choke on food caught in the throat.

To help meet your loved one's nutritional needs:

- Be aware that your loved one's appetite may decrease as the day goes on. Offer food when he or she has the most energy and make the most of favorite mealtimes.
- Serve meals in a relaxed, comfortable place. If possible, eat at the same time that your loved one does.
- Make every effort to let your loved one feed himself or herself.
- Don't force your loved one to eat. Follow his or her wishes.

- If your loved one becomes full after a few bites, serve small amounts of food more frequently, or serve foods higher in calories and protein.
- Mix foods in a food processor to make them easier to swallow.
- Use straws and cups with lids to make drinking easier.
- Use finger foods if the person struggles with utensils.
- Avoid tasks before mealtimes that upset or frustrate your loved one. The emotions may carry over and interfere with eating.

Failing to eat

- In early stages of Alzheimer's, provide simple meal reminders. For example, phone your loved one when it's about time to eat.
- If your loved one lives alone, leave step-by-step instructions on how to prepare simple meals.
- Stay with your loved one through an entire meal. If you provide help, do so with simple commands or demonstrate the steps.
- Provide adequate time for meals. Avoid rushing.
- Serve simple foods that don't require utensils.
- Leave finger foods within easy reach throughout the day.
- Serve several small meals during the day.

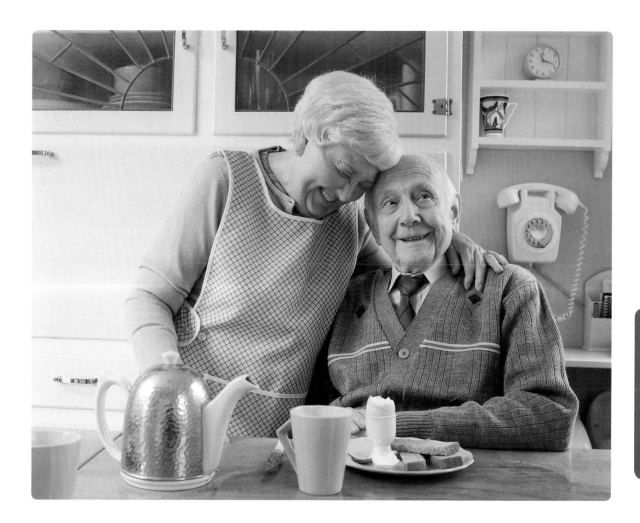

- Make sure the eating area is well lit.
- Reduce background distractions such as television or loud music.
- Display foods on attractive table settings. Serve familiar foods that have varied textures, colors and flavors.
- Use contrasting colors in the table setting to help your loved one locate food. For example, use a white plate with dark foods. But avoid putting mashed potatoes on a white plate.

- Unless weight is a significant problem, don't discourage eating sweets.
- Blend nutritional shakes with fresh fruit and ice cream to improve flavor.
- Have the person smell lemon or peppermint oils before a meal because this may stimulate appetite.
- Schedule a medical checkup to see if depression, ill-fitting dentures, illness or medication may be causing a decrease in appetite.

- Be aware that in late-stage dementia, some people's refusal to eat may signal a desire to end their journey.

Eating too much
- Keep food items out of sight except for at mealtimes.
- Serve food on plates instead of in serving bowls to control portions.
- Cut food into bite-size pieces to help avoid choking from eating too fast.
- Remove small nonedible items from the eating environment.
- Be patient if your loved one eats from others' plates.

Toileting

As with other activities of daily living, your loved one will eventually require help with toileting. A caregiver faces special challenges when providing assistance due to the inherently private nature of the activity as well as to sanitary concerns.

The same rules apply in this situation as for providing any kind of help: patience, calmness and understanding.

Many people with Alzheimer's begin to experience incontinence — the inability to physically control bladder or bowel function. If this is a new behavior, consider what may be the cause: Has your loved one forgotten where the bathroom is located, or is he or she having difficulty with unfastening clothing? Could bladder infection, medication change or prostate difficulty be responsible? If not, it may be a result of the disease. Here are ways to help you cope:

- Closely follow a routine for bathroom use. Provide regular reminders. Generally, a pattern of use every one to two hours works well. You may need to bring the person to the bathroom and provide hands-on assistance to unfasten clothing.
- Attach a picture of a toilet, accompanied by the word *toilet*, to the bathroom door. Avoid words like *restroom* or *bathroom*, which may be taken literally.
- Allow the bathroom door to stand open. Nightlights or motion sensor lights may help your loved one locate the room easily.
- Remove all throw rugs from the bathroom and from corridors leading to the bathroom. Some caregivers put reflective tape on the floor in the shape of arrows that point to the bathroom's location.
- Watch for nonverbal signs indicating a need to use the toilet. Your loved one may not recognize the feeling of a full bladder or lack the

If your loved one has incontinence

A variety of products can help ease your loved one's discomfort with incontinence. Check on their availability at a local pharmacy or drugstore.

- Small pads similar to those used for female menstruation may be placed in underpants if your loved one is experiencing urinary incontinence only. Specially designed incontinence briefs are best if your loved one has fecal incontinence or if the small pads don't adequately hold the urine. Depending on the incontinence pattern, some people use pads during the day and wear briefs at night. Your doctor or pharmacist can help you select the products best suited for your loved one.
- Place a plastic or rubber pad under a fitted bedsheet for nighttime incontinence. Disposable underpads, which are highly absorbent with waterproof backing, also can be used to reduce frequent bed changes.
- At night, you may find it is easier to change pads or briefs while the person is lying in bed rather than seated in the bathroom. During the day, changing may be easiest when the person is seated on the toilet.

verbal skills to state an urgent need. You may find your loved one tugging on his or her pants, pacing, or showing other signs of agitation.

- Often, there's little time between your awareness of a bathroom need and the incontinence episode. Accidents are going to happen. Be understanding and reassuring if your loved one is upset about the incident.
- Avoid clothing with complicated fasteners. Elastic waistbands and fabric fasteners usually work well.

Women may fare better with knee-high stockings instead of pantyhose.

- Dehydration is fairly common and can be dangerous for people with dementia. Don't decrease fluid intake unless the person is drinking excessive amounts of liquid — more than eight to 10 glasses a day.
- Discourage having more than one drink after dinner to decrease nighttime incontinence.
- Any new episode of incontinence should be carefully evaluated by a doctor. Routine tests can determine

whether or not the episode was caused by an infection of the urinary tract or the bladder.

Special occasions

Celebrations and holidays can be extremely stressful and emotionally wrenching for the family when a loved one with dementia is attending.

In such a case, you may wonder how to plan for the special occasion. If your loved one can't participate in large gatherings, should the gatherings be held at all? Should you modify favorite traditions or try something completely new? The following strategies may help you prepare for celebrations:

Set realistic expectations. You probably can't celebrate in the same way you did before the diagnosis — but you can still make the holiday meaningful.

- You may feel guilty if a loved one can't take part in every activity, but it's best to limit participation to a reasonable level.
- Mingle seasonal activities into your loved one's usual routine. Completely changing the routine or altering the environment will likely confuse the person.

- Expect to feel varying emotions throughout the event or the season. The occasion can be as painful as it is pleasurable. Work through fluctuating emotions by taking a break or by sharing them with a friend or support group.

Participate only in what you feel comfortable doing. Caregivers may feel pressure to participate in many activities, visit people or travel when they really don't want to. Share your time only with the people you love.

- It may be easier for your loved one to take part in several small gatherings of short duration rather than attend one big party.
- If you've planned a large family gathering, control the amount of stimulation arising from music, television, conversation and meal preparation.
- Reserve a quiet room for your loved one to get away from the celebration and to relax in. If the group gets too noisy or active, tone things down.
- Don't be afraid to enjoy quiet time by yourself or to attend events without your loved one.

Simplify your plans. As a caregiver, you probably won't have the time or energy to do all the preparations and participate in all the activities you once did. Likewise, your loved one won't be able to handle lots of stimulation.

- Planning a home-cooked meal for the family at your house can be an option if you ask people to help out and bring potluck.
- Limit your baking, for example, by making two or three kinds of goodies rather than a dozen varieties.
- Consider sending a single holiday letter to everyone rather than individual cards.

Identify which traditions are important and which you can live without. You may need to modify some activities:

- Your loved one may get stressed and worn out as the day progresses, so consider having your holiday meal earlier in the day.
- If religious services are overwhelming for your loved one, family members can alternate attending early or late services with staying at home.
- Avoid holiday shopping with your loved one when stores are most crowded. You may choose to shop from a catalog or online instead.
- Do holiday baking together. Have your loved one stir batter, roll dough into balls or simply watch as you work.

- Wrap gifts together. Have your loved one attach the bows.
- Read through the cards, letters and messages you receive with your loved one. Reminisce about the people who sent them.
- Take a drive around town to look at seasonal decorations.
- Plan simple entertainment. Sing holiday songs together or ask a family member to read favorite stories or verses aloud. Play simple games such as guessing song names.
- Avoid setting out nonedible decorations or ornaments in the shapes of

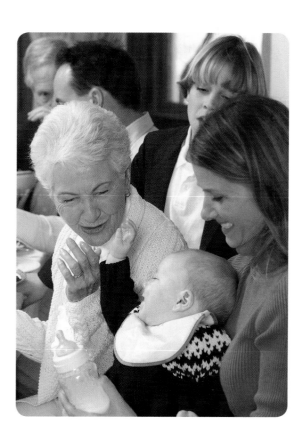

food, for example, artificial fruits. These can be mistaken as snacks.
- Avoid blinking decoration lights because they can increase confusion.

Deciding whether or not to take your loved one away from an assisted living facility or nursing home and to your residence during the holiday is difficult. Try a small outing beforehand as a test to see how it goes.

Some people accustomed to their living quarters begin to feel anxious when they're away from familiar environments. Having small family groups visit the facility for one or two hours over several days may work better. Consider joining holiday activities planned at the facility.

Good communication

Communication involves more than just speaking and listening — it includes the tone of your voice, facial expressions, gestures and demeanor. All factors are necessary to fully convey news, facts, ideas, opinions, needs, desires, feelings and emotions.

New ways of communicating will be necessary as Alzheimer's progresses in your loved one. Remember that a person with dementia is not trying to be difficult or troublesome. What you see and hear, and the changes in behavior, are a result of the disease. Your loved one's symptoms are caused by severe changes in the brain.

Early problems your loved one may experience often include finding the right word, and thoughts that are left hanging in midsentence. Most often these minor frustrations can be overcome, and you and your loved one can continue to communicate.

In moderate stages of dementia, it becomes more difficult to understand what your loved one is saying. Words and sentences become jumbled. In return, you may find it difficult to communicate to your loved one in ways that he or she understands. This situation may frustrate your loved one, leading to embarrassment, agitation and even aggressive behavior.

How do you communicate better with a person who has Alzheimer's? It starts when you're able to accept the reality of his or her disease and the symptoms that develop because of it. When that happens, you begin to shift and adapt how you communicate.

The interaction is better when you allow your loved one's reality, and not yours, to drive communication. It requires you to enter your loved one's world — a reality that's quite different from your own.

In your loved one's reality, the distinctions between past and present are often blurred. The person may be worried about situations that no longer apply, involving children (who are now grown up), parents (who may have passed on) or going home (to places he or she lived many years before).

Convincing your loved one of the truth is generally fruitless and produces anxiety. A better approach is to try and make his or her world a less frightening, more reassuring place. What you're attempting to do is join with and support your loved one, not to return him or her to your reality.

When you're communicating with your loved one, focus conversations on feelings and emotions. Your goal is providing comfort, warmth and security. Don't allow conversations to get caught up in facts — names, dates, places and numbers — which will only frustrate your loved one. Use nonverbal means to communicate, such as facial expressions, gestures and touch.

Basic techniques

No matter what stage of the disease, basic communication techniques can help you understand and interact with your loved one.

Be an active listener. Eyes and ears play important roles in good communication. The goal of active listening is to understand not only spoken words but also the underlying meaning — even if it's not expressed very well.

Establish a calm environment. Some environments are good for communication while others aren't so good. Be sensitive to the sights, sounds and hubbub around you. Converse in places that are free from distractions. Too much noise and activity hinders good communication.

Set the tone. The manner in which you present yourself to your loved one is critical for good communication. Are you nervous or frowning? Are you speaking clearly and simply? Is your facial expression or body language sending negative undertones?

People with dementia may struggle to understand spoken words but can be highly attuned to nonverbal signals. They will respond to them in kind.

When speaking to your loved one:

- Talk naturally with a relaxed tone and pleasant, positive manner.
- Keep your loved one's attention. Face the person before speaking. Saying the person's name or using a gentle touch may help.
- Speak at normal levels, or a little louder if listening conditions are difficult. Politely ask if you're being heard and understood.
- Maintain eye contact and relaxed body language. Let the person know you care about what is being said.
- Speak directly, using familiar words, short sentences and simple concepts. Avoid complicated questions. Avoid logic and reason in lengthy responses.
- Respond to emotions in your loved one's voice. If he or she is clearly upset, it's enough to give a hand squeeze or hug and say, "I know you're upset. I'm sorry."
- Use nonverbal cues, such as smiling or giving a reassuring touch. Don't hesitate to repeat what you've said.

More communication tips

- Give instructions in a few simple steps. After one step is completed, give instructions for the next step.

- Ask direct questions, one question at a time. Avoid leading questions that include the answer with it — "You're comfortable, aren't you?" The person will likely agree with anything you say.
- Allow plenty of time for your loved one to respond. Two or three minutes may be needed before he or she can answer a question. Rephrase your question if the person seems unsure of what has been asked.
- Don't interrupt your loved one's speech. A person with dementia may require extra time to express what he or she wishes to say. Gently offer a word or phrase if the person is struggling to express a thought.
- Use a best-guess strategy if you don't understand what's being said. Reassurance may count for more than learning the absolute truth.
- Your loved one may confabulate, that is, provide details of fictitious events that he or she will steadfastly swear are true. Consider whether it's really necessary to "correct" the truth or simply to let it slide.
- Take note of the facial expressions and hand gestures that your loved one uses when speaking, as they may be replacing forgotten words.
- Avoid criticizing, confronting or arguing with your loved one. This tends to make a bad situation

Communication challenges

There are days when my husband is alert and we communicate fine. Then there are days when it's difficult to make any connection with him.

One of the best ways to make him more responsive is with body language. I demonstrate this with my tone of voice, gestures and posture. If I appear calm, he generally is calmer and our interactions are more positive — at least most of the time. Nothing is ever certain with this disease.

Keep in mind, calm is how I appear — it may not be how I feel. It's like a duck swimming on a pond. To an observer, the duck is floating calmly on the surface of the water but underneath it's paddling like mad.

Allowing my husband time to talk without interruption is also important. I will offer words if he's grasping for an idea and seems to want the help. It's like a fill-in-the-blank game. I want to be helpful and work with the clues he gives me but, ultimately, I want him to express his needs.

I also try to cue my husband with short, simple sentences, without speaking down to him. My technique is to use sentences that convey one idea at a time. A command like, "We're going to go to the store, so please use the bathroom and get your shoes on and be ready in five minutes," will not get the desired results — at best, he'll remember to use the bathroom. It's more effective to start with, "Please go to the bathroom," and point in the right direction. After that task is complete, I give him the next step.

It can feel overwhelming sometimes to try and communicate with someone who has dementia. My support group helps me work through the frustrations. I also have a respite volunteer who stops by each week to play cards with my husband. He loves the company. I need the time away.

worse. A person with dementia struggles to be rational or logical, so it's unlikely that he or she will see things the way you do.

- When giving instructions, avoid statements with the words "don't," "you can't" and "that's not what I said." Instead of saying "You can't sit there," try saying "This other seat is more comfortable."

- Avoid quizzing your loved one or asking questions that depend on his or her memory. Instead of asking "Do you know who this is?" try saying "Here is your granddaughter Susan, who has come to visit you."

- Don't talk down to or condescend toward your loved one. Treat him or her as an adult.

Creating a positive atmosphere

Employ your home environment as another means of communicating with your loved one. In the same way that a person with dementia responds to mood and emotion, so too a person with dementia relates to the home environment. If your loved one feels relaxed, comfortable and safe at home, it increases the likelihood that you will be able to communicate and interact in a positive manner.

- If a noisy room seems to overwhelm your loved one, shut off the television and limit background noise to quiet music — preferably without interruption by commercials.

- If your loved one gets agitated by groups of visitors, try to limit their number or encourage shorter visits. Advise visitors to call before they come. If you or your loved one is having a bad day, don't be afraid to reschedule the visit.

- A long hallway with lots of doors may baffle someone looking for a place to nap or to use the bathroom. Provide cues to help your loved one navigate the space. Place arrows made of masking tape on the floor, pointing the way to special places. Attach a picture of a toilet on the bathroom door and a picture of your loved one (as a younger person) on the bedroom door — for someone having trouble reading, the pictures indicate personal space.

- Be accepting of your loved one, no matter what changes the disease brings. Scolding because he or she can't find the bathroom won't help. Gently guide rather than force your loved one to the right location. Remind yourself that the disease is the cause, not the person.

- Outside the home, you may prefer to avoid large, noisy settings such as amusement parks, stadiums or playgrounds with many young children. Familiar destinations make it easier for your loved one to feel relaxed. Try not to cram too many activities into a single excursion. Plan rest periods between activities, and locate a quiet spot to retreat to if necessary.

What's behavior telling you?

When dementia limits your loved one's cognitive and verbal skills, behavior often becomes his or her way to communicate needs to others. While these behaviors are meaningful, they may not be intentional — your loved one isn't doing harmful or embarrassing actions on purpose. More likely, a message is being conveyed that he or she can no longer express in words.

Consider what the gestures and actions may be telling you in addition to words. Try to view the situation through your loved one's eyes. Keep his or her reality to time and place in mind.

A bit of detective work may help you understand the message behind a behavior. Agitation, for example, can have many causes. Look for clues in the environment — is it too noisy or too drafty in the room? Perhaps a task your loved one is trying to accomplish is too difficult. Maybe your tone of voice sounds too demanding.

Stubbornness and lack of cooperation can be expressions of embarrassment, fear or not understanding the directions that you're providing. Your loved one may be sensing a loss of control over his or her life.

For example, your husband may be restless and repeatedly asking to go home. He may no longer recognize the place where he is as "home." In his reality, he may believe he's younger and be immersed in memories of childhood.

Home often is associated with comfort, familiarity, safety and belonging. Can you find other ways to help your husband feel that way? Paging through a book of old photos while wrapped in a familiar blanket and holding hands, for example, may provide some of the comforts he seeks.

Correcting your loved one

Sometimes, your loved one will say things that aren't true. This is a common symptom of dementia. The statement may be relatively minor, such as a wrong name or date, or it may feel disturbing, hurtful or embarrassing to you and to others.

Perhaps your wife tells a visitor that you force her to stay at home, never allowing her to leave the house. Do you attempt to correct your wife directly? How do you let other people know the statement is incorrect? Does "truth" really matter in this situation?

Consider the primary goals you've set for yourself as a caregiver. How does the offending statement affect your relationship with your loved one? Which is more important: insisting on the absolute truth or helping your loved one feel accepted and reassured? Are you simply tired of being on constant alert for the misstatements?

You may try a gentle correction, but pay close attention to your loved one's reaction. For example, if your wife laughs and says, "Oh yes, that's right, we went for a walk this morning," then your correction was not a big deal. If she continues to contradict you or becomes angry, then your correction may be doing more harm than good.

You may also wait until later — when you're out of your loved one's hearing range — to correct or clarify the misstatement with others. A glance or subtle shake of your head at the time the statement is made also may set the record straight for your friends. Most people probably realize that your loved one is confused.

If the incorrect statements are being made during an interview with a doctor that may lead to a diagnosis, mentally note your concerns and ask for time alone with the doctor to express them.

Surviving social situations

Bustle, activity, noise, large groups, unfamiliar faces — all of these factors can disorient and intimidate a person with Alzheimer's. Reassure your loved one in social settings by staying close by and stepping in when he or she is unsure of what to do or to expect.

Preparation beforehand may help. If possible, review the names of attendees with your loved one before going to an event. Don't hesitate to give prompts that ease concerns, for example, "You remember our neighbor Joe from across the street? He'll be there."

Some caregivers carry a card that reads, for example, "The person accompanying me has Alzheimer's disease. Thanks for your patience." This card can be shown to clerks, cashiers, waiters and others to quietly explain your loved one's behavior without making a public announcement and without embarrassment to him or her.

Some people with dementia may feel smothered if you're overly protective. Consider beforehand how much assistance your loved one requires. Also recognize that no matter how much or how little you do, he or she may never be satisfied with the assistance you're providing — and you may bear the brunt of that dissatisfaction.

Visiting

Some people find the experience of visiting a person with dementia to be frightening or emotionally wrenching. This may be, in part, because they don't understand the condition or have not interacted before with individuals who have symptoms of dementia.

Generally, the more information you have about the person before a visit, the more at ease you're likely to feel during the visit. Learn as much as you can about family and friends, personality traits, lifestyle, work history, and daily routines. This information will provide you with conversation topics and opportunities to share your own story.

Bring activities that can be shared — if they're at the level of the person's ability to participate in them. Reminiscence is an excellent way to connect with someone. This can come from looking at a photo album, telling a familiar story, talking about a favorite pet or listening to music.

People with dementia are sensitive to other people's moods, expressions, body language and tone of voice. Project a positive presence and don't carry the stress of your daily life with you on the visit. Gain their trust with warmth, reassurance and a confident smile.

Challenging behaviors

Some of the most perplexing signs and symptoms of Alzheimer's disease or related forms of dementia are brought on by changes in personality and behavior. The easygoing, trusting person that had existed before the disease may now be withdrawn and suspicious. A person who had been gentle and polite to others may now appear irritable, short-tempered and physically aggressive as the disease progresses.

Family, friends and caregivers must recognize and accept that the ways they may have interacted with their loved one in the past — before the disease took hold — may no longer be appropriate or effective. They will need to adapt their roles in the relationship in response to severe personality changes and learn new strategies for dealing with challenging behaviors.

This section can help caregivers better understand the nature of these changes and offer practical strategies for managing them. Challenging behaviors are normal and to be expected — it's a part of Alzheimer's disease. A person with dementia does not have the capacity to alter his or her actions. However, caregivers can help reduce the occurrence and lessen their impact.

Understanding challenging behaviors

For the purpose of this section, *behavior* is defined as "any action that can be seen and described." Being able to see a behavior allows you to collect information about it — how often it happens, for how long it occurs and what factors seem to trigger it.

Behavior is generally considered challenging if, for some reason, it's not deemed acceptable to you or to others. This could mean a behavior that's dangerous to someone (such as hitting or slapping) or damaging to something (such as throwing or breaking objects) or unpleasant to experience (such as yelling and arguing). Several challenging behaviors may happen at once.

People with dementia often lose their ability to verbally express themselves before they lose their ability to understand others. Behavior becomes an increasingly important way to compensate for this loss of verbal expression and to have urgent needs understood.

When your loved one exhibits an undesirable behavior — let's say, he or she resists bathing — your reaction will naturally be to stop or change that behavior. However, due to cognitive changes taking place in his or her brain, you can't reason with your loved one or teach new skills. A more reasonable, constructive goal would be to reduce the frequency or intensity of that behavior.

As you consider ways to respond, remember that your loved one isn't acting like this on purpose. Although you may feel angry or upset, do your best not to react negatively. Try not to label the person as "bad" or a "problem" — this only fosters a sense of futility in your loved one.

The following factors may contribute to many undesirable behaviors:

Physical discomfort. Behavior may be provoked by pain, fever, infection, a need to go to the bathroom or other discomforts.

Environment. Behavior may be provoked by the surroundings — an unfamiliar place, noise or lighting, or an uncomfortable temperature. An environment can be overstimulating or understimulating, either of which may lead to challenging behaviors.

Tasks. Behavior may be provoked by your loved one's inability to perform an activity or task that has become too complicated or misunderstood.

Managing challenging behaviors

Your loved one's behavior does have a purpose, although sometimes it may seem out of place or illogical. You may need to go along with it, and there may be little you can do to change it

Key questions to ask about challenging behaviors

People with Alzheimer's disease have a brain disorder that changes whom they have been and shapes whom they are now. Instead of trying to control their behavior, the question to ask is:

1) Can I accommodate the behavior?

If that is not possible, the question becomes:

2) What can I change that lessens this behavior — the physical environment, the activity, my behavior or approach?

anyway. For example, if your loved one insists on sleeping on the floor, sometimes it makes sense to accommodate him or her by making the environment comfortable and safe to do so.

Look to the following strategies to help you deal with challenging behaviors.

Identify the trigger. It's important to understand that challenging behavior is triggered — it doesn't happen out of the blue. The trigger can be pain or a need for sleep. It can be something that a visitor did or said. It can be something in the environment, such as an unwelcome air draft. It can be related to a task your loved one is trying to do. If you can identify the trigger, you may be able to avoid some episodes entirely.

Be proactive, not reactive. Your approach to a challenging behavior makes a significant difference to how it's resolved — you can establish the emotional tone. When your loved one becomes anxious or can no longer make sense of what's going on, he or she may respond to the confusion based on your demeanor and tone of voice. If you're tense or frustrated, your loved one will likely mirror that mood.

- Maintain a calm, matter-of-fact manner.
- Don't confront or argue with your loved one.
- Don't speak in a condescending manner.
- Avoid negative phrases using "don't," "can't," and "stop."

Relate life history to everything.
The more you know about your loved one's past, the more you may comprehend his or her behavior of the present. Sometimes, actions that don't seem to make sense stem from something that happened a long time ago. For example:

Problem — A woman with Alzheimer's disease always grows restless around 4 o'clock in the afternoon. As a young adult, she had loved entertaining and attending small social gatherings.

Solution — Establishing a 4 o'clock teatime as a daily event makes the restlessness easier to handle.

Set the right amount of stimulation.
Regularly review your loved one's response to his or her surroundings. Early in the disease, a person will generally benefit from some structured activity and social stimulation. Not having enough to do can lead to boredom — and dementia mixed with boredom increases the risk of challenging behaviors.

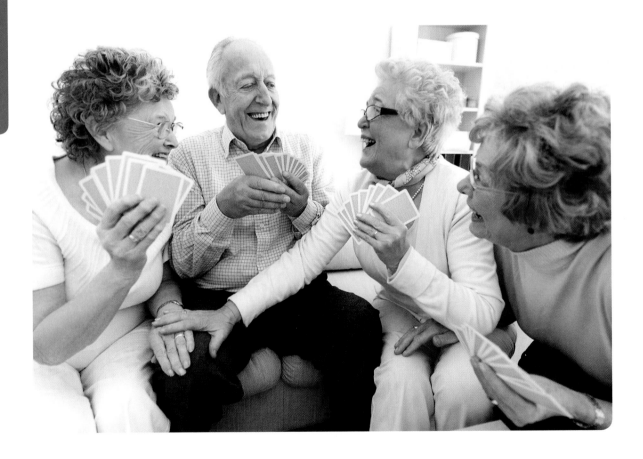

At later stages, stimulation becomes a trickier issue because too much can produce challenging behaviors. A calmer, quieter environment with minimal activity may work better. Tactile stimulation (based on touch) often is successful — a warm blanket or a stuffed toy animal to hold and stroke.

Offer an illusion of control. Nobody likes the feeling of someone ordering them around all of the time — and this applies to people with dementia. If caregivers communicate in ways that make loved ones feel they have no control over their own decisions, anger often follows. Caregivers can adapt to new ways of communicating that offer a greater sense of dignity and control.

Don't take shortcuts to distract. A successful approach to dealing with challenging behaviors is known as "join, validate, distract" — join their reality, validate their feelings, and then find ways to distract their attention. Don't jump ahead in the sequence to distract before you've taken time to connect with your loved one.

Distraction is not effective unless your loved one feels as if he or she has been understood and his or her concern is being addressed. Once you've provided that reassurance, you're more likely to redirect your loved one successfully to a new activity.

Avoid creating a behavior vacuum. It's too easy to focus on the behaviors you don't want your loved one to do. Sometimes what you overlook are the ways in which your loved one is supposed behave — what are the alternatives? This requires encouraging the behaviors that you want your loved one to be engaged in. If you can find meaningful activities to do, it's unlikely that your loved one will respond with behavior that's challenging.

Accept your loved one's reality. Remember that you, as a caregiver, must learn to accept your loved one's reality — a reality that's unlikely to be anchored in present time. Logic and reason typically don't work as ways to reconnect your loved one to the "truth." Acceptance means allowing your loved one to experience the disease and to love his or her reality.

Reassure. Don't hold back efforts to comfort your loved one. The emotions that drive a challenging behavior, no matter how extreme or ill-founded they are, can feel very real to your loved one. Respond to those emotions positively with reassuring words, expressions, gestures and touch.

Resolving anger and agitation

Ted, in the early stages of Alzheimer's disease, was accompanying his wife, Maureen, to a family wedding that was a two-day drive from home. After the rehearsal dinner, sitting in the car in the hotel parking lot, Ted informed Maureen that he was ready to go home. Maureen explained that it was already late in the evening and the wedding was tomorrow afternoon. They would not be going home. Ted became angry and said to his wife, "I'm sleeping in the car!" He refused to budge.

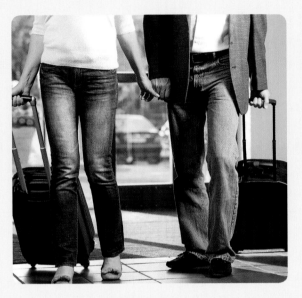

It's not surprising that after a long day in a hectic environment, Ted would be worn out and susceptible to agitation. Ted wanted to return to the comfort and familiarity of his own home. Maureen's response only made Ted more determined to stay in the car. Maureen could change her approach by saying:

"Ted, I understand that you want to go home. It's been a long day, and I'm tired, too. It's OK if you want to sleep in the car tonight. Why don't we get a blanket and pillow from the hotel room so you'll be comfortable?"

Hearing this, Ted is more likely to follow Maureen into the hotel room. He knows his emotions have been heard, his wife understands his request, and he feels more in control. Once in the hotel room, Maureen can say, "It feels good to relax. Would you like to watch TV and order room service before you go back outside? I know I'm a little hungry." After a short time in a calm environment, Ted likely will forget his demand to go home and want to stay right where he is in the hotel room.

Challenging symptoms of dementia

Aggression. Aggressive behavior involves confrontation and belligerent action in the form of hitting, grabbing, pushing or threatening. Aggression can occur as a caregiver assists with the activities of daily living, such as bathing or dressing. It's important to try and ease this behavior before the person can cause injury to himself or herself or to someone else.

Agitation. Agitation involves urgent talk and movement that signals the person with dementia is experiencing some sort of distress. The behavior can be disruptive and unsafe. Signs of agitation include shouting, complaining, cursing, fidgeting and pacing.

Anger and frustration. People who are angry and frustrated seem to be in a chronic state of tension and insecurity, caused by their inability to resolve problems. The feelings often show themselves in a desire to fight back at the cause of displeasure.

To reduce these emotions, you can try to anticipate troublesome incidents before they occur. However, it's important to remember that anger and frustration are natural responses to the mental and physical losses caused by dementia. You will not be able to prevent all occurrences.

Anxiety. Anxiety generally involves an extreme fear about an impending event in the near future — the dangers can be real or imagined. A person with dementia may worry needlessly about family, work or things left undone, even if these elements are no longer his or her responsibility. Someone with anxiety may feel restless and unable to sleep.

Apathy. Apathy is the challenging behavior that's most commonly reported by the caregivers of people with dementia. The behavior is characterized by indifference, often in situations that would normally arouse strong feelings or reactions from the person. Apathy may include lack of motivation, sitting and staring blankly into space, and disengagement from the world.

Delusions. Delusions are false beliefs that your loved one may have that you can't change, no matter how much you reason with him or her. Delusions often occur with Alzheimer's disease, and may lead to suspicion and paranoia.

Depression. Depression is common in people with Alzheimer's disease or

Managing confusion and paranoia

Katherine was in the moderate stage of Alzheimer's disease. One evening at dinner, Katherine glanced over at George, her husband of 46 years, and abruptly asked, "Who are you?" Although startled by the question, he replied, "I'm George, your husband." Katherine said, "Oh, that's what I thought" and seemed to be reassured.

Later that week, Katherine was very upset as she approached George and said, "The kids aren't home yet! They should be home by now. Something must have happened to them!" Katherine and George's three children were grown-up, and the last one had left home almost 18 years earlier. George took a deep breath and replied, "The children just called to say that they're staying with friends tonight. I'm sorry I forgot to tell you. They're having a good time and said that they'll see you tomorrow." "Oh," said Katherine, "That's sounds nice!"

People with Alzheimer's disease often experience delusions and paranoia. In Katherine's situation, she may not have recognized her husband because dementia had moved her reality to an earlier time in her life. Katherine may now believe she is a young mother with children at home. When she looks across the table at her aged husband, she doesn't recognize him as the person she's married to. And it makes sense that she has become worried that the children aren't home.

Although his wife's confusion has saddened George, he responded in a way that she could understand and accept. To Katherine, the belief that she has young children was absolutely real to her — and anyone saying otherwise would only increase her agitation and produce more paranoia. When George told Katherine that the children were safe, he had accepted the realities of her disease and offered the comfort and reassurance that she needed. Minutes later, Katherine forgot her worries about the children.

a related form of dementia. The medical illness causes a persistent feeling of sadness and a variety of emotional and physical problems. Signs and symptoms include anger and irritability, frequent crying spells, changes in appetite and sleep patterns, and apathy.

Hallucinations and misperceptions. A hallucination is seeing or hearing something that's not there, such as seeing a child in an empty backyard or hearing disconnected voices. A misperception is seeing an object and mistaking it for something else, such as seeing a chair and thinking it's an animal or trying to pick the flowers from a floral pattern in the carpet. Misperceptions are generally harmless. Hallucinations may be harmless but also may indicate a reaction to medication or an illness.

Hiding and hoarding things. People with Alzheimer's disease may hide objects in unusual places for a variety of reasons. Your loved one may hide items out of fear that they may be stolen, or tuck them away for safekeeping out of concern they will be lost. The behavior may be reassuring for a person who hoards objects that he or she finds comforting.

Inappropriate sexual activity. Sexual needs and feelings are a natural part of

adult life. Although the sexual needs of someone with dementia may change, a need for human contact and touch will likely stay consistent. Some behavior exhibited by your loved one may be sexual in nature, but often the cause is misinterpreted.

Problem behavior can include accusations of infidelity, sexual advances, masturbation in public, and vulgar or obscene language. Lack of inhibition may cause your loved one to touch his or her genitals or undress in public — perhaps because he or she feels uncomfortable or needs to use the bathroom. Although these actions may not be sexual in nature, they can be considered as such by onlookers.

Repetition. Individuals with dementia may ask the same question over and over again or repeat the same activity over and over again. Due to memory loss, they may not be aware that they are repeating themselves. The behavior may also be caused by misunderstanding or anxiety.

Restlessness and wandering. Wandering may include pacing back and forth, walking aimlessly from place to place, or leaving the house entirely. It may be caused by an unsettled environment, physical discomfort, frustration or

Dealing with shadowing

Mark became a dedicated caregiver after his wife was diagnosed with Alzheimer's disease in her early 50s. After a year of struggle accepting the diagnosis, Mark arranged for early retirement to care for his wife. He had a wonderfully supportive family. He participated in a support group that offered advice and helped him manage his own emotions.

His wife loved reading and would spend significant amounts of time occupied with books. As long as Mark provided for her reading activities, he was free to manage other aspects of care. However, as his wife's disease progressed, Mark noticed that she began to "puppy dog" or "shadow" him. She became anxious whenever he left the room and would follow him around the house as he went about his chores. Directing her to read became more difficult as she became less able to sustain her attention.

Eventually, Mark noticed himself becoming angry that he had no personal space. He could barely go to the bathroom without his wife knocking on the door and calling for him. Members of the support group also noticed Mark's frustration and directed him to respite programs. They encouraged him to exploit his role as a "security blanket" by identifying familiar objects that might substitute for him for a short time — family photo albums, music, even stuffed animals or dolls that could provide his wife with a sense of security and contentment. They reminded Mark to increase the reassuring messages he provided — messages as simple as "I love you."

On his own, Mark remembered that his wife enjoyed dancing. Although he himself had never liked to dance, Mark put on music and tried dancing with her one evening. He noticed that his wife seemed especially relaxed. He took it upon himself to begin a regular evening activity of dancing with his spouse. This seemed to provide her with a great deal of reassurance and relief. And, he said, "I'm finally getting a little exercise myself."

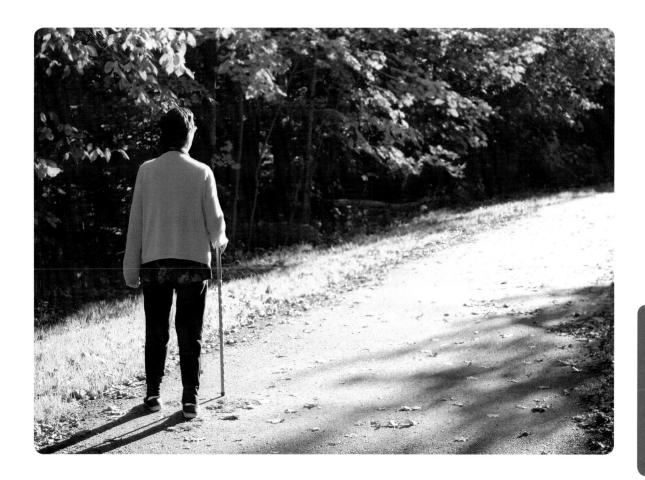

boredom. Your loved one may be looking for a family member or attempting to perform what was once a career-related task. You may register your loved one in an emergency-response program that helps locate your loved one should he or she wander away.

Rummaging. People with dementia may spend long periods of time searching through their belongings or someone else's belongings in what may seem like an undirected, haphazard manner. Sometimes, the person may not know what he or she is looking for. Sometimes, the thing being looked for doesn't exist.

Shadowing. Sometimes, people with dementia will closely follow caregivers wherever they go, imitate their actions, and continuously talk or interrupt conversations. Shadowing often results from a fear of abandonment or sense of uncertainty. Your loved one may want to be by your side constantly and rely on you completely to maneuver through the day. Your loved one may also watch your moods and expressions for clues on how to react to situations.

Suspicion and paranoia. Lack of trust often increases as your loved one's memory loss worsens due to dementia. For example, your loved one may forget where he or she placed a purse or wallet and automatically assume that someone has stolen it. You may even be accused of being the thief. Also due to dementia, your loved one may develop paranoia — a very strong sense of persecution — believing, for example, that people are "out to get me." Keep in mind that these emotions are very real to your loved one. Don't ignore, confront or attempt to impose your reality on him or her. Rather, try to offer reassurance and comfort.

Action Guide 8

Housing and care options

Today there's a wide array of community services and residential care facilities that allows you, as a primary caregiver, to provide a comfortable, safe and secure living environment for your loved one. And you can arrange this environment so that it will be adaptable to the changes that inevitably occur as the disease progresses.

Sometimes, having too many options only confuses caregivers. Other times, caregivers are aware of only one option — for example, a nursing home — that they may consider unsuitable for their loved one's needs. The best course of action is to become aware of all of the resources available in your community and take full advantage of what they have to offer. This section outlines the care options and provides tips that may help guide your decisions.

The living arrangement you decide on should blend the needs and comforts of your loved one with your needs and capabilities as a caregiver. What stage of the disease is your loved one in? What tasks do you require help with? Do you still work outside the home or have other, noncaregiving responsibilities?

Regardless of your situation, caregivers generally perform better having several hours of respite every week. Respite is a period of time when the responsibilities of caregiving are shifted temporarily to someone else. Respite can be arranged through family members, friends or neighbors, or through formal channels, such as community services or elder care programs. Some assisted living facilities and nursing homes may allow short-term stays for your loved one to give you a rest.

Living at home

Many people in the early, moderate and even late stages of dementia continue living at home, typically with a spouse or caregiver present. People with dementia usually find it easier to live in a familiar, routine environment. Additional assistance can often be obtained from family members, friends and neighbors. Some communities have volunteers or professional caregivers who can be contacted as needed.

As the disease progresses, keeping someone with Alzheimer's disease or another form of dementia at home becomes increasingly difficult. People in the moderate or late stages of dementia may no longer be able to perform essential functions and require constant supervision. They run the risk of injury to themselves or causing household damage. Caregiving at home eventually requires a total commitment of time and deep reserves of energy and physical strength.

While some caregivers are able to manage these demands, almost all recognize that they cannot and should not do everything alone. Caregivers cope better with the demands by relying on services such as respite care and adult day care programs. They may need regular visits by a home health aide or need to move a loved one into a facility that provides 24-hour medical care. Whatever decisions are made to get assistance, the changes don't mean a caregiver has failed in any way.

Getting respite care

Research indicates that caregivers who arrange regular breaks from their responsibilities and who seek supportive services in their homes can cope better with stress and keep their loved ones at home longer. These general strategies can guide your decision about getting respite help.

The earlier, the better. Establish respite care early — well before it's absolutely necessary. This can be a trial period when the risks are low, and if the arrangement doesn't quite work out, you can try something else.

In the early stages of dementia, a respite caregiver can be more of a companion to your loved one and less of a "sitter." There's greater opportunity for them to develop a meaningful connection. As the disease progresses, the respite caregiver transitions to a more direct caregiving role.

Coping with the emotions of caregiving

Many caregivers feel guilty when asking friends and family for help, hiring help, or taking a break from caregiving. Keep these points in mind:
- You do many things in your life very well.
- You are entitled to have a life of your own.
- Your feelings about asking for help are normal.
- Taking care of yourself is a gift to your loved one.
- You can't meet every demand.
- You feel guilty because you care.

Don't look for permission from your loved one. If you're expecting approval from your loved one for respite caregiving, you may not get it at first. A person with dementia generally lacks the ability to understand his or her own needs and limitations, much less your needs. The decision to get respite caregiving should be yours, and only yours, to make. Rest assured that you're making the best decision on behalf of your loved one.

Introduce a respite caregiver carefully into the daily routine. Frame the arrival of a respite caregiver in a way that makes sense to your loved one. If you only say, "Someone new is coming to stay with you while I'm out," you'll likely face a great deal of resistance. Your loved one will often feel anxious about new people, new situations and any changes to the familiar routine. Nobody likes to feel like they're giving up personal control of their lifestyles, and it's better to soothe any misgivings as best you can.

Consider introducing a respite caregiver with something like, "I really need help so Martha is going to spend a little time at the house." Or, "I'm so excited that you can meet John. He's a college student who really wants to hear about your ... (hobby, career, family home or trip)."

Some caregivers have suggested that it's best to not say anything at all in advance. When the respite caregiver arrives, simply invite him or her in, have lunch, get acquainted, and then, after a moment, casually mention that you need to run an errand.

Action Guide 8

Safety concerns

These warning signs may signal that your loved one should no longer be left alone in the residence:

- Persistent feelings of anxiety and fear of being alone
- Wandering away from home and becoming disoriented
- Stove burners left on in the kitchen
- Food left sitting out on the kitchen counter
- Food in the refrigerator not fresh and well covered
- Medications not taken reliably
- Strong odors or evidence of incontinence
- Dressing inappropriately for the weather when leaving home

Accept guilt feelings as normal. One reason, among many, that caregivers may feel guilty about the decisions they make is that they set unreasonably high standards for themselves and the care they provide. They feel that anything less than 100 percent devotion is somehow a failure.

Your decision to get respite support doesn't mean that you love the person any less. You're simply choosing to let other people help you provide care. This decision will be the best for your loved one as well as for you.

It's simply not practical to think that you can eliminate all feelings of guilt — guilt comes with loving.

Home-based services

If your goal is to keep your loved one at home for as long as possible, you'll likely need extra support, occasionally at first and regularly later on. A variety of services are available from home health agencies to assist you. The services vary from one agency to the next, and may include skilled medical and nonmedical care and companion services. A range of support options may include personal care such as bathing and dressing, light housekeeping, meal preparation, and running errands.

Some of the most helpful services involve bringing someone new into the home. Caregivers can be reluctant to invite strangers to help. However, in-home assistance may be the most effective, efficient and safest way to get caregiving respite, reduce the risk of burnout and delay the move of your loved one to a care facility. Many caregivers also find that their loved one will benefit from the relationship that he or she establishes over the long term with an in-home worker.

Because home is familiar, safe and predictable, it may be an ideal place to arrange for other people to provide the care for your loved one. The following

are skilled professionals who may be available for a variety of in-home services, depending on your need:

- Nonmedical home companions provide supervision and companionship to your loved one. They may assist in activities and outings. They can do housecleaning, meal preparation, laundry, shopping, and medication reminders (although they cannot administer drugs).
- Home health aides provide hands-on assistance with bathing, grooming, toileting, dressing and feeding.

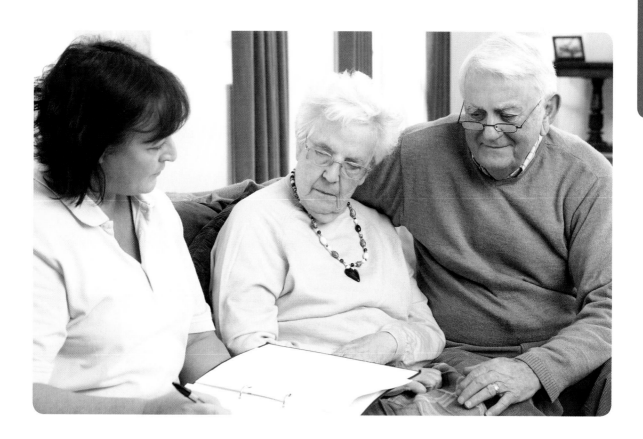

- Nurses may assist with injections, medications and intravenous therapies; wound care; applying ointment or lotion; assessing blood pressure; and using equipment.
- Occupational therapists may be available to assess home safety, recommend equipment such as grab bars and shower chairs, and create an activity schedule.
- Physical therapists may help with recovery from a secondary condition such as stroke or hip fracture.

Medical equipment may be available through home health agencies. You

If you consider a home-based service

The following questions may help you evaluate whether a particular home-based service is right for you:

- How long has the agency been in business?
- Is the agency certified by Medicare, meeting federal requirements for health and safety?
- Is the agency licensed by the state? Most states — but not all — require agencies to be licensed and reviewed regularly. These reviews can be obtained from the state health department upon request.
- What is the professional training of the staff?
- What are the duties of the person working in your home?
- Is there an explanation of what services will be provided and what fees are charged? Documents should be given to you before service begins.
- What procedures does the agency have for emergencies? Are caregivers available around-the-clock?
- How does the agency protect personal information?
- Is the agency approved by a health maintenance organization or supplemental insurance?
- To locate home-based services anywhere in the country, contact the Eldercare Locator at 800-677-1116 or *www.eldercare.gov*, or your local Alzheimer's Association chapter at 800-272-3900 or *www. alz.org*.

may need bedpans, commodes, walkers, wheelchairs, incontinence products, oxygen respirators and nebulizers, all of which may be helpful in the disease process. Handyman services, including minor house repairs and yardwork, may be provided by certain agencies.

Specialized services

The Meals on Wheels Association of America delivers hot, nutritious food directly into your home. Meals generally are provided once each day on weekdays. Some communities offer a group meal at senior centers or religious centers. Contact Meals on Wheels at 703-548-5558 or *www.mowaa.org*.

Senior companion programs may be available that provide a volunteer friend to socialize with your loved one, keep him or her safe, and provide respite for you. Companions may engage your loved one by going for a walk, reminiscing with a photo album, bringing a pet for a visit or listening to music.

Adult day care

Adult day care provides individualized services and therapeutic activities in group settings for adults who are cognitively and physically impaired, frail, and socially isolated. These services include supervision and assistance with the activities of daily living. Some programs are specifically designed for individuals with dementia.

This is an opportunity to take time off while giving your loved one a chance to be with other people in a safe, structured environment. Even if you feel guilty about dropping your loved one off for a few hours during the week, remember that the respite will allow you to be a better caregiver in the long run.

The staff generally consists of a team of professionals, usually with nurses and sometimes with social workers and therapists. Most centers are open from morning until early afternoon, five days a week. You generally can schedule time according to your needs. Most centers provide lunch, and some offer transportation to and from your home.

Some centers have weekend or nighttime hours. Night service offers supervision for individuals in the later stages of Alzheimer's, providing a night of rest for the caregiver.

You may wonder if your loved one would really like being left among strangers. The answer isn't always easy

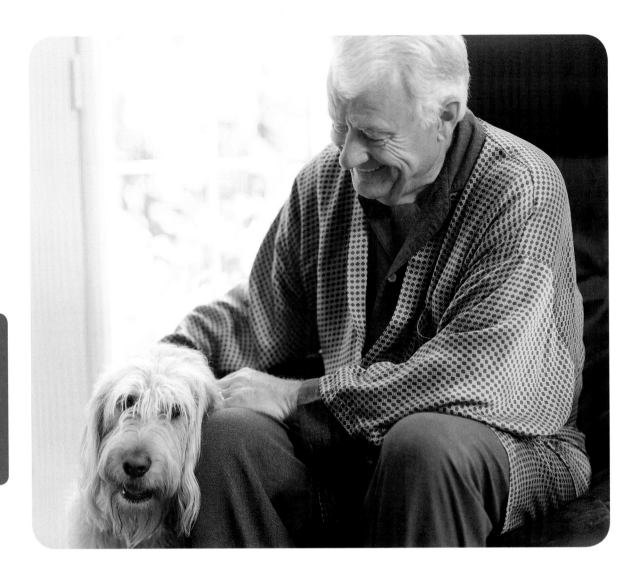

to gauge, but you may be pleasantly surprised to find that your loved one will enjoy and be entertained by caring, supportive individuals.

Following is a list of services that adult day care centers may offer. One center may not provide all services but then, not all services are always needed.

- Activities that may include sing-alongs, games, arts and crafts projects, movies, trivia, and pet therapy
- Counseling support for clients and their families
- Some health services
- Meals and snacks
- Personal care such as grooming, toileting and showering

- Management of challenging behaviors such as wandering, incontinence and hallucinations
- Physical, occupational and speech therapy
- Accessibility for those with wheelchairs or special equipment

Contact the National Adult Day Services Association at 877-745-1440 or *www.nadsa.org* to learn more about different adult day care opportunities in your community.

Emergency response service

People with dementia are at high risk of wandering and becoming lost. Due to cognitive loss, many in this situation are incapable of finding their way back home or providing a home address should they receive assistance.

The MedicAlert + Safe Return program is a source of identification for these individuals. The program is formed from an alliance of the MedicAlert Foundation and the Alzheimer's Association.

Here's how it works: After a family registers with the program, basic information about the person with dementia is placed in a confidential database, accessible 24 hours a day nationwide.

Both care receiver and caregiver receive identification bracelets or necklaces with a name, identification number and 24-hour emergency response telephone number. Key chains, wallet cards, pins and clothing labels are also available with this information.

The care receiver and caregiver wear or carry at least one of these items with them at all times. Should the care receiver ever become lost or missing, the caregiver can immediately call the response number (800-625-3780).

On notification, a responder at Medic Alert + Safe Return activates a community support network, including local Alzheimer's Association chapters and law enforcement agenices, to help find the person and reunite him or her with caregiver and family. Medical information can be provided to emergency responders, if or when it's required.

Anyone attempting to help a lost care receiver can call the emergency response number. The identification number helps assure the identity of the lost individual. MedicAlert + Safe Return will notify the caregiver and family members from a list of contacts.

If, for whatever reason, a caregiver becomes incapacitated, the identification jewelry will indicate that a person with dementia will need assistance.

There's an initial registration fee for both care receiver and caregiver to join the program, as well as an annual renewal fee.

For more information on the Medic Alert + Safe Return program, contact the MedicAlert Foundation at 888-633-4298 or *www.medicalert.org* or the Alzheimer's Association at 800-272-3900 or *www.alz.org*.

Living outside of the home

The reality for people diagnosed with Alzheimer's disease is that many will ultimately need to be moved to care facilities that offer greater assistance. Due to the progressive nature of the disease, a person with dementia will need more care than any one caregiver can realistically manage at home.

You may be put in a position of having to decide at what point to make that change. This can be one of the most difficult decisions you face throughout the entire disease process. And under-

standably, you may resist the thought of moving a loved one, at least initially.

In making the decision, there are no absolute indicators — no right or wrong answers — of when to move. All care receivers and caregivers are unique individuals. They live and function in different environments. You know your situation better than anyone else. Rely on your own instincts, but don't be afraid to ask for the help of family, friends and professionals.

Find out what local housing resources are available. It's critical to do your homework as early as possible — well before your loved one needs long-term care. Don't wait for a crisis to erupt before looking at other alternatives. Your loved one's health and your own health are unpredictable — don't let a crisis make the plans for you.

For most people, the decision to move a loved one will be based on a combination of physical, emotional and medical reasons that may include one or more of the following:

- Caregiver's own health is deteriorating (including sleep deprivation)
- Caregiver's own physical limitations for caregiving (including lifting and mobility)

- Caregiver's inability to manage primary work, household and family responsibilities
- Sufficient respite support or home care is unavailable or unaffordable
- Disease symptoms of loved one are too challenging to manage at home (incontinence, aggression, paranoia, wandering)
- Loved one needs more supervision than can be provided at home
- Home environment is no longer safe for loved one (negotiating stairs and doorways, getting in and out of the bathroom)
- Loved one is becoming more dependent on others for activities of daily living (feeding, dressing, bathing)
- Medications for loved one no longer properly managed
- Loved one is experiencing weight loss, dehydration or simply refusing to eat
- Loved one no longer recognizes home as home

Family members, friends and health care professionals may each offer a different opinion about what you should do. Balance their collective advice with what you think is the best course of action. As the time to move a loved one nears, it's most often the family, especially the children, who influence the decision most.

Even when a thoughtful decision is made, it is often heart-wrenching and met with uncertainty, fear and guilt on the part of the family and the caregivers involved in the process. These feelings are normal.

Caregivers may feel guilty about not upholding promises made to parents or spouses, or they may fear what others will think. Or they may fear that care at the new facility will be inferior. The decision underscores the inevitable decline of their loved one, resulting in further sadness and grief.

Many families claim the move is harder than they could have ever imagined. Some families will think they probably waited too long to make the move. How well you may reasonably adjust to the transition is often associated with how well you think you planned before the move. In other words, the experience may seem less painful if families feel that they took the time to explore all the options and made the best decision they could.

Keep in mind that the role of a caregiver doesn't end abruptly once a loved one moves out and lives elsewhere. The role just changes. You are still your loved one's primary advocate, but without direct care responsibilities.

If you love someone with Alzheimer's disease, remember that you are still entitled to a life of your own. Because of the heavy demands, primary caregivers often have more health problems than the person they're caring for.

Consider taking good care of yourself as a gift to your loved one as well as to yourself. You simply cannot meet every demand. The guilt you feel is because you love.

Finding a housing option

So what long-term care do you look for in the context of someone who has Alzheimer's disease or another form of dementia? You're looking for specialized care in a residential setting other than the home. There are generally two types of residential care available in many communities: assisted living and nursing homes.

Currently, 27 states have legislation requiring assisted living residences and nursing homes to state what special services they provide. The requirements include providing you with written information about trained staff, fees, specialized activities, and care for residents with behavioral or memory needs.

Assisted living. Assisted living includes a wide spectrum of residential programs that are not licensed as a nursing home. The definition of what is assisted living and the specific regulations for operating a facility differ from state to state. Typically, a facility offers independence to its residents but can also provide support for basic needs, if and when they're needed. The facility tries to operate more as a home than as a hospital.

Assisted living services involve a variety of options including adult foster care homes, congregate housing and memory-care assisted living. The facilities generally provide 24-hour staff, recreational activities, meals, housekeeping, laundry and transportation. Although some facilities accept state funding such as Medicaid, assisted living is ordinarily paid for privately.

Adult foster care homes provide meals and help with some daily activities, such as money management, transportation scheduling, medication reminders, laundry and housekeeping. These residences may also be called board and care homes, elder care homes, or residential care homes. Some foster homes are dementia specific, providing round-the-clock supervision, assistance with daily care and social activities.

Evaluating housing options

Arrange site visits of more than one facility. Find out how the centers operate. Try to visit each site more than once and at different times of day. Bring a family member or friend to help you evaluate.

As you tour, observe the following:

- Does the facility appear properly staffed? Do staff members seem harried or overly rushed? Is there backup support in case an employee cannot come to work?
- How are emergency situations handled?
- What is the facility's philosophy of dementia care? How do staff members handle challenging behaviors? Is the facility secure in case your loved one wanders?
- How do staff members interact with residents? Do they smile and call residents by name? Do they talk to residents during meals?
- Ask to see an activity schedule. Ask if you can sit in on a program or activity during one of your visits.
- Examine the environment. Is the facility clean and well cared for? Does background noise from sources such as televisions, radios, intercoms and alarms appear under control?

Memory-care assisted living is a step beyond basic assisted living, with the needs of a person with dementia in mind. Residents live in a supervised, sometimes secured, facility. Meals and activities of daily living, including medications, are managed by staff.

Most people with dementia can live in the facility throughout the course of the disease unless medical conditions require the skilled services offered in nursing homes.

Nursing homes. Nursing homes provide a full range of skilled care needs, including acute medical care and long-term care, both for dementia and for coexisting medical conditions. Some nursing homes offer Alzheimer's

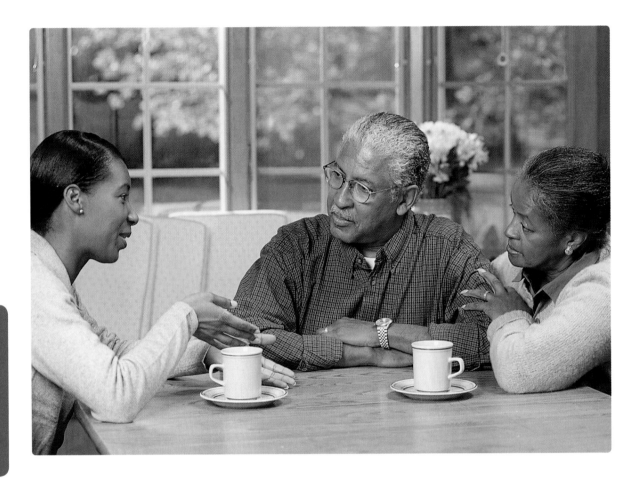

special-care or memory-care units to meet the special needs of residents with dementia. Special-care units are usually contained within a floor or section of the nursing home.

Helpful resources. What kind of residence might work best for you and your loved one? Try the Alzheimer's Association CareFinder at *www.alz.org/carefinder*, or call 800-272-3900. This useful tool walks you through the following:

- What types of care are available at different institutions
- How to recognize good care
- What the Alzheimer's Association recommends
- How to decide what care you need
- How to make sure you've found quality care

To locate care centers anywhere in the country, use the CareFinder or the Eldercare Locator at *www.eldercare.gov*, or call 800-677-1116.

Making a decision

A variety of housing options may be available, and some of these options will suit your needs better than others. The question becomes how to narrow your choice. Consider these issues when choosing your options:

- Your choices, especially in rural areas, may be limited by proximity. Decide how far you're willing to travel to a location.
- Consider how you'll pay for care. It may help to consult a financial planner or social worker. Compare payment options at each type of facility. Ask if additional fees are charged for specific services.
- Consider which of your loved one's needs are of greatest concern. Match these priorities to available services.
- What steps are involved in the admissions process? Ask for specific admission and discharge criteria.
- Is there a waiting list to get in? How long is the wait? Under no circumstances are you obligated to take an opening when it becomes available, even if you're on a waiting list.

Look for a facility that is efficiently run, clean, safe and comfortably suits the needs of your loved one and you. Decide on a top choice or choices.

Once you've made a decision, carefully review the terms of the contract and the financial arrangements before signing. It may be useful to have a lawyer review these documents with you.

Moving day

When you've decided on a new living arrangement, you can begin the process of adjustment. You are indeed letting go of some control over your loved one's care. Although others may care for your loved one differently than you, you still have a tremendous influence over the new system.

Here are tips for handling the move to a new living facility:

- Beforehand, share with your loved one as much or as little information about the move as you deem appropriate. Experts vary on their advice to families about how much to say. You should do what you feel is best. There's no single, correct way to handle the process.
- You may consider breaking the news on the day of the move. Avoid providing too much explanation. Keep the statement simple: "Mom, today you're moving to a new home." Lengthy explanations often

lead to frustration and argument. You're unlikely to convince your loved one of the need to change his or her living situation.

- Try projecting a positive attitude. Explain the move in terms the person can understand. Use statements such as, "We want you to be safe, and I'm sure you want that too," or "The home is going to help you make new friends." Help your loved one feel secure. You might introduce an in-house caregiver as a nurse or just a new friend. You might describe going to an elder care center as going to work or staying with friends.

- Acknowledge your loved one's feelings of anger, grief and loss. You may find it helpful to apologize. Thank your loved one for understanding why the move is so important.

- Try to stay calm and reassuring during the move. Sometimes, families discover the process is harder for them than it is for the person with dementia. Your loved one may be watching you closely for signs that the situation is safe. If you're tense, the person may sense this and also become anxious.

- Try to fill out all admissions paperwork in advance so that you can focus your attention on the move and on reassuring your loved one. Ask the facility staff in advance for advice. You may be an expert on your loved one, but staff members have probably helped many families through this difficult process. Work together to create a plan.

- Help the staff get to know your loved one by providing information about his or her personal history and current care needs. A written list is more likely to be passed along to all staff, as opposed to telling one staff member. Bring a photo album or scrapbook that describes important events, friends, trips and hobbies. You may want to leave a video or an audio recording of your voice for the staff to play, giving reassuring messages to your loved one.

- Be aware that Monday through Thursday tend to be the best days for moving, when care facilities are more likely to be fully staffed. Fridays may be too close to the weekend, when there are more visitors.

- If possible, bring your loved one to the new facility before lunch or dinner. The meal provides a distraction and good excuse for leaving.

- Think about decorating the living quarters before your loved one moves in. Arrange familiar items, such as photographs and knickknacks, to provide a sense of identity, security and comfort.

- Decide ahead of time how long you'll stay at the new facility. Hovering over your loved one may provide a sense of security but doesn't allow for him or her to become acclimated to the environment. Your loved one and the staff need time to become familiar with each other.
- When it's time to leave, proceed according to a plan you've made with the new caregivers. You may excuse yourself to run errands or simply say, "I'll be back soon." To avoid calling attention to your absence, you may decide to slip out without saying goodbye.
- Be gentle with yourself. This is often the most difficult thing a person has to do with a family member. Take some time to do whatever you need to do to feel better.

Evaluating quality of service

As you try to gauge the quality of care that a professional service provides, try to strike a balance between being an advocate and not overwhelming the staff with minor concerns. You may be limited in how much control you have over certain issues. Be willing to let go of the issues that have a minimal effect on your loved one's experience.

At the same time, it's important that you're included in decisions that ensure your loved one's needs are met. Keep lines of communication open. Offer your input as a team member, approach staff members in a gentle, assertive manner, and be prepared to listen to the reasons behind a particular approach.

Before addressing a concern with a care provider, ask yourself:

- Which person does this issue concern the most?
- Is my loved one at risk of being physically harmed?
- How much will my loved one's quality of life improve?

For example, if your father and a nursing home roommate often wear each other's clothes, who is this practice really bothering? On the other hand, if your father becomes aggressive during bath time when in the care of a particular staff member, raising this concern can help defuse the situation.

When change is necessary

Your loved one's safety and well-being are of primary importance. If you're seriously concerned about either, you may need to find a new environment or new facility. If you have grave concerns about a specific care provider, seek help immediately. Report signs of physical, emotional or financial abuse to the proper authorities.

Each state has an advocacy organization to investigate concerns about care providers. To contact your state's ombudsman — a public official appointed to investigate your complaints — look in the phone directory or check with your Area Agency on Aging or local Alzheimer's Association chapter. Or you may contact a social worker in adult protective services at your local social services department.

Visiting your loved one

Bear in mind that during visits, you are not expected to continue providing care for your loved one. And you are no longer required to protect the staff from your loved one's challenging behaviors. You're now part of a team of caregivers at the facility. Allow the staff to be in charge. Focus on enjoying the visit and providing love, comfort and reassurance to your loved one.

- Work with the staff to determine when and how often to visit. Use this arrangement to recharge your energy and enthusiasm and to resume some neglected aspects of your life outside of caregiving.

- When you visit, expect that there may be changes in your loved one. It's naturally going to be a challenge getting used to a new environment. With time, your loved one will almost always adjust.

- Try to plan visits during times of the day when your loved one is most alert, active and feeling at his or her best. You might bring along something familiar to show or do with your loved one, such as looking at photographs or playing music. You can use these items and activities during the visit, or skip them if they're not needed.

- Your loved one often cannot remember how frequently you visit or for how long. Expect to hear comments like "Where have you been?" or "Why don't you ever visit?" no matter how short it has been between visits.

- When it's time to leave, family members may know the best way to say goodbye. A simple "Goodbye, Mom. I have errands to do. I'll come back soon" is usually best.

- Giving a personal item such as a scarf or cap to "keep for me until I come back" may be reassuring to your loved one.

Preparing for the inevitable

My mother is in the early stages of Alzheimer's disease. She lives alone in the home that she and my father shared for 40 years. My father died last year. I'm worried about mother living alone, but the thought of moving her is very painful. How do I prepare her for this possibility?

Moving can trigger anxiety for almost anyone, especially when it's a move from a home you've lived in for many years. For people with Alzheimer's disease, relocating to an unfamiliar environment can be extremely stressful, even though doing so is often in their best interests.

In making decisions about when and where to move a loved one, there are no right or wrong answers. Friends and neighbors will have opinions, but the decision rests with the family. And the best decision is the one made by informed family members.

Plan ahead now for the day you decide to move your mom. Explore all housing options, and talk to your mom — while she can still make choices — about what she wants. The best approach may not be to directly ask if your mom would like to move because the answer will inevitably be no. Instead, bring up the topic in a casual way. For instance, if your mom says she isn't eating because she doesn't feel like cooking for herself, you may say, "Wouldn't it be helpful to have someone cook your meals?" This might begin to ease her into the benefits of an alternative living arrangement.

As moving day draws near, don't dwell on it too much. Don't remind your mom that she's "moving in a week." On the actual day, move your mom during the best time of her day — whether that's in the morning or the afternoon. This can make the transition go more smoothly. Allow for time during the day to reminisce with your mom, looking at photo albums or memory boxes. This activity is helpful in relieving anxiety not only for her but also for you.

Support groups

Caregivers and family members often appreciate the opportunity to talk to others about their caregiving experiences and how the disease has impacted their lives. One place this can happen is in a support group. Support groups provide a safe forum for individuals to share emotions, changes and concerns with people in similar situations. Support groups can be a place to vent frustrations, problem solve challenging behaviors, learn from other's experiences or even share a laugh to lighten the burden of the disease.

Support groups may be offered in a variety of locations, such as medical clinics, nursing homes, churches, community centers and senior centers. A facilitator, who may be a professional or a trained volunteer, typically runs the support group. Meetings may be weekly, biweekly or monthly, generally for about an hour.

Support groups may exist in your community for family caregivers and for people in the early stages of dementia. Typically you don't have to live with the family member who has dementia in order to participate in a support group. For more information on sup-port groups in your area, contact the Alzheimer's Association at 800-272-9300 or *www.alz.org*.

If you're looking to share experiences but aren't comfortable in a group setting, try talking with a trusted friend, family member, clergyperson or trained professional. The Alzheimer's Association can refer you to family counselors who can discuss your situation with you.

You may also ask to speak with a social worker or nurse at your local clinic. Even regularly going out for lunch or coffee with a friend can help reduce the stress of caregiving.

Hospice care

Hospice care is designed for people in the final phase of a terminal illness — many may have no more than six months to live. It's a special kind of care that focuses on comfort rather than treatment and on quality of life rather than length of life.

Emphasis is no longer on curing disease. Rather, it addresses two fears that a dying person may have — the fear of pain and the fear of being alone.

In order to use hospice services, you must decide to stop any life-prolonging treatments for your loved one and focus only on comfort measures. For example, you may choose to no longer employ ventilators, cardiopulmonary resuscitation (CPR), antibiotics, and artificial nutrition and hydration (tube feeding and intravenous hydration).

This doesn't mean you're providing assisted suicide. Rather, it's a planned decision not to aggressively treat medical illness. You can still provide pain medication and oxygen to help your loved one stay comfortable.

The instructions provided in advance directives, such as a living will or health care power of attorney, can help you make these important decisions according to your loved one's wishes.

Many hospice programs are run by nonprofit, independent organizations. Some programs are affiliated with hospitals, nursing homes or home health care agencies.

Hospice care can take place in the home or in a specially designated hospice facility under the direction of a medically trained staff. Support of the entire family — not just the person who is ill — is a core element of hospice care.

Predicting the remaining length of life can be difficult for someone with dementia. Even people with severe Alzheimer's disease may have a prognosis of up to two years. Their survival often depends on the presence of coexisting diseases and on the comprehensiveness of the care they are receiving. To qualify for hospice care, a physician must certify that the person is in the end stage of the disease.

Most hospice programs offer the following types of service:

Giving comfort. In many cases, the individual remains in his or her home or in homelike surroundings instead of at a hospital. Care is designed to relieve or decrease pain, control other symptoms, and provide as much quality time as possible with family and friends.

Providing comfort is a cooperative effort involving the primary caregiver, family and friends with a team of professionals and volunteers working together to meet your loved one's needs. This team supplies all necessary medications and equipment.

Providing support. Individuals in the last stages of life often prefer receiving basic care from family and friends. A nurse may lead the team and coordinate the day-to-day care. A doctor is also part of the team. Chaplains and social workers are available to counsel the family and make sure emotional, spiritual and social needs are being met.

Trained volunteers perform a variety of tasks as needed, such as companionship, doing light housekeeping, preparing meals and running errands.

Improving quality of life. Caring for someone who is dying is emotionally and physically demanding. But primary caregivers and family members can take comfort knowing that hospice is an act of love that can improve the quality of life for everyone involved.

Action Guide 9

Travel and safety

Safety becomes a greater concern as your loved one becomes increasingly dependent on others for care. The impairment of cognitive functions, such as memory, judgment and attention, due to dementia, coupled with the impairment of mobility, balance, vision and hearing that sometimes accompanies aging, puts your loved one at high risk of injury.

It's also true that every person moves through the disease process at his or her own pace. Safety concerns vary widely from individual to individual, influenced by that unique combination of genetic inheritance, medical history and lifestyle patterns that each person carries. As a caregiver, you must adapt to the changes that occur, based on what's safest for, and in the best interests of, your loved one.

While there's no precise template to follow that can ensure a "safe" environment for your loved one, these guidelines should apply to most situations:

Anticipate problems. Don't wait for accidents to happen before taking steps to remedy problems. If you're aware of the potential but take no action, you'll be in a perpetual state of high alert.

Modify the environment, not the behavior. Caregivers often face the choice of changing a loved one's potentially harmful behavior or the environment in which this behavior takes place. Generally, changing the environment is a better remedy. For example, if stairs are a growing concern, you may consider converting a downstairs room into a bedroom so that your loved one doesn't need to use the stairs at all.

Keep it simple. Devices and supports should be easy to use and accessible — not complex or requiring new learning. It's better if these relate in some way to the person's past skills and knowledge.

Do routine checks. Schedule regular times — perhaps three or four times a year — when you do a room-by-room check for potential safety concerns.

Driving

Do you remember how great it felt to drive a car all by yourself for the first time? Driving provides a sense of independence and self-sufficiency that you become accustomed to through the years — and rarely will people with dementia voluntarily choose to surrender their car keys. But driving and dementia make a risky combination.

People with dementia often can't recognize when is the right time to stop driving. They often feel driving is the last thing they can do by themselves, and they want to hang on to that opportunity for as long as they can. The final decision of taking away the keys generally falls to caregivers, and it's among the most difficult decisions they have to make.

Some caregivers allow their loved one to drive only in familiar neighborhoods or only when the caregiver rides along. This approach doesn't address how your loved one will respond if an unexpected detour arises or a child darts into the road.

Other caregivers employ a wait-and-see method, thinking, "He hasn't had any trouble till now, so we're keeping our fingers crossed." If this is your plan, ask yourself what sign you're waiting for. A fender bender may, indeed, be the time for you to intervene, but a catastrophic accident could happen before that minor one does.

Fact is, driving is a privilege, not a right. Dementia impairs judgment, planning, visuospatial skills and reaction time, all of which are essential to maneuver a ton of steel down the road. Families who wait too long risk injury and death to themselves and their loved ones as well as to others.

Most specialists feel it's important to help the person with dementia stop driving as soon as possible. A rule of thumb is to ask yourself whether you feel safe riding in a car that your loved one is driving. If the answer is no, then you know it's time to take away that driving privilege.

When is it time to stop driving?

Carefully observe your loved one's driving habits for signs of potential trouble and changes from previous behavior. Intervene quickly if you notice any of the following:

- Failing to yield or observe traffic signals
- Getting lost in familiar locations
- Problems with changing lanes or making turns
- Driving at inappropriate speeds
- Confusing the brake pedal and the gas pedal
- Being confused about directions or detours
- Hitting the curb while driving
- Making poor or slow decisions

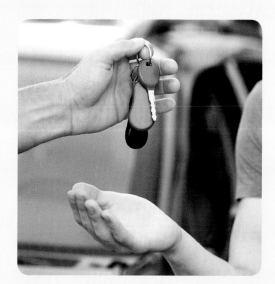

Making the decision

When you decide that it's time for your loved one to stop driving, stay committed to that decision. It's not your fault — blame the disease. You're only ensuring your loved one's safety. Here are tips to ease the transition for your loved one:

- Elicit the support of family, friends and neighbors.
- When you inform your loved one of the decision, remember that de-

mentia affects the ability to reason. Don't spend too much time trying to convince the person why he or she can no longer drive — you're unlikely to succeed.

- A simple statement of fact may work best, but others should offer a similar explanation to yours: "The doctor says you can no longer drive," or "It's not safe because of your memory problems."
- You may decide not to tell your loved one about the decision. Some families remove the car without

discussion or with an explanation such as "Your car needs repairs at the mechanic's shop."

- Your doctor may be willing to prescribe "no driving" in an official letter to confirm your decision.
- You or the doctor may request that your loved one take a driver's test. The test results can bolster your case. Some states require doctors to report diagnoses of dementia to state transportation officials.
- Allow your loved one time to grieve and adjust to the loss of driving privileges. It may provoke frustration and anger. Try to remember that, although these feelings are directed at you, they actually relate to the disease.

Sticking with the decision

Even after you've made the decision to take away the keys, you may still need to come up with clever ways to prevent your loved one from driving:

- When your loved one asks to drive, avoid giving a straightforward no. Tell the person that you would like to drive, or you're taking a new route, or the doctor doesn't recommend driving because of a heart condition or other illness.

- Out of sight means out of mind. Park the car where your loved one can't see it. Hide the keys, and if the person insists on carrying a set of keys, provide substitutes that don't work in the car.
- If your loved one has used a particular mechanic in the past, be sure to alert the mechanic in case your loved one asks for help in getting the car started.
- Ask for assistance from a mechanic to disable the car. Older cars may be disabled easily by removing the distributor cap. Of course, you can always disconnect the battery. A mechanic may be able to install a kill switch that must be deactivated in order to start the car.
- Your loved one will probably continue enjoying car rides after the keys are taken away. If a familiar vehicle prompts a desire to drive, you may need to sell the car and replace it with a different model. Your loved one may be less likely to drive if the car is unfamiliar.
- Always offer to drive when your loved one needs transportation. During the drive, find other ways to make the person feel active and useful, like identifying landmarks along the way.
- Look for alternative means of transportation, such as senior buses

and taxis. Very often, friends will be happy to help out by giving rides. Check with your local Area Agency on Aging or an Alzheimer's Association chapter to learn about transportation options.

- Keep in mind that as the symptoms of dementia become more severe, your loved one will likely have less desire to leave his or her safe, familiar home environment. Eventually, it will be more common for you to be running errands for your loved one rather than providing transportation to the store.

Traveling

Traveling to different locations, even ones that are close by, and participating in events outside the familiar home environment will grow increasingly difficult for your loved one as dementia progresses. If you decide to travel with your loved one, here are suggestions for making those times easier:

- If you're uncertain how your loved one will react to a long stay away from home, do a "trial run" of day-long or overnight trips beforehand.

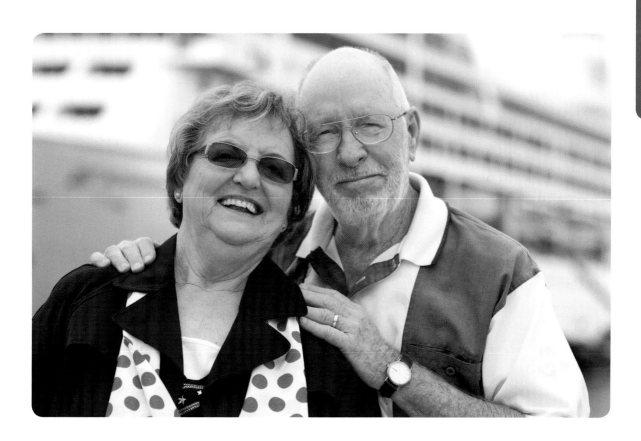

- Simplify your vacation plans. Avoid cramming too many activities into a single day and try to keep changes throughout the day to a minimum. Plan for rest periods between activities and, if possible, set aside a quiet haven for your loved one to retreat to if necessary.
- Alert travel or hospitality staff ahead of time that your loved one has dementia. Special arrangements can be made to board planes early for seating or to use wheelchairs to alleviate fatigue in places that involve a lot of walking.
- Your loved one may become confused about when the trip is taking place and what preparations are required. You may find it easier to simply not talk about the trip until just before leaving. Provide reassurance: "Tomorrow we're going to visit our daughter Susan in Wisconsin. Don't worry. We've packed everything we need, and I'll be with you the whole time."
- Before leaving home, consider registering in the MedicAlert + Safe Return program in case your loved one should wander away from you. Contact the Alzheimer's Association for more information.
- You may find it helpful to alert people you meet of your loved one's condition in a discreet manner. Bring a small card with you that states, "The person with me has dementia. Thank you for your patience." Show the card to restaurant staff, flight attendants, store clerks, cashiers and others who should be aware of your situation.
- Consider bringing along another person on the trip to assist you. This may be particularly helpful at locations with public restrooms, if you and your loved one aren't of the same sex.
- Create a backup plan in case there's a need for your loved one to return home quickly.
- Give your loved one a small amount of money to put in a wallet or purse, but no more money than you would be comfortable losing if he or she misplaces it.
- Bring an updated medications list, insurance information and emergency contacts. Know the locations of medical facilities for each destination you're going to — information that's available from the Alzheimer's Association.
- Provide family members with your travel itinerary and contact information.
- Bring snacks and simple, fun activities like magazines with bright colorful pictures, music and film recordings, or a deck of cards.

- Allow your loved one to wear comfortable shoes and familiar clothes when traveling. New, unfamiliar apparel will only add to apprehension that your loved one is feeling.
- On airplanes, buses or trains, take the aisle seat and have your loved one sit away from the aisle to control wandering. A window seat may help keep your loved one engaged.
- Keep meal times similar to those at home. If crowded restaurants confuse your loved one, consider taking advantage of room service.
- Bring a waterproof sheet and extra pads if your loved one experiences incontinence.
- Caregivers often find trips with their loved ones to be extremely stressful and exhausting. The person with dementia typically experiences anxiety and confusion away from home, then quickly forgets about the trip afterward. Consider an alternative: using respite care that allows your loved one to stay home while you travel may be easier on both of you.

Wandering

People with Alzheimer's disease are at increased risk of wandering away from home and getting lost. The wandering may be a result of hunger, fatigue or boredom. Here are ways to reduce the risk of wandering:

- Install a slide bolt at the top of doors to the outside or to stairwells, or use a deadbolt that requires a key.
- Install alarms that alert you when a door is being opened. These can be purchased for a reasonable cost.
- Some caregivers disguise doors to the outside by covering them with curtains, wallpaper or paint, or by posting a "Stop" or "Do not enter" sign on the door.
- Take daily walks with your loved one, or allow him or her to wander in safe areas with supervision, such as a fenced backyard.
- Alert neighbors of your loved one's condition so that they can notify you if they see that your loved is outside alone.

Making the home environment safe

There are many ways to modify your home environment that can help your loved one stay safe, feel comfortable and move easily from room to room. Following is a list of general precautions you may take to keep you and your loved one safe:

- Keep a list of emergency numbers by all telephones, including family contacts, doctor's office, first responders and fire department.
- Use an answering machine or voice mail when you're unavailable to answer the phone — and turn off the phone ringer when the machine is on. You don't want your loved one subjected to possible exploitation by solicitors.
- Make sure you have a fire extinguisher and an updated first-aid kit in your home.
- Install smoke alarms at strategic locations throughout the house.
- Install locks on all outside doors and windows.
- Keep a spare key hidden outside your home in case your loved one accidentally locks you out.
- Post a "No solicitation" sign on your outside door.

Securing living spaces

- Keep living spaces picked up. Clutter creates potential problems and disguises many others.
- Make sure there's adequate lighting throughout the house, particularly in areas that have little natural light, such as hallways and stairwells or walk-in closets.
- Place childproof locks on cupboards and drawers to prevent chance access to sharp utensils, matches, small appliances and household cleaning products.
- Install plugs, covers and plates on unused electrical outlets.
- Keep medications — both prescription and over-the-counter products — locked away or at least out of sight, especially if your loved one is prone to taking medications more frequently than prescribed.
- Store household-cleaning products and poisons in secure locations, preferably away from living spaces.
- Remove poisonous plants from the home. A list of poisonous plants can be obtained from nurseries or poison control centers. Similarly, remove artificial fruits, vegetables and other food-shaped items that can be mistaken as edible.
- Be careful with electric blankets and heating pads, which are capable

Preventing falls

A person with dementia may be at higher risk of falls due to tripping, losing his or her balance, slipping on a wet or uneven surface, or misjudging the height of a step. You may not be able to prevent falls completely but the following advice may reduce your loved one's risk:

- Provide well-fitting, low-heeled shoes with nonslip soles.
- Keep walkways and stairways free of clutter.
- Make sure there's at least one handrail in all stairways. If possible, steps should be carpeted or have safety grips.
- Place night lights in hallways, bathrooms and bedrooms.
- Get rid of throw rugs or secure the edges with carpet tape.
- Move electrical cords under furniture or tape them to walls. Avoid the use of extension cords, if possible.
- Arrange furniture so that walkways aren't obstructed. Avoid moving the furniture once it's in place, as this may disorient your loved one.
- If your loved one habitually falls out of bed, move the bed against a wall or put the mattress on the floor.
- Immediately clean up any spills on the floor.
- Place nonskid decals in bathtub units.
- Install grab bars in the shower and use a specialized shower chair.

of causing burns if the controls are tampered with. Avoid the use of portable space heaters.
- Never leave your loved one alone with an open fire in the fireplace. Keep matches and cigarette lighters out of sight.
- Use curtains or decals on sliding glass doors and picture windows to indicate the presence of glass.

In the kitchen and bathroom

- Install single faucets that mix hot and cold water together in all sinks and the tub. Adjust the thermostat on your water heater to 120 F to avoid the possibility of burns. If you have double faucets, consider color-coding them red and blue to help prevent confusion.

- Install drain traps in sinks to catch materials or valuable items that may fall in and clog the plumbing.
- Regularly clean the refrigerator, removing out-of-date or spoiled food that your loved one might eat.
- Limit stove use if necessary. Whenever the stove is not in use, throw the circuit breaker or unplug the unit. You also can remove stove knobs that control heating or cover them with bubble lenses.
- Use small appliances equipped with automatic shut-off devices.
- Consider removing metal bowls from the kitchen. They could start a fire if placed in the microwave.
- Store all electrical appliances outside the bathroom and, if possible, use the appliances outside the bathroom as well.
- Remove the lock from the bathroom door to prevent your loved one from being locked in.

Health concerns

This section discusses many common health concerns experienced by people with dementia, especially in later stages of the disease. The list is by no means a complete one. On the other hand, your loved one may not experience some of the conditions described. Contact your doctor for further information regarding these problems.

Choking

As dementia progresses, your loved one may have difficulty chewing or swallowing food. Choking is often the result of inadequately chewed food becoming lodged in the throat or windpipe, which blocks the passage of air. Most often, solid foods such as meat are the cause of the choking.

- If food "goes down the wrong pipe," the coughing reflex often resolves the problem. A person isn't choking if he or she is able to cough freely, has normal skin color and can continue to speak.
- A universal sign for choking is hands clutched to the throat, with thumbs and fingers extended. The person's face will assume a look of panic. He or she may wheeze or gasp and be unable to communicate except by hand motions. A person who displays these symptoms requires emergency treatment.
- Be prepared for emergencies. Ask a nurse or the Red Cross for techniques to help your loved one if he or she is choking.
- To reduce the risk of choking, serve soft, thick foods to ease the process of swallowing.

- If you mix foods in a blender, use a product called a food thickener, which is tasteless and helps to even out the texture. For example, fruit may separate into pulp and liquid, increasing the likelihood of choking. Using a thickener will smooth the texture and make swallowing easier for your loved one.
- Try to make sure your loved one's head is tilted slightly forward while eating. Leaning back increases the risk of choking.

Dehydration

People with dementia may forget to drink enough fluids. Signs of dehydration include dry mouth, little or no urination, weakness, dizziness or lightheadedness. Dehydration can also increase confusion and cause constipation, fever and rapid pulse.

- Encourage your loved one to drink fluids. Most healthy people meet their daily hydration needs by letting thirst be their guide. As a caregiver for someone with dementia, you'll need to monitor fluid intake closely because your loved one may have lost that sense.
- Keep a glass of water or a favorite beverage near your loved one throughout the day. Provide gentle reminders to drink — for example, by asking, "Is your water still cold enough for drinking?"

The Heimlich maneuver

This maneuver is the best-known method of removing an object from the airway of a person who is choking.

1. Stand behind the choking person and wrap your arms around his or her waist. Bend the person slightly forward.
2. Make a fist with one hand and place it slightly above the person's navel.
3. Grasp your fist with the other hand and press hard into the abdomen with a quick upward thrust. Repeat this procedure until the object is expelled from the airway.

- Drinking caffeinated beverages in moderate amounts is fine, but be aware that caffeine may increase anxiety and sleeplessness. If you choose to decrease your loved one's caffeine intake, phase out caffeinated beverages gradually to reduce the risk of caffeine-withdrawal symptoms, such as headaches.
- If your loved one was accustomed to drinking coffee throughout the day, serve noncaffeinated beverages in a coffee mug.
- If incontinence is a problem, discourage drinking fluids after the evening meal. However, don't discourage fluids altogether because of incontinence. This may cause dehydration, bladder infections and other serious complications.

Dental care

People with dementia may neglect dental hygiene and develop oral infections. Poor dental care can also affect good nutrition.

- Inform your dentist about the diagnosis of dementia. Some dentists have experience working with people with dementia. Ask a support group for referrals.

- Make sure the dentist is aware of all medications that your loved one is taking. Some medications can cause dry mouth or other conditions that could affect dental health.
- Help your loved one brush after each meal. Your dentist may be able to provide dental aids such as mouth swabs that can be used in place of a toothbrush. Ask your dentist for suggestions if your loved one refuses to open his or her mouth for cleaning.
- Give simple one-step instructions for brushing teeth: "Take the cap off the toothpaste. Good. Now squeeze the tube. Good. Now brush your top teeth."
- Brush your own teeth at the same time to model the process.
- Help your loved one grip the toothbrush by making the handle thicker. You can do this by wrapping aluminum foil around the handle or by attaching it to a plastic bicycle handlebar grip. Or try wrapping a strip of fabric fastener around the person's hand and tucking the toothbrush inside the strap.
- If you're helping your loved one brush, use a spoon to gently pull the cheek away from gums. This helps you see the teeth.
- Encourage eating raw fruits and vegetables at meals. Suggest rinsing

the mouth with water after meals, particularly if the person has difficulty with brushing teeth.

- Some caregivers choose to no longer have their loved ones use dentures as the disease progresses. A dietitian can help you meet the specific needs of a soft diet.
- Refusal to eat is often a clue that a person has mouth sores or poorly fitting dentures. Ask your dentist for assistance.

Falls

Studies suggest that people with Alzheimer's disease will experience at least one fall during the course of the disease. They're also twice as likely to experience a hip fracture as people their age who don't have Alzheimer's.

- Physically restraining your loved one may not prevent falls — and may actually increase the likelihood of injury. Some falls may simply not be preventable.
- Your loved one may not remember to call for assistance whenever he or she wants to get up, even with frequent reminders. Try putting a sign on a lap tray that says, "Stay in your chair. I'll be right back."

- Have your loved one sit on the edge of the bed for a few moments before trying to stand.
- The use of bedrails is controversial. Some people believe bedrails can prevent their loved ones from rolling out of bed or from standing up and falling. However, people with Alzheimer's have been known to climb over bedrails and fall or to injure themselves after becoming stuck between the rails. The state where you live may have specific guidelines about bedrail use.
- In case of a fall, try to remain calm. Sit with your loved one to determine if an injury has occurred. Look for signs of redness, swelling, bruises or broken bones. If you believe a bone is broken or a head injury has occurred, call for emergency medical assistance. If your loved one seems uninjured, eventually encourage the person to stand independently rather than trying to lift him or her up.
- If you do try to lift your loved one, put your hands in the armpits and use your legs, rather than your back, for strength. Try to have a neighbor or family member on call to lend assistance. Remember that you'll not be able to care for your loved one if you get a back injury from overexertion.

- A physical therapist can help determine whether your loved one could benefit from the use of a walker or other device.

Hospitalization

Hospitalization may be necessary, but even an overnight stay can be very disruptive for a person with dementia. Find out whether care can be provided on an outpatient basis or at home instead of at the hospital.

- If hospitalization is unavoidable, speak to staff members about the current stage of your loved one's condition. This may be helpful if some of the staff are unfamiliar with dementia. Express your loved one's needs but try not to overwhelm the staff with too many demands. A written list of important information may prove helpful.
- Try to have family or friends on call to reassure your loved one and answer questions from the staff at times when you may not be available to do so. Give yourself breaks.
- See if a private room at the hospital is an option. Bring familiar items to the room, such as pictures of family and favorite quiet music.

- You may need to ask for the services of a social worker who can help answer your questions, be your loved one's advocate and plan for discharge. Social workers are trained to help you communicate with the hospital staff and maneuver the various professional networks involved in caregiving.
- Check with the doctor frequently about how long your loved one is expected to stay in the hospital. If you receive conflicting information from doctors and nurses on the discharge date, ask your social worker to help you clarify the information.
- Make sure you communicate with the hospital staff about your goals for care, quality of life and pain management.

Surgery and medical treatment

When your loved one has received a diagnosis of dementia, it may be difficult deciding whether to treat other conditions that require intervention, such as heart surgery or chemotherapy. Here are some considerations:

- Specialists in a particular field of medicine, such as cardiology or cancer, may recommend treatments for the conditions they know best. When an invasive treatment is recommended, you may want to discuss other options with a general practitioner or neurologist.

- General anesthesia, which is used to render a person unconscious during surgery, usually makes cognitive impairment worse. Sometimes people bounce back from the decline, but often this isn't the case. Ask your doctor if local anesthesia is possible to use instead.
- Asking the following questions to a specialist may help you make a well-informed decision.
  - What is the goal of treatment?
  - What are some benefits that treatment could provide?
  - Would treatment affect the person's cognitive skills?
  - How may treatment affect the person's quality of life?
  - Is the person likely to experience pain or nausea from treatment?
  - How frightening or confusing might treatment be for the person?
- Responses to these questions may help you weigh the pros and cons of treatment. Consider your caregiving goals: Do you want to lengthen your loved one's life at the risk of decreasing his or her quality of life? For example, electroconvulsive therapy (ECT) for depression may

impair your loved one's memory, but his or her quality of life may improve. Surgery may lengthen a person's life but decrease quality of life because of pain or diminished cognitive skills from anesthesia.

Medications

Your loved one may be taking medications for more than one condition at different times throughout the day. Here are suggestions to keep your loved one on track:

- Keep an updated list of medications, along with dosages and times, posted inside a cupboard door. Carry a list with you whenever you leave the house.
- Place contact information for your doctor's office and poison control center next to the phone in case of an accidental overdose.
- Use a pillbox to help keep track of medications.
- If your loved one lives alone, you may need to provide a reminder phone call. Stay on the phone to ensure that the person takes the medications.
- When a new medication is prescribed, ask your doctor or nurse to

provide the following information: drug name, purpose, dosage, time of day given and potential side effects.

- If your loved one experiences changes in behavior, demeanor or physical condition, consider whether any medications have been changed recently. Contact your doctor with concerns.

- Make sure every specialist who examines your loved one is aware of all medications, especially supplements and over-the-counter products. These substances may interact with prescribed medications and cause harmful side effects.

- Don't change dosages without the consent of your physician.

- Throw out old prescriptions, and don't use medications for anyone other than the person for whom they're prescribed.

- If your loved one refuses a medication or spits it out, provide a simple explanation for its purpose. For example, "Mom, the doctor says you need to take blood pressure medication for your heart." If she continues to refuse, ask your doctor if you can crush the medication and hide it in food or juice. You may also be able to obtain it in liquid form.

- Medications used to control challenging behaviors can have particularly harmful side effects. You may

want to try using nonmedication interventions first.

Pain

Although dementia may not cause pain, your loved one can experience stomach cramps, pressure sores and sprains. Problems arise as your loved one loses the ability to understand why something hurts and to tell you when something is wrong.

- Watch facial expressions and body language for signs of pain. Wincing, grimacing, tugging at clothes or pulling away from touch may indicate that your loved one is feeling uncomfortable.

- Your loved one may be unable to indicate where pain is occurring. Use bathing and dressing times to look for swelling, redness, warmth, bruising, and other signs of inflammation or injury.

- Complaints of pain may indicate emotional distress — such as depression, boredom or fatigue — rather than physical injury.

- If pain is experienced frequently, talk to your doctor about a pain management plan that is safe for your loved one.

Pressure sores

Pressure sores may develop if your loved one sits or lies in the same position for hours at a time. Bones wear away muscle and skin at pressure points when the body isn't regularly readjusted.

- A warning sign of pressure sores is red and swollen skin, particularly at places where the body is in contact with the chair or bed. Common locations include knees, elbows, hips, heels, shoulder blades, spine, buttocks and ankles. Eventually the red areas will become open sores if they're not treated.
- If your loved one is sedentary for extended periods, reposition him or her every two hours. Place pillows between the knees and ankles when the person is lying on his or her side. Use foam pads or gel pads to cushion vulnerable areas.
- A home health agency can help you provide personal care and move your loved one. Ask nursing home staff how often your loved one is repositioned throughout the day and night.
- Ill-fitting clothes can put people at risk of pressure sores. Make sure clothes are comfortable and adequate in size.

Sleep disturbance

Disrupted sleep patterns and poor quality sleep are common in people with dementia. Disturbances may be caused by the dementia. Or they may be caused by other illnesses, medication use or a poorly adapted environment. Be careful of sleep medications, which may only make confusion worse. If your loved one has difficulty sleeping, consider one of the following strategies:

- Try to maintain a regular bedtime in the daily routine.
- To indicate that it's bedtime, yawn and stretch. Turn off the lights together as a bedtime ritual.
- Don't discuss tomorrow's plans before bedtime. Your loved one may confuse time and start to worry.
- Avoid loud television before bedtime. Instead, try reading aloud, playing soft music or offering a light snack to help calm your loved one.
- Have your loved one use the bathroom before bedtime.
- If changing into pajamas upsets your loved one, use a cotton sweatsuit that can be worn day and night.
- Allow your loved one to sleep wherever he or she prefers, including in a recliner chair or on a couch.
- Give the person an activity to do at night if sleep seems unlikely.

- Avoid giving your loved one alcohol or caffeine, especially in the late afternoon or early evening. Be aware that quitting caffeine abruptly can cause headaches and irritability.
- Encourage regular exercise to burn off excess emotions.
- If background noise is keeping your loved one awake, try a white noise generator that creates a quiet hum to counteract the noise.
- Don't discourage napping during the day, especially if it's the only sleep your loved one gets. A little sleep is better than no sleep at all.
- Excessive sleep is generally not a problem unless it's caused by depression, boredom or medications.

Bladder and bowel conditions

Urinary tract infection

A urinary tract infection (UTI) occurs when bacteria take hold in the bladder or the urethra — the tube that transports urine from the bladder — and multiply into a full-blown infection. UTIs are more common in older adults, but people with dementia may not be able to communicate how they feel. The caregiver will need to look for indications.

- Signs and symptoms of a UTI may include frequent or urgent urination, burning pain during urination, blood or pus in the urine, and fever.
- Consider the possibility of a UTI if your loved one experiences a sudden change of behavior, such as increased anger, drowsiness, confusion or fatigue.
- In late-stage Alzheimer's disease, UTIs are a leading cause of death. That is because the immune system is unable to fight off infection when the person becomes bedridden.
- If you suspect your loved one has a UTI, your doctor can perform a urinalysis exam and treat the infection with antibiotics.

Constipation

Constipation occurs when a person has uncharacteristically infrequent bowel movements or difficulty passing stools. Your loved one may become constipated as the effects of dementia make him or her more sedentary and immobile. Avoiding constipation is important in preventing bowel obstruction, pain and fatigue — all of which can only increase confusion.

- A person with dementia often isn't able to keep track of bowel movements, even in early stages of the disease. Pain, bloating or gas may be signs of constipation.
- Provide a balanced diet with high-fiber foods such as vegetables, fruits and whole-grain products.
- Encourage your loved one to drink plenty of fluids.
- Establish a routine for your loved one to attempt bowel elimination.
- The use of laxatives is generally not recommended for relieving constipation in a person with dementia.

The final stages of Alzheimer's disease

Sometimes it's difficult to know when someone is experiencing the symptoms of late-stage dementia. Typically, your loved one will be bedridden, no longer able to walk and totally dependent on the caregiver in all activities of daily living. Other changes may include:

- Loss of weight
- Disinterest in eating or refusal to eat
- Loss of bowel and bladder control

- Sleepiness
- Being mute, extremely quiet or difficult to understand
- Groaning, mumbling loudly or crying out when touched
- Inability to recognize family, friends, caregivers and self
- Seizures and frequent infections

You'll face many complex care decisions at this time. It's important that you follow your loved one's wishes, if these are known from an advance directive. If no specific directions are known, you will need to depend on the knowledge of your loved one's values and beliefs for guidance.

You'll also need to consider the progress of the disease, the overall health of your loved one, and the risks or benefits that may be obtained from certain procedures or medications. In the late stages of dementia, options for end-of-life care generally include:

- Treatment to prolong life using all available resources, such as tube feeding for nutrition
- Treatment to maintain health, such as blood pressure medication for hypertension and insulin for diabetes
- Treatment intended to provide comfort (palliative care), primarily pain control and emotional support

Whatever option you may decide to follow, you'll want to continue maintaining the dignity and privacy of your loved one. Advice from your doctor, other specialists and members of a hospice team are important at this time.

You may wonder if your loved one is aware of what's going on around him or her in this last stage of the illness. Although the body and mind are in the process of shutting down, your loved one still may be aware of your care and affection. Hold hands. Stroke his or her forehead. Say what you need to say to bring closure to your relationship.

The process of grief

Grief can be defined as the process of adjusting to loss. Grief brings on powerfully intense feelings and emotions. For some, the grieving process begins long before death occurs.

The grieving process is a gradual one. There are many emotional ups and downs. Don't try to avoid the process or to simply "wait it out." You must grieve in order to bring about emotional healing and adjust to your new life situation.

- Don't try to rush through the grieving process. Remember that most people need at least two years to begin feeling "normal" after the death of a loved one.
- Be open with others about what you're experiencing. Your family and friends may avoid the topic, believing this will be easier on you.
- Avoid making major decisions for at least one year. This is a period of time when you may still be feeling unsettled and in shock.
- Follow your normal routine as much as possible, but let others help you with daily tasks. People will want to help you, but they may not know how.
- Try to confront the reminders of your loved one. Be aware of situations when you would expect to see your loved one, and make an effort to remind yourself of his or her death at those times.
- Identify the source of any anger you feel and find ways to cope with it. Crying, shouting or punching a cushion may help relieve some tension. Physical activity often helps release anger. You may also direct your anger into something constructive such as volunteer work.
- Expect to experience feelings of relief now that the responsibility of caregiving is gone.

- Try to keep a realistic view of your past actions and present emotions to reduce any guilt you may feel. Don't focus on what you wish could have been better or could have been done differently.
- Accept fear as a normal part of the grieving process. Remaining involved socially rather than isolating yourself helps ease fear.

In the final stage of the grieving process, you'll quit focusing on the past and seeking an explanation for death. Instead, you can begin concentrating on living life to the fullest in spite of death and looking for ways to grow from this experience.

Additional resources

AARP
601 E Street NW
Washington, D.C. 20049
888-687-2277
www.aarp.org

Administration for Community Living
One Massachusetts Ave. NW
Washington, D.C. 20001
202-619-0724
www.acl.gov

Agency for Healthcare Research and Quality
Office of Communications and Knowledge Transfer
540 Gaither Road, Suite 2000
Rockville, MD 20850
301-427-1104
www.ahrq.gov

Alzheimer's Association
National Office
225 N. Michigan Ave., 17th Floor
Chicago, IL 60601
312-335-8700 or 800-272-3900
www.alz.org

Alzheimer's Disease Education and Referral (ADEAR) Center
800-438-4380
www.nia.nih.gov/alzheimers

Alzheimer's Disease International
64 Great Suffolk Street
London SE1 0BL
United Kingdom
44-20-79810880
www.alz.co.uk

Alzheimer's Foundation of America
322 8th Ave., 7th Floor
New York, NY 10001
866-232-8484
www.alzfdn.org

The Association for Frontotemporal Degeneration
Radnor Station Building 2, Suite 320
290 King of Prussia Road
Radnor, PA 19087
267-514-7221 or 866-507-7222
www.theaftd.org

BrightFocus Foundation
22512 Gateway Center Drive
Clarksburg, MD 20871
800-437-2423
www.brightfocus.org

Center for Drug Evaluation and Research (CDER)

Office of Medical Products and Tobacco
Food and Drug Administration
855-543-3784 or 301-796-3400
www.fda.gov/Drugs

Centers for Medicare and Medicaid Services

7500 Security Blvd.
Baltimore, MD 21244
800-633-4227 or 800-447-8477
www.cms.gov

CenterWatch

Clinical Research and Drug Information
10 Winthrop Square, 5th Floor
Boston, MA 02110
617-948-5100 or 866-219-3440
www.centerwatch.com

Department of Health and Human Services

200 Independence Avenue, SW
Washington, D.C. 20201
877-696-6775
www.alzheimers.gov

Eldercare Locator

(Administered by the
Administration on Aging)
800-677-1116
www.eldercare.gov

Family Caregiver Alliance

785 Market St., Suite 750
San Francisco, CA 94103
415-434-3388 or 800-445-8106
www.caregiver.org

Lewy Body Dementia Association

912 Killian Hill Road, SW
Lilburn, GA 30047
404-935-6444 or 800-539-9767
www.lbda.org

MedicAlert Foundation

2323 Colorado Ave.
Turlock, CA 95382
888-633-4298
www.medicalert.org

National Association of Area Agencies on Aging

1730 Rhode Island Ave., NW,
Suite 1200
Washington, D.C. 20036
202-872-0888
www.n4a.org

National Association of States United for Aging and Disabilities

1201 15th Street NW, Suite 350
Washington, D.C. 20005
202-898-2578
www.nasuad.org

National Council on the Aging
1901 L Street, NW, 4th Floor
Washington, D.C. 20036
202-479-1200
www.ncoa.org

**National Hospice and
Palliative Care Organization**
1731 King Street
Alexandria, VA 22314
703-837-1500
www.nhpco.org

**National Institute of
Mental Health (NIMH)**
Science Writing, Press,
and Dissemination Branch
6001 Executive Blvd.,
Room 6200, MSC 9663
Bethesda, MD 20892
301-443-4513 or 866-615-6464
www.nimh.nih.gov

**National Institute of Neurological
Disorders and Stroke (NINDS)**
National Institutes of Health
P.O. Box 5801
Bethesda, MD 20824
301-496-5751 or 800-352-9424
www.ninds.nih.gov

**National Institutes of Health
Clinical Center**
10 Center Drive
Bethesda, MD 20892
301-496-2563 or 800-411-1222
www.clinicalcenter.nih.gov

National Institute on Aging
31 Center Drive, MSC 2292
Bethesda, MD 20892
301-496-1752 or 800-222-2225
www.nia.nih.gov

National Library of Medicine
Reference and Web Services
8600 Rockville Pike
Bethesda, MD 20894
888-346-3656
www.nlm.nih.gov

Society for Neuroscience
1121 14th Street NW, Suite 1010
Washington, D.C. 20005
202-962-4000
www.sfn.org

Image credits

NAME: HANDS.EPS/PAGE: COVER/CREDIT: © MFMER — NAME: 3278729_0002.JPG/ PAGE: V/CREDIT: © MFMER — NAME: CH01_BRAIN.JPG/PAGE: 19/CREDIT: © MFMER — NAME: CH01_BRAIN STRUCTURES.JPG/PAGE: 20/CREDIT: © MFMER — NAME: CH01_BRAIN FUNCTIONS.JPG/PAGE: 22/CREDIT: © MFMER — NAME: CH01_NERVES.JPG/PAGE: 23/CREDIT: © MFMER — NAME: CH01_NEURON.JPG/PAGE: 25/CREDIT: © MFMER — NAME: 77900164.JPG/PAGE: 26/CREDIT: © DESIGN PICS/THINKSTOCK — NAME: 119582317.PSD/PAGE: 28/CREDIT: © ISTOCKPHOTO/THINKSTOCK — NAME: 139986326.PSD/ PAGE: 30/CREDIT: © ISTOCKPHOTO/THINKSTOCK — NAME: STK113717RKE.PSD/PAGE: 34/CREDIT: © STOCKBYTE/THINK-STOCK — NAME: AGING GRAPHFIG01.1.PSD/PAGE: /CREDIT: © MFMER — NAME: 200271541-001.JPG/PAGE: 45/CREDIT: © MICHAEL MATISSE/PHOTODISC/THINKSTOCK — NAME: CH03_NORMAL_CT_AXIAL COPY.JPG/PAGE: 55/CREDIT: © MFMER — NAME: CH03_NORMAL_MRI_AXIAL COPY.JPG/PAGE: 55/CREDIT: © MFMER — NAME: AXIAL.PSD/PAGE: 55/CREDIT: © MFMER — NAME: CH03_NORMAL_MRI_SAGITTAL.TIF/PAGE: 55/CREDIT: © MFMER — NAME: SAGITAL.PSD/PAGE: 55/CREDIT: © MFMER — NAME: CH03_NORMAL_MRI_CORONAL.JPG/PAGE: 55/CREDIT: © MFMER — NAME: CORONAL.PSD/PAGE: 55/ CREDIT: © MFMER — NAME: CH04_EARLYSTAGEAD.JPG/PAGE: 68/CREDIT: © MFMER — NAME: CH04_NEURONPHOTO.JPG/ PAGE: 70/CREDIT: © MFMER — NAME: CH04_PLAQUEFORMATION.JPG/PAGE: 72/CREDIT: © MFMER — NAME: CH04_TANGLE-FORMATION.JPG/PAGE: 74/CREDIT: © MFMER — NAME: CH04_TANGLEPHOTO.JPG/PAGE: 75/CREDIT: © MFMER — NAME: 124972266.PSD/PAGE: 76/CREDIT: © ISTOCKPHOTO/THINKSTOCK — NAME: CH04_BRAINATROPHY.JPG/PAGE: 81/CREDIT: © MFMER — NAME: 56385359.JPG/PAGE: 83/CREDIT: © STOCKBYTE/THINKSTOCK — NAME: AGING GRAPHFIG02.2.PSD/ PAGE: /CREDIT: © MFMER — NAME: CH05_MILDAD.JPG/PAGE: 89/CREDIT: © MFMER — NAME: CH05_MODERATEAD.JPG/ PAGE: 89/CREDIT: © MFMER — NAME: CH05_SEVEREAD.JPG/PAGE: 89/CREDIT: © MFMER — NAME: 137227738.PSD/PAGE: 90/CREDIT: © ISTOCKPHOTO/THINKSTOCK — NAME: 126870071.PSD/PAGE: 95/CREDIT: © ZOONAR/THINKSTOCK — NAME: AGING GRAPHFIG03.2.JPG/PAGE: 102/CREDIT: © MFMER — NAME: 105614672.JPG/PAGE: 111/CREDIT: © ISTOCKPHOTO/ THINKSTOCK — NAME: AGING GRAPHFIG04.2.JPG/PAGE: 114/CREDIT: © MFMER — NAME: AGING GRAPHFIG05X.JPG/PAGE: 116/CREDIT: © MFMER — NAME: CH07_NORMAL_MRI_CORONAL.JPG/PAGE: 118/CREDIT: © MFMER — NAME: CH07_MCI_MRI_CORONAL.JPG/PAGE: 118/CREDIT: © MFMER — NAME: CH07_AD_MRI_CORONAL.JPG/PAGE: 118/CREDIT: © MFMER — NAME: SLIDE08.JPG/PAGE: 149/CREDIT: © COPYRIGHT ELI LILLY AND COMPANY. ALL RIGHTS RESERVED. USED WITH PERMISSION. — NAME: SLIDE08.JPG/PAGE: 149/CREDIT: © COPYRIGHT ELI LILLY AND COMPANY. ALL RIGHTS RESERVED. USED WITH PERMISSION.— NAME: CH09_DSI_NEURAL_PATHWAYS.TIF/PAGE: 149/CREDIT: © IMAGE COURTESY OF VAN J. WEEDEN, M.D., AND LAWRENCE L. WALD, PH.D., ATHINOULA A. MARTINOS CENTER FOR BIOMEDICAL IMAGING, 2013. USED WITH PERMISSION. — NAME: CH10_FTD.PSD/PAGE: 158/CREDIT: © MFMER — NAME: CH10_NORMAL_MRI_CORONAL.JPG/ PAGE: 164/CREDIT: © MFMER — NAME: CH10_FTD_MRI_FRONTAL_CORONAL.JPG/PAGE: 164/CREDIT: © MFMER — NAME: CH10_FTD_MRI_TEMPORAL_CORONAL.JPG/PAGE: 164/CREDIT: © MFMER — NAME: CH11_DAT_NORMAL.TIF/PAGE: 176/ CREDIT: © MFMER — NAME: CH11_DAT_DLB.TIF/PAGE: 176/CREDIT: © MFMER — NAME: CH11_DAT_AD.JPG/PAGE: 176/ CREDIT: © MFMER — NAME: CH11_NORMAL_MRI_CORONAL.JPG/PAGE: 177/CREDIT: © MFMER — NAME: CH11_AD_MRI_CORONAL.JPG/PAGE: 177/CREDIT: © MFMER — NAME: CH12_E1037742-002-1.PSD/PAGE: 185/CREDIT: © MFMER — NAME: CH12_NORMAL_WITH_STROKE.JPG/PAGE: 189/CREDIT: © MFMER — NAME: CH12_VCI_MRI.JPG/PAGE: 189/CREDIT: © MFMER — NAME: CH12_BINSWANGERS_MRI_AXIAL.JPG/PAGE: 189/CREDIT: © MFMER — NAME: CH13_HYDROCEPHALUS. JPG/PAGE: 194/CREDIT: © MFMER — NAME: CH13_PARKINSONS.JPG/PAGE: 202/CREDIT: © MFMER — NAME: CH13_MUL-TIPLESCLEROSIS.PSD/PAGE: 207/CREDIT: © MFMER — NAME: 121118593.JPG/PAGE: 212/CREDIT: © ISTOCKPHOTO/ THINKSTOCK — NAME: 161145149.JPG/PAGE: 216/CREDIT: © WAVEBREAK MEDIA/THINKSTOCK — NAME: DV1540017.JPG/ PAGE: 225/CREDIT: © DIGITAL VISION/THINKSTOCK — NAME: 104238441.PSD/PAGE: 232/CREDIT: © ISTOCKPHOTO/THINK-STOCK — NAME: 99894276.JPG/PAGE: 235/CREDIT: © HEMERA/THINKSTOCK — NAME: 90587059.JPG/PAGE: 240/CREDIT: © ISTOCKPHOTO/THINKSTOCK — NAME: 86482069.JPG/PAGE: 252/CREDIT: © THINKSTOCK IMAGES/COMSTOCK/THINK-STOCK — NAME: 151529016.JPG/PAGE: 258/CREDIT: © ISTOCKPHOTO/THINKSTOCK — NAME: 80380319.PSD/PAGE: 265/ CREDIT: © JUPITER IMAGES/BRAND X PICTURES/THINKSTOCK — NAME: 83162855.JPG/PAGE: 280/CREDIT: © RYAN MCVAY/ LIFESIZE/THINKSTOCK — NAME: 116978667.JPG/PAGE: 290/CREDIT: © ISTOCKPHOTO/THINKSTOCK — NAME: 78783348. JPG/PAGE: 293/CREDIT: © FUSE/THINKSTOCK — NAME: 86523725.JPG/PAGE: 295/CREDIT: © JUPITERIMAGES/POLKA DOT/ THINKSTOCK — NAME: 78727296.JPG/PAGE: 299/CREDIT: © FUSE/THINKSTOCK — NAME: 115737169.PSD/PAGE: 304/CRED-IT: © ISTOCKPHOTO/THINKSTOCK — NAME: 146790384.JPG/PAGE: 312/CREDIT: © ISTOCKPHOTO/THINKSTOCK — NAME: 162582099.JPG/PAGE: 314/CREDIT: © ISTOCKPHOTO/THINKSTOCK — NAME: 99112209.JPG/PAGE: 319/CREDIT: © HEMERA/ THINKSTOCK.COM — NAME: 114273954.JPG/PAGE: 325/CREDIT: © ISTOCKPHOTO/THINKSTOCK — NAME: 78768104.JPG/ PAGE: 328/CREDIT: © FUSE/THINKSTOCK — NAME: 78494580.JPG/PAGE: 334/CREDIT: © COMSTOCK/THINKSTOCK — NAME: STK150411RKE.JPG/PAGE: 345/CREDIT: © GEORGE DOYLE/STOCKBYTE/THINKSTOCK — NAME: 120264760.JPG/PAGE: 347/ CREDIT: © ISTOCKPHOTO/THINKSTOCK

THE IMAGES ON PAGES 56, 57, 107, 118 AND 163 APPEAR IN COOPERATION WITH GE HEALTHCARE MEDICAL IMAGING.

Index

A

ABC approach, 135–136

abnormal aging
  cognition changes, 34–37
  signs and symptoms,
    34–35

acetylcholine, 69, 126

Action guide for caregivers,
    247–364
  activities of daily living,
    289–300
  becoming a caregiver,
    257–266
  care plan, 267–274
  challenging behaviors,
    309–320
  communication, 301–308
  diagnosis, 249–256
  health concerns, 353–364
  housing and care options,
    321–342
  self-care, 275–288
  travel and safety, 343–352
  use instructions, 247

activities of daily living
  assisting loved one in, 290
  bathing and grooming,
    291–292
  defined, 289
  dressing, 292–293
  eating and nutrition,
    293–296
  severe Alzheimer's, 94

special occasions, 298–300
  taking time with, 290
  toileting, 296–298

AD signature, 117–118

adult day care
  defined, 327
  resource contact, 329
  services, 328–329
  staff, 327

adult foster care homes, 332

advance directive, 268,
    269–270

aggression, 315

aging
  abnormal, 34–37
  on brain function, 213–214
  as dementia risk factor, 42
  process, 14
  as risk factor, 141–142
  typical, 13–32

agitation
  causes of, 306
  as behavior, 314-315

alcohol
  in moderation, 241–242
  strokes and, 191

alpha-synuclein protein, 171

Alzheimer's disease
  apolipoprotein E (APOE)
    gene and, 78
  basics of, 67–84
  contributing factors, 77–83
  defined, 67
  dementia due to, 13–14,
    39–40, 85–100
  dementia with Lewy bodies
    and, 176–177

diagnosis, 249–256
  final stages, 362–363
  frontotemporal
    degeneration and, 168
  genetics and, 77–78
  inflammatory response and,
    79–80
  insulin resistance and, 82
  mild cognitive impairment
    due to, 102
  oxidative stress and, 79
  pattern of degeneration,
    68–69
  plaques and, 70–73
  preclinical, 68, 113–122
  protective factors, 82–83
  tangles and, 74–77
  treatment of, 123–138
  vascular brain injury and,
    80–81
  VCI combined with, 186
  warning signs of, 88

Alzheimer's vaccine, 150–151

amnestic MCI, 104

amygdala, 19, 22

amyloid imaging, 57, 147

amyloid plaques, 143

amyloid precursor protein
    (APP), 71, 72, 77

amyloid-beta
  buildup, 107, 115–116, 120
  defined, 71
  in MCI diagnosis, 109
  in preclinical Alzheimer's
    disease, 115–116
  toxicity, 71–73, 77
  See also plaques

visiting, loved one, 308, 338

visual hallucinations, in DLB, 172, 173

vitamin E, 111–112

vitamins, 129–130

W

wake-promoting drugs, 182

walking
  difficulty, 194
  program, 233

wandering, 317–319, 349

Wilson's disease, 207-208

Y

yoga, 239, 282

Z

zinc acetate (Galzin), 208

Visit our online store

for a wide selection of books, newsletters and DVDs developed by Mayo Clinic doctors and editorial staff.

Discover practical, easy-to-understand information on topics of interest to millions of health-conscious people like you ...